T0227127

Biomarkers in the Critically Ill Patient

Guest Editor

MITCHELL M. LEVY, MD

CRITICAL CARE CLINICS

www.criticalcare.theclinics.com

Consulting Editor
RICHARD W. CARLSON, MD, PhD

April 2011 • Volume 27 • Number 2

SAUNDERS an imprint of ELSEVIER, Inc.

W.B. SAUNDERS COMPANY

A Division of Elsevier Inc.

Elsevier Inc. ● 1600 John F. Kennedy Blvd., ● Suite 1800 ● Philadelphia, Pennsylvania 19103-2899

http://www.theclinics.com

CRITICAL CARE CLINICS Volume 27, Number 2
April 2011 ISSN 0749-0704, ISBN-13: 978-1-4557-0432-3

Editor: Patrick Manley

Critical Care Clinics (ISSN: 0749-0704) is published quarterly by Elsevier Inc., 360 Park Avenue South, New York, NY 10010-1710. Months of issue are January, April, July, and October. Business and Editorial Offices: 1600 John F. Kennedy Blvd., Suite 1800, Philadelphia, PA 19103-2899. Customer Service Office: 6277 Sea Harbor Drive, Orlando, FL 32887-4800. Periodicals postage paid at New York, NY and additional mailing offices. Subscription prices are $179.00 per year for US individuals, $435.00 per year for US institution, $87.00 per year for US students and residents, $222.00 per year for Canadian individuals, $539.00 per year for Canadian institutions, $257.00 per year for international individuals, $539.00 per year for international institutions and $127.00 per year for Canadian and foreign students/residents. To receive student/resident rate, orders must be accompanied by name of affiliated institution, date of term, and the *signature* of program/residency coordinator on institution letterhead. Orders will be billed at individual rate until proof of status is received. Foreign air speed delivery is included in all *Clinics* subscription prices. All prices are subject to change without notice. POSTMASTER: Send address changes to *Critical Care Clinics*, Elsevier Periodicals Customer Service, 11830 Westline Industrial Drive, St. Louis, MO 63146. **Customer Service: 1-800-654-2452 (US). From outside of the US, call 1-314-447-8871. Fax: 1-314-447-8029. E-mail: journalscustomerservice-usa@elsevier.com (for print support) or journalsonlinesupport-usa@elsevier.com (for online support).**

Reprints. For copies of 100 or more of articles in this publication, please contact the Commercial Reprints Department, Elsevier Inc., 360 Park Avenue South, New York, NY 10010-1710. Tel.: 212-633-3813; Fax: 212-462-1935; E-mail: reprints@elsevier.com.

Critical Care Clinics is also published in Spanish by Editorial Inter-Medica, Junin 917, 1er A, 1113, Buenos Aires, Argentina.

Critical Care Clinics is covered in *MEDLINE/PubMed (Index Medicus), EMBASE/Excerpta Medica, Current Concepts/Clinical Medicine, ISI/BIOMED, and Chemical Abstracts.*

Printed and bound by CPI Group (UK) Ltd, Croydon, CR0 4YY

Transferred to Digital Print 2011

Contributors

CONSULTING EDITOR

RICHARD W. CARLSON, MD, PhD
Chairman Emeritus, Department of Medicine, Maricopa Medical Center; Director,
Medical Intensive Care Unit; Professor, University of Arizona College of Medicine;
Professor, Department of Medicine, Mayo Graduate School of Medicine,
Phoenix, Arizona

GUEST EDITOR

MITCHELL M. LEVY, MD
Division of Pulmonary and Critical Care Medicine, Rhode Island Hospital, The Warren
Alpert Medical School of Brown University, Providence, Rhode Island

AUTHORS

CHARLES A. ADAMS Jr, MD, FACS
Assistant Professor of Surgery, Warren Alpert School of Medicine of Brown University;
Chief, Division of Trauma and Surgical Critical Care, Rhode Island Hospital; Medical
Director, Surgical and Trauma Intensive Care Units, Rhode Island Hospital,
Providence, Rhode Island

ANTONIO ARTIGAS, MD, PhD
Critical Care Center, Hospital de Sabadell, Sabadell; CIBER Enfermedades Respiratorias,
Instituto Universitario Parc Tauli, Universidad Autónoma de Barcelona, Barcelona, Spain

DAMIEN BARRAUD, MD
Medical ICU, University Hospital of Nancy, Nancy, France

BRIAN CASSERLY, MD
Assistant Professor, Division of Pulmonary and Critical Care Medicine, The Memorial
Hospital of Rhode Island, Pawtucket, Rhode Island

PHIL DELLINGER, MD
Professor of Medicine, University of Medicine and Dentistry of New Jersey, Robert Wood
Johnson Medical School; Head, Division of Critical Care Medicine, Cooper University
Hospital, Camden, New Jersey

KATIA DONADELLO, MD
Department of Intensive Care, Erasme Hospital, Universitè Libre de Bruxelles,
Brussels, Belgium

LANCE D. DWORKIN, MD
Professor of Medicine, Division of Kidney Diseases and Hypertension, Rhode Island
Hospital, Alpert Medical School of Brown University, Providence, Rhode Island

RICARD FERRER, MD, PhD
Critical Care Center, Hospital de Sabadell, Sabadell, Spain; CIBER Enfermedades
Respiratorias, Instituto Universitario Parc Tauli, Universidad Autónoma de Barcelona,
Barcelona, Spain

HERWIG GERLACH, MD, PhD
Professor and Director of Anesthesiology, Department of Anesthesia, Critical Care
Medicine, and Pain Management, Vivantes Clinics Neukoelln; Lecturer, Charitè, Medical
Faculty of the Universities of Berlin; Klinik fuer Anaesthesie, Operative Intensivmedizin
und Schmerztherapie, Vivantes – Klinikum Neukoelln, Berlin, Germany

SÉBASTIEN GIBOT, MD, PhD
Medical ICU, University Hospital of Nancy, Nancy, France

STEVEN P. LAROSA, MD
Assistant Professor of Medicine, Warren Alpert School of Medicine, Brown University;
Division of Infectious Diseases, Rhode Island Hospital, Providence, Rhode Island

MARCEL LEVI, MD
Department of Vascular Medicine and Internal Medicine, Academic Medical Centre,
Amsterdam, The Netherlands

L.J. MARK CROSS, MRCP, PhD
Centre for Infection and Immunity, The Queen's University of Belfast, Belfast, Northern
Ireland, United Kingdom

MITCHELL M. LEVY, MD
Division of Pulmonary and Critical Care Medicine, Department of Medicine,
Rhode Island Hospital, The Warren Alpert Medical School of Brown University,
Providence, Rhode Island

MICHAEL A. MATTHAY, MD
Cardiovascular Research Institute; Division of Pulmonary and Critical Care, Department
of Medicine; Department of Anaesthesia, University of California San Francisco,
San Francisco, California

MICHAEL MEISNER, Dr Med Habil
Clinic of Anaesthesiology and Intensive Care Medicine, Staedtisches Krankenhaus
Dresden-Neustadt, Dresden, Germany

OKORIE NDUKA OKORIE, MD
Assistant Clinical Professor of Medicine, Florida State University school of Medicine;
Department of Critical Care Medicine, Orlando Regional Medical Center,
Orlando, Florida

STEVEN M. OPAL, MD
Professor of Medicine, Warren Alpert School of Medicine, Brown University,
Providence, Rhode Island; Division of Infectious Diseases, Memorial Hospital,
Pawtucket, Rhode Island

RICHARD READ, MD
Pulmonary Fellow, Rhode Island Hospital, Alpert Medical School of Brown University,
Providence, Rhode Island

KONRAD REINHART, Dr Med Habil
Clinic of Anaesthesiology and Intensive Care Medicine, Friedrich-Schiller-University Jena, Jena, Germany

XAVIER SCHMIT, MD
Department of Intensive Care, Erasme Hospital, Universitè Libre de Bruxelles, Brussels, Belgium

MARCUS SCHULTZ, MD
Academic Medical Centre, Department of Intensive Care Medicine, University of Amsterdam, The Netherlands

DOUGLAS SHEMIN, MD
Associate Professor of Medicine, Division of Kidney Diseases and Hypertension, Rhode Island Hospital, Alpert Medical School of Brown University, Providence, Rhode Island

SUSANNE TOUSSAINT, MD, MA, DEAA, EDIC
Klinik fuer Anaesthesie, Operative Intensivmedizin und Schmerztherapie, Vivantes – Klinikum Neukoelln; Chair, Interdisciplinary Intensive Care Unit, Department of Anesthesia, Critical Care Medicine, and Pain Management, Vivantes Clinics Neukoelln, Berlin, Germany

TOM VAN DER POLL, MD
Laboratory for Experimental and Molecular Medicine; Center for Infection and Immunity Amsterdam, Academic Medical Center, University of Amsterdam, The Netherlands

COREY E. VENTETUOLO, MD
Division of Pulmonary, Allergy, and Critical Care Medicine, Department of Medicine, College of Physicians and Surgeons, Columbia University, New York, New York

JEAN-LOUIS VINCENT, MD, PhD
Professor, Department of Intensive Care, Erasme Hospital, Universitè Libre de Bruxelles, Brussels, Belgium

Contents

> Biomarkers are frequently used in critically ill patients, especially during inflammatory and/or infectious diseases such as severe sepsis and septic shock. The rationale of when to measure laboratory parameters, which marker may be useful, and how to interpret the results is not well defined. Terms like sensitive, predictive, or significant to describe the capabilities of specific markers are often mixed up or misused, which may have fatal consequences regarding diagnosis and treatment. This review reflects some statistical basics with clinical examples, showing possibilities as well as limitations of how data for biomarkers may be used in critically ill patients.

> Sepsis generates an overwhelming host response characterized by changes in physiologic parameters. Monitoring these parameters can help identify and stratify septic patients. Recognizing sepsis early and identifying septic patients at risk of worsening are keys to successful treatment. Several studies have analyzed the independent physiologic parameters associated with the diagnosis of sepsis or bacteremia, with the development of severe sepsis or septic shock, and with mortality. Physiologic variability of heart rate and body temperature is reduced in sepsis and measuring the variability of these parameters can be useful for the diagnosis and prognosis of sepsis.

> Levels of C-reactive protein (CRP), an acute phase protein, are elevated in many inflammatory conditions and are used to detect and follow disease in many fields of medicine, including rheumatology, gastroenterology, and cardiology. CRP concentrations are also used in critically ill patients, notably because they are increased during the inflammatory response to infection, that is, sepsis. However, CRP is not specific for sepsis, and serum CRP concentrations need to be interpreted in the context of a full clinical examination and the presence of other signs and symptoms of sepsis.

> Infection and/or sepsis biomarkers should help to make the diagnosis and thus initiate therapy earlier, help to differentiate between infectious and

sterile inflammation, allow the use of more-specific antimicrobials, shorten the time of antimicrobial use, and ideally identify distinct phenotypes that may benefit from specific adjunctive sepsis therapies. Procalcitonin (PCT) was proposed as a sepsis and infection marker more than 15 years ago. Meanwhile, PCT has been evaluated in various clinical settings. In this review the present use of PCT on the ICU and in critically ill patients is summarized, included it's role for diagnosis of severe sepsis and septic shock and antibiotic stewardship with PCT.

Sepsis is a common cause of morbidity and mortality in intensive care units. There is no gold standard for diagnosing sepsis because clinical and laboratory signs are neither sensitive nor specific enough and micro-biological studies often show negative results. The triggering receptor expressed on myeloid cell 1 (TREM-1) is a member of the immunoglobulin superfamily. Its expression is upregulated on phagocytic cells in the presence of bacteria or fungi. This article reports on the potential usefulness of the assessment of the soluble form of TREM-1 in biologic fluids in the diagnosis of infection.

This article discusses coagulation biomarkers in critically ill patients where coagulation abnormalities occur frequently and may have a major impact on the outcome. An adequate explanation for the cause is important, since many underlying disorders may require specific treatment and supportive therapy directed at the underlying condition. Deficiencies in platelets and coagulation factors in bleeding patients or patients at risk for bleeding can be achieved by transfusion of platelet concentrate or plasma products, respectively. Prohemostatic treatment may be beneficial in case of severe bleeding, whereas restoring physiological anticoagulant pathways may be helpful in patients with sepsis and disseminated intravascular coagulation.

Lactate levels are frequently elevated in critically ill patients and correlate well with disease severity. Elevated lactate levels are prognostic in prehospital, emergency department, and intensive care unit settings. This review discusses the role of lactate as a biomarker in diagnosing and assessing the severity of systemic hypoperfusion, as well as the role of serum lactate measurements in guiding clinical care and enabling prognosis in critically ill patients.

Cardiac biomarkers have well-established roles in acute coronary syndrome and congestive heart failure. In many instances, the detection of cardiac biomarkers may aid in the diagnosis and risk assessment of critically ill patients. Despite increasing interest in the use of cardiac bio-markers in noncardiac critical illness, no clear consensus exists on how and in which settings markers should be measured. This article briefly describes what constitutes an ideal biomarker and focuses on those that have been most well studied in critical illness, specifically troponin, the natriuretic peptides, and heart-type fatty acid–binding protein.

Despite continual advances in medical care and injury prevention efforts, traumatic injury remains a leading cause of death of Americans with these deaths occurring in a tri-modal pattern. The early phases of this pattern are characterized by immune activation whereas the last phase is marked by profound immune dysfunction. It is during this last phase that many trauma patients die of septic complications pointing to a dire need for a specific biomarker for post-traumatic infection. This article discusses several biomarkers, including emerging ones, for infection and sepsis following trauma including inflammatory cytokines, intracellular proteins, and cellular biomarkers.

Studies of potential biomarkers of acute lung injury (ALI) have provided information relating to the pathophysiology of the mechanisms of lung injury and repair. The utility of biomarkers remains solely among research tools to investigate lung injury and repair mechanisms. Because of lack of sensitivity and specificity, they cannot be used in decision making in patients with ALI or acute respiratory distress syndrome. The authors reviewed known biomarkers in context of their major biologic activity. The continued interest in identifying and studying biomarkers is relevant, as it provides information regarding the mechanisms involved in lung injury and repair and how this may be helpful in identifying and designing future therapeutic targets and strategies and possibly identifying a sensitive and specific biomarker.

Based on information to date, although limitations in the accuracy of NGAL in predicting AKI persist, the preponderance of published studies demonstrate that NGAL, when measured in the plasma and in the urine, is a reliable biomarker for the subsequent development of clinically apparent AKI. If very early detection of AKI, via the measurement of plasma or urinary NGAL, can be followed by effective treatment to abort the development or limit the severity of AKI, and therefore decrease the rate of RRT, length of hospitalization stay, and/or mortality risk, NGAL measurement will become a critically important diagnostic tool in critical care medicine, pediatrics, and surgery.

Biomarkers differentiate between 2 or more biologic states. The complexity of diseases like sepsis makes it unlikely that any single marker will allow for precise disease specification. Combining several biomarkers into a single classification rule should help to improve their accuracy and, therefore, their usefulness. This article reviews several studies using multimarker panels, and highlights the potential of more sophisticated diagnostic and prognostic techniques in future multimarker panels. More complex algorithms should accelerate the adoption of multimarker panels into the routine management of patients with sepsis, provided that clinicians understand the multimarker approach.

The future application of biomarkers in critical illness will be to select and guide therapy. Specific biomarkers could identify a pathophysiologic perturbation or noxious mediator to counteract or the need to replete a deficient protective protein. Functional genomics could identify patients at risk for illness or at risk for a poor outcome in critical illness. Genetic expression studies could help differentiate patients with sepsis from those with noninfectious inflammation and could also help to monitor illnesses over time. Expressional and functional proteomics could lead to the identification of new biomarkers and organ-specific therapies.

THE CLINICS ARE NOW AVAILABLE ONLINE!

Access your subscription at:
www.theclinics.com

Preface

Biomarkers in Critical Illness

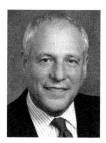

Mitchell M. Levy, MD
Guest Editor

Prompt diagnosis and early intervention in critically ill patients have come to be appreciated as perhaps the primary determinant in good outcomes across several critical disease states: Early institution of appropriate antibiotics for sepsis, minimizing time to balloon dilatation for acute coronary syndrome, initiation of rapid, aggressive fluid resuscitation in severe sepsis and shock have all been shown to improve outcomes in critically ill patients.[1–4] In addition, accurate risk assessment to guide treatment and disposition, such as identifying and treating patients with right ventricular failure or submassive and massive pulmonary embolism, has also been recognized as a crucial ingredient in the early management of the critically ill patient. Of course, the daunting challenge that bedside critical care practitioners face daily is how to identify these patients rapidly and with precision. Increasingly, the use of biomarkers in critically ill patients is being recognized as essential adjuncts in this process.[4] Cardiac biomarkers have long been established as the driving force, along with ECG monitoring, to dictate immediate therapies for acute coronary syndrome. More recently biomarkers are now being incorporated in algorithms that guide the management of pulmonary embolism and sepsis.[5–10] The use of biomarkers for diagnosis is also under active investigation and several published reports, discussed in this issue of *Critical Care Clinics*, have demonstrated the value of procalcitonin (PCT), and triggering receptor expressed on myeloid cells (TREM)-1, as well as composite markers or biomarker panels (PCT, TREM 1) for the diagnosis of bacterial infection.[11]

Another important aspect in the management of critically ill patients is early risk assessment to guide triage and therapeutic intervention. Lactate and neutrophil gelatinase associated lipocalin are two such biomarkers that will be reviewed in this issue. There is also potential benefit in using biomarkers to limit therapy. Limiting exposure when infection is absent will become exceedingly important as drug resistance increases. There are several published studies that suggest that PCT may be effective in reducing the duration of antibiotic therapy, which will also be reviewed in this issue.[12]

Crit Care Clin 27 (2011) xiii–xv
doi:10.1016/j.ccc.2011.01.001
0749-0704/11/$ – see front matter © 2011 Elsevier Inc. All rights reserved.

criticalcare.theclinics.com

Finally, and just as important, the use of vital signs and the routine variation in vital signs must not be forgotten in the search for the "holy grail" of biomarkers. Vital signs, which will also be reviewed in this issue, present a readily accessible portrait of the physiology of the critically ill and the change in variation in these vital signs is often ignored.

DEFINITIONS AND CRITERIA

A biomarker is defined as "a characteristic that is objectively measured and evaluated as an indicator of normal biological processes, pathogenic processes, or pharmacologic responses to a therapeutic intervention."[13] What do clinicians and clinical trialists expect from an "ideal" biomarker? Several characteristics come to mind: to be highly sensitive and specific for the disease state being evaluated, to have prognostic value, to indicate the severity and the course of illness, and to be biologically plausible. In septic patients, biomarkers should ideally allow the differentiation between infectious and noninfectious causes of inflammation and predict the onset of the clinical signs of organ dysfunction and shock. Biomarkers are an appealing addition to the care of the critically ill patient since they are noninvasive and ideally rapidly available and may be followed over a patient's course.

Prior to the widespread use of a marker of interest, it must endure *validation* (ie, have known characteristics, be well-standardized and accurate) and *qualification* (ie, be integral to the disease process and clinical endpoints).[14] Depending on the intended use, the validation and qualification process may be more or less rigorous. Assay reliability, the establishment of cutoffs, and timely, affordable processing must be considered and addressed prior to the widespread adoption of a given marker. This important concept is also covered later in this issue. As more studies on biomarkers in the critically ill are published, it becomes essential for clinicians to be cognizant of how to interpret these studies and so make a careful clinical judgment as to the value of incorporating the use of these markers into routine bedside practice.

CONCLUSION

Convincing evidence now exists that biomarkers may become useful adjuncts to the clinician and may ultimately serve as targets in large, randomized, controlled trials for new therapeutic agents and management strategies. New understanding of inflammatory mediators and pathways, immunity, and genetic variability in critical illness will further inform and enhance the search for appropriate biomarkers.

With this issue, we hope to offer the clinician a summary of the current biomarker literature and to identify the markers most likely to prove useful in clinical practice. No single marker has been shown to possess all the ideal qualities mentioned here, but there are encouraging signs in the literature that we are on the right path toward finding a marker or set of markers that will facilitate diagnosis, risk assessment, and management in critically ill patients.

Mitchell M. Levy, MD
Division of Pulmonary and Critical Care Medicine
Rhode Island Hospital
The Warren Alpert Medical School of Brown University
593 Eddy Street, MICU Main 7
Providence, RI 02903, USA

E-mail address:
mitchell_levy@brown.edu

REFERENCES

1. Rivers E, Nguyen B, Havstad S, et al. Early goal-directed therapy in the treatment of severe sepsis and septic shock. N Engl J Med 2001;345:1368–77.
2. Levy MM, Macias WL, Vincent JL, et al. Early changes in organ function predict eventual survival in severe sepsis. Crit Care Med 2005;33:2194–201.
3. Kumar A, Roberts D, Wood K, et al. Duration of hypotension before initiation of effective antimicrobial therapy is the critical determinant of survival in septic shock. Crit Care Med 2006;34:1589–96.
4. Marshall JC, Vincent JL, Fink MP, et al. Measures, markers, and mediators: toward a staging system for clinical sepsis. A report of the Fifth Toronto Sepsis Roundtable, Toronto, Ontario, Canada, October 25–26, 2000. Crit Care Med 2003;31:1560–7.
5. Konstantinides S, Geibel A, Olschewski M, et al. Importance of cardiac troponins I and T in risk stratification of patients with acute pulmonary embolism. Circulation 2002;106(10):1263–8.
6. Meyer T, Binder L, Hruska N, et al. Cardiac troponin I elevation in acute pulmonary embolism is associated with right ventricular dysfunction. J Am Coll Cardiol 2000;36(5):1632–6.
7. Kostrubiec M, Pruszczyk P, Bochowicz A, et al. Biomarker-based risk assessment model in acute pulmonary embolism. Eur Heart J 2005;26(20):2166–72.
8. Douketis JD, Leeuwenkamp O, Grobara P, et al. The incidence and prognostic significance of elevated cardiac troponins in patients with submassive pulmonary embolism. J Thromb Haemost 2005;3(3):508–13.
9. Pruszczyk P, Bochowicz A, Torbicki A, et al. Cardiac troponin T monitoring identifies high-risk group of normotensive patients with acute pulmonary embolism. Chest 2003;123(6):1947–52.
10. Christ-Crain M, Stolz D, Bingisser R, et al. Procalcitonin guidance of antibiotic therapy in community-acquired pneumonia: a randomized trial. Am J Respir Crit Care Med 2006;174:84–93.
11. Gibot S, Cravoisy A, Kolopp-Sarda MN, et al. Time-course of sTREM (soluble triggering receptor expressed on myeloid cells)-1, procalcitonin, and C-reactive protein plasma concentrations during sepsis. Crit Care Med 2005;33:792–6.
12. Reinhart K, Brunkhorst FM. Meta-analysis of procalcitonin for sepsis detection. Lancet Infect Dis 2007;7:500–2.
13. The Biomarker Definitions Working Group. Biomarkers and surrogate endpoints: preferred definitions and conceptual framework. Clin Pharmacol Ther 2001;69:89–95.
14. Wagner JA, Williams SA, Webster CJ. Biomarkers and surrogate end points for fit-for-purpose development and regulatory evaluation of new drugs. Clin Pharmacol Ther 2007;81:104–7.

Sensitive, Specific, Predictive... Statistical Basics: How to Use Biomarkers

Herwig Gerlach, MD, PhD[a,b,c,*],
Susanne Toussaint, MD, MA, DEAA, EDIC[c,d]

KEYWORDS

- Biomarkers • Infection • Inflammation • Sensitivity
- Specificity • Prediction

What is the rationale of using biomarkers in critically ill patients? This seems to be an easy question: we want to use objective parameters to enable or at least support the diagnosis of a disease, or to monitor the state of the patient to guide treatment strategies. This strategy requires a clear difference between healthy and sick individuals for the biomarker. However, how is a clear difference defined, and is it sufficient to have a difference? This question leads to the first simple example:

> Situation: We have the objective and correct information that a person has a height of 172 cm (approximately 5.7 ft) and a weight of 68 kg (approximately 150 lb).
> Question: Is this person a man or a woman?

The question is impossible to answer, and **Fig. 1** shows why. Although males are significantly taller ($P<.001$) than females (based on the Statistical Microcensus 2009 in Germany[1]), the ideal cutoff of 172 cm (ie, the value that differentiates males and females in an optimal manner) does not differentiate or predict gender, because there is a 1:1 distribution exactly at this value (see **Fig. 1**, arrow). The data for weight are

The authors have nothing to disclose.
[a] Department of Anesthesia, Critical Care Medicine, and Pain Management, Vivantes Clinics Neukoelln, Rudower Strasse 48, D-12313 Berlin, Germany
[b] Charité, Medical Faculty of the Universities of Berlin, Augustenburger Platz 1, D-13353 Berlin, Germany
[c] Klinik fuer Anaesthesie, Operative Intensivmedizin und Schmerztherapie, Vivantes – Klinikum Neukoelln, Rudower Strasse 48, D-12313 Berlin, Germany
[d] Interdisciplinary Intensive Care Unit, Department of Anesthesia, Critical Care Medicine, and Pain Management, Vivantes Clinics Neukoelln, Rudower Strasse 48, D-12313 Berlin, Germany
* Corresponding author. Klinik fuer Anaesthesie, Operative Intensivmedizin und Schmerztherapie, Vivantes – Klinikum Neukoelln, Rudower Strasse 48, D-12313 Berlin, Germany.
E-mail address: herwig.gerlach@vivantes.de

Crit Care Clin 27 (2011) 215–227
doi:10.1016/j.ccc.2010.12.007
0749-0704/11/$ – see front matter © 2011 Elsevier Inc. All rights reserved.

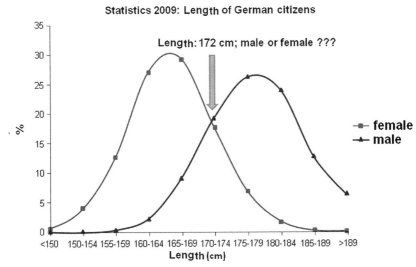

Fig. 1. Distribution of height in Germany 2009 for male and female citizens. The histograms show the percentage of citizens within ranges of body height. The data for male and female individuals are significantly ($P<.001$; t test) different. x-axis: range of length in cm; y-axis: percentage of persons within ranges. (*From* Statistisches Bundesamt: Mikrozensus–Fragen zur Gesundheit. Körpermaße der Bevölkerung. Wiesbaden, Germany: Statistisches Bundesamt; 2010; with permission.)

similar (not shown). This simple example already provides 2 important conclusions: first, significant differences do not necessarily enable prediction, and second, the question "Which cutoff is used for a parameter" is crucial.

STEP 1: EVALUATING SIGNIFICANCE

When a new biomarker is introduced, most clinical studies follow a similar design: 2 cohorts (eg, healthy vs sick patients, survivors vs nonsurvivors) are part of the investigation, and the new marker is measured at a specific time point. Afterwards, the data of the 2 groups are compared (independent samples, me vs you) using statistical tests such as a t test or a Mann-Whitney U test.[2] Alternatively, measurements may be part of a time series in the same group of patients (dependent samples, before vs after), in which other tests are applied (amended t test for dependent samples, Wilcoxon test). Because this review is not dedicated to the description of statistical methods, the interested reader should use standard literature to obtain more detailed information about the specific tests.

We look again at 2 examples for a virtual marker from 2 independent cohorts (**Figs. 2** and **3**). Whereas the first set of data seems to be a convincing example for a good biomarker (see **Fig. 2**), the second one seems to be poor in differentiating between the 2 cohorts (see **Fig. 3**). The same statistical test reveals highly significant differences (nonparametric tests are similar, data not shown) for both examples. This result shows that a significant difference, which is used in most scientific publications, is no guarantee that the biomarker is useful in any way for differentiating between groups, or for predicting if a single patient belongs to one of the 2 groups, regardless if this corresponds to a diagnosis (sick vs healthy) or a prognosis (survivor vs nonsurvivor).

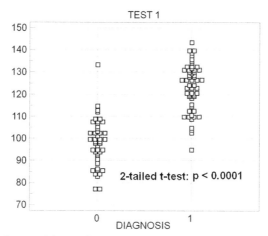

Fig. 2. Example of a good biomarker. Two samples of virtual biomarker levels; the first group has no diagnosis (= 0), the second group is sick (diagnosis = 1). Two-tailed *t* test for independent data revealed a highly significant difference between the 2 groups. x-axis: level of the virtual biomarker; y-axis: 2 subsets of data (healthy, diagnosis = 0 vs sick, diagnosis = 1). (*Data from* an artificial data set, analysis and plot were generated using MedCalc software, Version 11.3.6, Mariakerke, Belgium.)

A second way to describe a biomarker is using a 2 × 2 contingency table: the 2 cohorts refer to the first level, and the results of the biomarkers to the second level, using a threshold or cutoff that differentiates between subgroups (**Fig. 4**). In this case, the statistical tests are different: for the 2 × 2 table, the Fisher exact test is frequently used, which describes if there is a significant association between the level of the marker and the group of the patient (see **Fig. 4**). In this example, a total of 100 patients are part of the analysis, 40 are sick (eg, critically ill patients with infections), 60 are healthy (patients without infections). Serum levels of a biomarker (eg, procalcitonin [PCT]) was measured, using a cutoff of 1 (eg, in case of PCT, 1 ng/mL). A total of

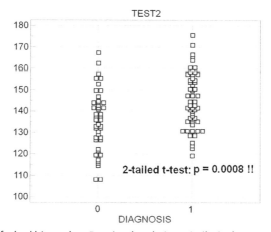

Fig. 3. Example of a bad biomarker. Despite the obvious similarity between the 2 subgroups, a 2-tailed *t* test for independent data revealed a highly significant difference. For more information, see caption for **Fig. 2**.

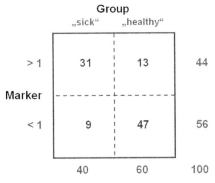

Fisher's exact test: p < 0.000001

Fig. 4. 2 × 2 contingency table for a virtual biomarker. x-axis: 2 patient cohorts (sick vs healthy patients); y-axis: 2 subgroups (positive >1 vs negative <1) for the results of the biomarker. The Fisher exact test revealed a highly significant association of the marker and the diagnosis.

44 patients had serum levels of the marker more than 1, of whom 31 were sick and 13 were healthy; 56 patients had levels less than 1, of whom 9 were sick and 47 were healthy. The Fisher exact test reveals a highly significant association between serum levels of the marker and the state of the patients (see **Fig. 4**). On first view, this result seems to be positive; however, the question arises of why a cutoff of 1 was arbitrarily chosen to define the 2 groups for the biomarker (high vs low).

STEP 2: DEFINING SENSITIVITY, SPECIFICITY, AND THE IDEAL CUTOFF

Sensitivity and specificity are the most common quality parameters for biomarkers, and **Fig. 5** shows their definitions. Sensitivity describes how many of the sick patients (or survivors, and so forth) provide positive results for a biomarker. If the marker is

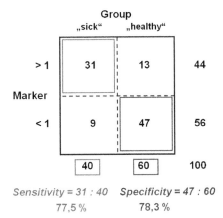

Sensitivity = 31 : 40   Specificity = 47 : 60
77,5 %   78,3 %

Fig. 5. Calculation of sensitivity and specificity, using the data set from **Fig. 4**. Sensitivity is defined by the percentage of correctly positive data divided by the sum of correctly positive and false-negative data of the marker. Vice versa, specificity is the percentage of correctly negative data divided by the sum of correctly negative and false-positive data.

lower in healthy persons (as in our example), positive means higher values; this may be reversed for other laboratory parameters (eg, hemoglobin levels for hypovolemic patients). In our example, 31 of the 40 sick patients have positive (high) levels of the marker; hence, this equals a sensitivity of 31:40 or 77.5% (see **Fig. 5**, left side). In general, this means that the more sensitive a marker is, the fewer of the sick patients have false-negative results.

Vice versa, the definition of specificity uses only the data of the healthy patients: the number of healthy patients with negative results is divided by the total number of healthy patients. In our example, 47 of the 60 healthy patients provide negative (low) levels of the marker, which equals a specificity of 47:60 or 78.3% (see **Fig. 5**, right side). The higher the specificity, the lower the risk of defining healthy individuals in a false-positive manner by using the biomarker. Although in our virtual example, sensitivity and specificity have similar results (77.5 and 78.3%, respectively), both parameters are independent of each other, because they are based on 2 independent samples (sensitivity uses the sick patients; specificity uses the healthy patients). Other data sets may (and do) result in largely differing values for sensitivity and specificity (see later discussion).

Cutoff plays an important role in using biomarkers. For designing a 2 × 2 table, as in the previous example, a cutoff must be arbitrarily defined. If we ask for the best or ideal cutoff, we have to go back to the raw data as in **Figs. 2** and **3**. To start with **Fig. 2**, which contained a good marker, a cutoff of around 109 seems to differentiate both groups in an optimal manner. With a cutoff such as a horizontal line within the data, a virtual 2 × 2 table is created (eg, >109 vs ≤109, and diagnosis 0 vs 1), and both sensitivity and specificity can be calculated according to the definitions mentioned earlier. If the cutoff is set to higher values, data for sensitivity and specificity change: the higher the cutoff, the more sensitivity decreases, whereas specificity rises. In our example (**Fig. 6**), changing the cutoff from 109 to 125 decreases sensitivity from roughly 90% to 50% (ie, those 40% of the patients with values between 110 and 124 are no longer defined as positive for the marker). On the other hand, specificity increases, because fewer patients are defined in a false-positive way. Vice versa, a lower cutoff results in more positive patients for both groups, which means that the test is now more sensitive (more patients with the diagnosis are positive for the biomarker), but less specific (more positive patients without diagnosis, ie, false-positive results). Theoretically, this way of playing with the cutoff may lead to 100% sensitivity with 0% specificity and vice versa. Thus, definition of an ideal cutoff always remains arbitrary; usually, a value is taken for which sensitivity and specificity are more or less outweighed (ie, the sum of both sensitivity and specificity has its maximum with the lowest rate of false-positive and false-negative results). **Fig. 7** shows the data for the second example (bad biomarker); in contrast to **Fig. 6**, in which an optimal cutoff results in more than 90% sensitivity and specificity, the data from **Fig. 7** show that despite both groups (diagnosis 0 and 1) having significantly different data (see **Fig. 3**), sensitivity and specificity are no more than roughly 60% at an ideal cutoff of around 140 (see **Fig. 7**, red line). This last example shows that a marker with highly significant differences between patient subgroups may lead to roughly 40% false results, which is too much for clinical use in critical care medicine.

STEP 3: RECEIVER OPERATING CHARACTERISTICS CURVES: THE MAGIC BULLET?

So far, we learned that significance is important, but not sufficient for accepting a biomarker as a useful tool in critically ill patients. Moreover, the definitions of sensitivity and specificity show that (although per se both parameters in a given data set are

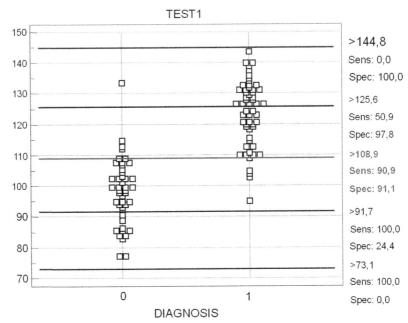

Fig. 6. Playing with the cutoff, example from **Fig. 2** (good marker). Changing the cutoff results in variation of sensitivity and specificity with a contrary trend (ie, the higher sensitivity, the lower specificity, and vice versa). The ideal cutoff is set at the point where the sum of sensitivity and specificity has its maximum. (*Data from* an artificial data set, analysis and plot were generated using MedCalc software, Version 11.3.6, Mariakerke, Belgium.)

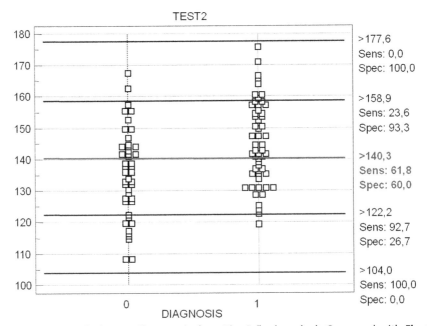

Fig. 7. Playing with the cutoff, example from **Fig. 3** (bad marker). Compared with **Fig. 6**, sensitivity and specificity are lower. For more information, see caption for **Fig. 6**.

independent of each other) there is a high association with the cutoff. To analyze this phenomenon in an objective manner, so-called receiver operating characteristics (ROC) curves have been used more and more within recent years. Historically, the ROC curve was first used during World War II for the analysis of radar signals before it was used in signal-detection theory. In the 1950s, ROC curves were used in psychophysics to assess human (and occasionally nonhuman animal) detection of weak signals.[3] Later, ROC curve analysis has been extensively used in the evaluation of diagnostic tests in medicine.[4]

The creation of ROC curves is the logical consequence of the facts that were presented earlier; it describes the association between sensitivity and specificity depending on different cutoffs and transfers it into a graph. Changing the value for the cutoff in **Fig. 6** results in different data for sensitivity and specificity. In **Fig. 6**, 5 examples for different cutoffs are shown; however, if this principle is extended to a step-by-step analysis (again using the data from **Figs. 2** and **6**, respectively), a table is created containing individual data sets for each possible cutoff and the related sensitivity and specificity (**Fig. 8**): Beginning from the left, the cutoffs are listed beginning with the lowest value of the marker (77.3) up to the highest value of 143.6. The next 2 columns show the related data for sensitivity and specificity. To make the graph easier to read, the next step is to subtract 100 minus the specificity (column 4); by this transformation, both sensitivity and specificity start with the value of 0 and end up with 100 (see **Fig. 8**). To complete the data, column 5 shows the sum of sensitivity and specificity; the ideal

Cut-off	Sensitivity	Specificity	100 - Specificity	Sum of Sens. + Spec.
>=77,3	100	0	100	100
> 94,9	100	37,8	62,2	137,8
> 95	98,2	37,8	62,2	136
> 102,5	98,2	66,7	33,3	164,9
> 102,7	96,4	66,7	33,3	163,1
> 103,2	96,4	73,3	26,7	169,7
> 104	94,5	73,3	26,7	167,8
> 104,5	94,5	75,6	24,4	170,1
> 104,9	92,7	75,6	24,4	168,3
> 108,3	92,7	86,7	13,3	179,4
> 108.9 *	90.9	91.1	8.9	182
> 110,7	81,8	91,1	8,9	172,9
> 112,2	81,8	93,3	6,7	175,1
> 112,7	80	93,3	6,7	173,3
> 112,9	80	95,6	4,4	175,6
> 114,6	76,4	95,6	4,4	172
> 114,8	76,4	97,8	2,2	174,2
> 133,1	14,5	97,8	2,2	112,3
> 133,4	14,5	100	0	114,5
> 143,6	0	100	0	100

Fig. 8. Setting up a table to generate an ROC curve. Each row refers to different cutoffs for the marker in the data set from **Fig. 6**. Columns (from left to right): (1) cutoff of the marker; (2) sensitivity; (3) specificity; (4) 100 minus specificity; (5) sum of sensitivity and specificity. Columns 2 and 4 are used for plotting the ROC curve (see **Fig. 9**). The ideal cutoff is at the maximum of column 5. (*Data from* an artificial data set, analysis and plot were generated using MedCalc software, Version 11.3.6, Mariakerke, Belgium.)

cutoff is the value at which this sum has its maximum (ie, the sum of false-positive and false-negative results is minimal) (see **Fig. 8**). The ROC curve is the graph created by columns 2 and 4 (ie, it shows the association between sensitivity and 100 minus specificity). **Fig. 9** shows the example for the good marker (data from **Fig. 2**); **Fig. 10** uses the data from **Fig. 3** (bad marker). The better the marker, the more the knee of the curve is at the upper left corner of the graph; as an additional tool, modern software for medical statistics calculates the area under the ROC curve (AUROCC), which may have values between 0.5 and 1.0.[5] There is no absolute value to define good and bad markers; a minimum of 0.7 is required, and values more than 0.8 are good, especially in the heterogeneous population of critically ill patients.

STEP 4: TRANSFERRING STATISTICS INTO CLINICAL RELEVANCE: THE PREDICTIVE VALUE

High significance, sensitivity, and specificity of more than 90%, AUROCC greater than 0.8 – done? A second example, based on historical data, shows that this strategy may lead to wrong conclusions:

Situation: An enzyme-linked immunoassay (ELISA) test for the human immunodeficiency virus (HIV) is available; both sensitivity and specificity are around 99.9%. This test is used by a company to screen individuals without any medical history during the employment process.
Question: If the test is positive for an individual without any symptoms or suspected medical history, what do you recommend to this person? What is the chance that the test is false-positive?

This kind of screening is also used in other fields of medicine, such as mammograms in women more than a defined age. But how can the data be interpreted? To answer this question, we have to go back to **Fig. 4**. Definitions of sensitivity and

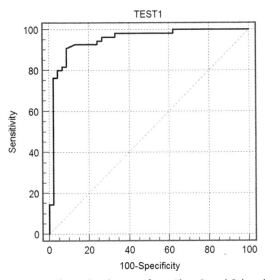

Fig. 9. ROC curve, generated from the data set from **Figs. 2** and **8** (see information in the caption for **Fig. 8**). The knee of the curve has a clear trend toward the upper left corner of the plot, which is associated with a good marker (high sensitivity, high specificity). (*Data from* an artificial data set, analysis and plot were generated using MedCalc software, Version 11.3.6, Mariakerke, Belgium.)

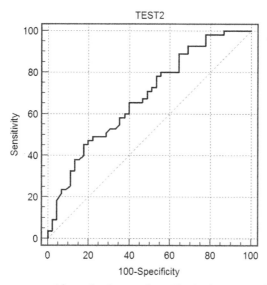

Fig. 10. ROC curve, generated from the data set from **Fig. 3**. The curve is flat compared with **Fig. 9**, which is associated with a bad marker (low sensitivity, low specificity). (*Data from* an artificial data set, analysis and plot were generated using MedCalc software, Version 11.3.6, Mariakerke, Belgium.)

specificity are based on a separate analysis of sick and healthy persons. Is this what the physician is doing when he applies a screening test? Did the company want to know if individuals with known HIV have a positive ELISA? Does the gynecologist want to know if the patient with known breast cancer has a positive mammogram? Of course not. In both cases, this would be a retrospective view (ie, superfluous). The key question is if a positive test can predict a disease, and not if sick persons have a positive test. The approach to calculating prediction is different from sensitivity and specificity. For assessment of predictive values, the subgroups of individuals with positive and negative tests are separately analyzed (not sick vs healthy).

   Fig. 11 shows how positive predictive value (PPV) and negative predictive value (NPV) are defined, using the same set of data as in **Figs. 3** and **4**. The PPV describes how many of the patients with a positive test are sick. In our example, 31 of the 44 patients with a positive test are sick, which equals a PPV of 31:44 or 70.5% (see **Fig. 11**, upper side). Vice versa, the definition of the NPV uses only the data of the patients with a negative test: the number of negative and healthy patients is divided by the total number of negative patients. In our example, 47 of the 56 negative patients are healthy, which equals an NPV of 47:56 or 83.9% (see **Fig. 11**, lower side). On first view, it may be concluded that PPV and NPV are based on different equations, but the results are similar to sensitivity and specificity. In our virtual example, this result is because the subgroups are more or less outweighed (ie, 60 healthy vs 40 sick patients, and 56 negative vs 44 positive patients). Again, PPV and NPV are independent of each other, because they are based on 2 independent subgroups of the patient cohort.

   For screening tests, this situation is often different: the quality of the HIV ELISA was measured comparing sick patients with healthy individuals with a comparable number of persons in each subgroup. For instance, if 1000 healthy individuals are compared with 1000 patients with known HIV, a sensitivity of 99.9% means that 1 of the 1000

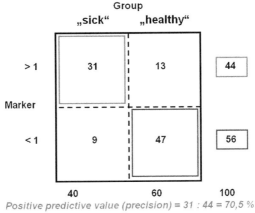

Positive predictive value (precision) = 31 : 44 = 70,5 %

Negative predictive value = 47 : 56 = 83,9 %

Fig. 11. Calculation of PPV and NPV, using the data set from **Fig. 4**. The PPV is defined by the percentage of correctly positive data divided by the sum of correctly and false-positive data of the marker. Vice versa, the NPV is the percentage of correctly negative data divided by the sum of correctly and false-negative data of the marker.

sick persons is measured false-negative. A specificity of 99.9% means that 1 of the 1000 healthy individuals is measured false-positive. Although this may look positive in the precision of the test, the conditions during screening tests are different: in 2008, HIV infection in Germany was estimated, with a result of 63,500 infected persons.[6] Compared with roughly 80 million citizens, this result reveals a prevalence of less than 0.1%. If 1000 individuals are screened using the HIV ELISA, 1 infected person is estimated among this cohort. Because sensitivity is 99.9%, it is probable that this person is discovered by a positive test. On the other hand, a specificity of 99.9% means that 1 of the 999 healthy persons is probably measured false-positive. Hence, there are 2 positive tests in the cohort, one of which belongs to the infected person, the other to a healthy individual (**Fig. 12**). The PPV of the HIV ELISA in a cohort of persons without any medical history is no more than 50%. The predictive values depend on the prevalence of the disease; the lower the prevalences, the lower the chance of detecting sick persons with a test.

APPLYING STATISTICAL BASICS IN CLINICAL PRACTICE: EXAMPLES IN CRITICALLY ILL PATIENTS

In this last section, an example is presented using the statistical basics that were presented in the previous sections. PCT is measured frequently in critically ill patients to detect infectious states and/or severe sepsis. For infectious patients, there are many publications reporting significantly higher values of PCT compared with nonseptic patients. In addition, ROC curve analyses revealed better data for sensitivity and specificity with higher AUROCC values compared with other clinical or laboratory parameters.[7,8]

In the last example, the difference in how to use sensitivity, specificity, and predictive values is shown. In **Fig. 13**, the raw PCT data from 100 patients in an intensive care unit with suspected infection are shown, 50 of whom had a positive blood culture (group 1), 50 of whom were negative (group 0). As expected, the difference was highly significant. Furthermore, ROC curve analysis (**Fig. 14**) revealed a sensitivity of 74% and a specificity of 92% at an ideal cutoff of 6 ng/mL (see **Fig. 13**). However, is this

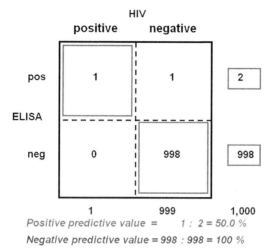

Fig. 12. Example for PPV and NPV in a virtual screening test. The prevalence of the disease is low (0.1%), which results in a low PPV, but a high NPV, even if the test is precise in terms of sensitivity and specificity. The wrong interpretation of tests like this may lead to fatal consequences.

the ideal base for screening patients? **Fig. 15** shows that this result differs from optimal predictive values. Moreover, as in the example for the HIV screening test, PPV and NPV may be different. If, instead of 6 ng/mL, a cutoff of around 1 ng/mL is chosen, this results in a higher sensitivity with a low specificity. More importantly,

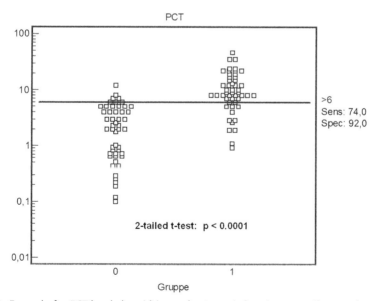

Fig. 13. Example for PCT levels (y-axis) in nonbacteremic (x-axis, group 0) versus bacteremic (group 1) patients (unpublished data). Two-tailed *t* test for independent data revealed a highly significant difference between the 2 groups. A cutoff of 6 ng/mL reveals the optimal sensitivity and specificity. (*Own data*, unpublished, analysis and plot were generated using MedCalc software, Version 11.3.6, Mariakerke, Belgium.)

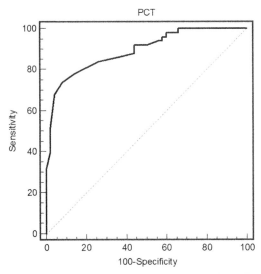

Fig. 14. PCT in critically ill patients, comparing bacteremic and nonbacteremic subgroups (unpublished data). ROC curve, generated from the data set from **Fig. 13**. (*Own data*, unpublished, analysis and plot were generated using MedCalc software, Version 11.3.6, Mariakerke, Belgium.)

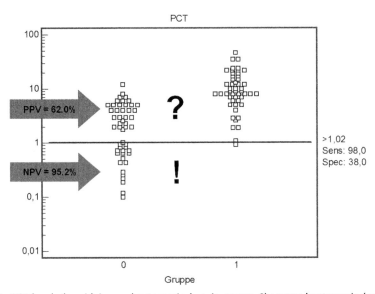

Fig. 15. PCT levels (y-axis) in nonbacteremic (x-axis, group 0) versus bacteremic (group 1) patients (own data, unpublished). A cutoff of roughly 1 ng/mL reveals a low PPV but high NPV. Hence, it is not possible to detect bacteremia with high PCT levels. On the other hand, the high NPV enables exclusion of nonbacteremic patients from extended diagnosis and unnecessary antibiotic therapy.

the PPV is poor (see **Fig. 15**, upper arrow, PPV = 62%). High PCT levels do not differ-entiate between bacteremic and nonbacteremic patients, because PCT values of more than 1 ng/mL are more or less equally distributed between both patient groups. However, a PCT value of less than 1 ng/mL is seen only in nonbacteremic patients (except in 1 bacteremic patient), which equals a high NPV (see **Fig. 15**, lower arrow, NPV = 95,2%). This example shows that PPV and NPV are independent parameters. Moreover, the NPV (like many other parameters for diagnosis and prediction in medi-cine) is often more relevant than the PPV, especially when the prevalence of diseases is low.

In a recent article,[9] gene-expression tests were used to predict septic complications after major surgery. Similar to the last example, a low prevalence of septic complica-tion of less than 10% was revealed in a low PPV for a combined set of 3 parameters. In contrast, the NPV was 98.1%.[9] It is important to understand what the frequently cited parameters for evaluating biomarkers really mean, how they are calculated, and how they can be interpreted. The NPV for screening tests is probably the key to assessing the capability for using biomarkers in clinical practice.

REFERENCES

1. Statistisches Bundesamt. Mikrozensus–Fragen zur Gesundheit. Körpermaße der Bevölkerung. Wiesbaden, Germany: Statistisches Bundesamt; 2010.
2. Reed JF III, Salen P, Bagher P. Methodological and statistical techniques: what do residents really need to know about statistics? J Med Syst 2003;27:233–8.
3. Green DM, Swets JM, editors. Signal detection theory and psychophysics. New York: John Wiley; 1966.
4. Zweig MH, Campbell G. Receiver-operating characteristic (ROC) plots: a funda-mental evaluation tool in clinical medicine. Clin Chem 1993;39:561–77.
5. Hand DJ, Till RJ. A simple generalization of the area under the ROC curve to multiple class classification problems. Machine Learning 2001;45:171–86.
6. Hoffmann C, Rockstroh J, Kamps B, editors. HIV 2009. 16th edition. Berlin. Medizin Fokus Verlag; 2010.
7. Charles PE, Kus E, Aho S, et al. Serum procalcitonin for the early recognition of nosocomial infection in the critically ill patients: a preliminary report. BMC Infect Dis 2009;9:49–57.
8. Mueller F, Christ-Crain M, Bregenzer T, et al. Procalcitonin levels predict bacter-emia in patients with community-acquired pneumonia. Chest 2010;138:121–9.
9. Hinrichs C, Kotsch K, Buchwald S, et al. Perioperative gene expression analysis for prediction of postoperative sepsis. Clin Chem 2010;56:613–22.

Physiologic Parameters as Biomarkers: What Can We Learn from Physiologic Variables and Variation?

Ricard Ferrer, MD, PhD[a,b,*], Antonio Artigas, MD, PhD[a,b]

KEYWORDS

- Sepsis - SIRS - Heart rate - Respiratory rate
- Body temperature - Physiologic variability

A consensus conference of the American College of Chest Physicians and the Society of Critical Care Medicine (ACCP/SCCM) in 1992 led to the publication of the first formally agreed upon definitions of sepsis, severe sepsis, and septic shock.[1] One notable result of this consensus conference was the introduction of a new term related to sepsis: systemic inflammatory response syndrome (SIRS). The development of this term was important because it placed a label on a complex set of findings that reflect a nonspecific inflammatory reaction to various insults. In sepsis, defined as SIRS triggered by infection, a complex network of mediators contributes to the clinical syndrome. The host response in sepsis is characterized by changes in physiologic parameters, and monitoring these parameters can help identify patients who might benefit from either conventional anti-infective therapies or from novel therapies targeting specific mediators of sepsis. **Table 1** lists the physiologic criteria associated with SIRS and sepsis, and the diagnostic criteria of severe sepsis and septic shock. An international consensus panel convened in 2001 to review the 1992 definitions essentially reconfirmed the definitions[2] but included a larger list of possible signs of systemic inflammation in response to infection (**Box 1**).

Disclosure: The authors have nothing to disclose.

[a] Critical Care Center, Hospital de Sabadell, Parc Tauli s/n, 08208 Sabadell, Spain
[b] CIBER Enfermedades Respiratorias, Instituto Universitario Parc Tauli, Universidad Autónoma de Barcelona, Barcelona, Spain
* Corresponding author. Critical Care Center, Hospital de Sabadell, Parc Tauli s/n, 08208 Sabadell, Spain.
E-mail address: rferrer@tauli.cat

Table 1
Definitions for SIRS, sepsis, severe sepsis, and septic shock based on the consensus conference of the ACCP/SCCM in 1992

Term	Definition
SIRS (at least 2 of these are needed to meet criteria for SIRS)	Body temperature $\geq 38°C$ or $<36°C$ Heart rate >90/min Respirations >20/min or $PaCO2$ <32 mm Hg White blood cell count >12.0 $\times$ 10^9/L or <4.0 $\times$ 10^9/L
Sepsis	SIRS plus infection
Severe sepsis	Sepsis associated with organ dysfunction, systemic hypoperfusion, or hypotension.
Septic shock	Sepsis with arterial hypotension despite adequate fluid replacement

SIRS

The term SIRS has been widely adopted by clinicians and investigators.[5,6] As SIRS criteria are not specific for sepsis, several studies have evaluated the usefulness of SIRS criteria for the diagnosis of sepsis. A subanalysis of the Sepsis Occurrence In Acutely Ill Patients (SOAP) study,[6] based on intensive care unit (ICU) patients, showed that critically ill patients often fulfill the criteria for SIRS, regardless of whether they are infected or not. At ICU admission, 87% of patients had at least two SIRS criteria, most commonly respiratory rate (84%) or heart rate (71%). There was, however, a higher frequency of three or four SIRS criteria versus two SIRS criteria in infected than in noninfected patients. Interestingly, all infected patients had at least two SIRS criteria. Thus, although the SIRS criteria are so sensitive and are present in so many ICU patients that their value in identifying infected patients is limited, patients fulfilling two or more SIRS criteria should be closely evaluated for infection.

The mortality attributable to infection seems to be similar in patients with sepsis and in those without (ie, those that fulfill the SIRS criteria and those that do not),[7] but some studies have demonstrated that an increasing number of SIRS criteria is accompanied by increasing mortality.[3,6,7] However, another study in patients with pneumonia found that SIRS criteria measured as early as the patient's presentation to the emergency department (ED) are poorly predictive of severe sepsis, shock, or death.[8]

The physiologic variables associated with SIRS and sepsis are not only important for the diagnosis and prognosis but also for guiding the treatment. In 1997, a ACCP/SCCM consensus group created a set of practice parameters for the hemodynamic management of patients in septic shock.[9] According to these practice parameters, the initial priority in managing septic shock should be to maintain mean arterial pressure (MAP) by adequate hemodynamic support. In fact, treatment with either MAP or systolic blood pressure as the main therapeutic endpoint is the most commonly recommended and supported clinical monitoring practice.[10] Maintenance of adequate MAP can help ensure adequate organ and tissue perfusion during the time required to detect and treat the infectious process causing the sepsis.

In 2004, an updated version of recommended clinical practice parameters was published.[11] In this publication, the continuous monitoring of physiologic parameters for early sepsis screening continued to center on hypoperfusion and the clinical definitions of hypoperfusion were expanded to include systolic blood pressure less than 90 mm Hg, MAP less than 65 mm Hg, a decrease in systolic blood pressure of more than 40 mm Hg, and a decrease in urine output.

Box 1
Diagnostic criteria for sepsis based on 2001 Society of Critical Care Medicine/European Society of Intensive Care Medicine/American College of Chest Physicians/American Thoracic Society/Surgical Infection Society International Sepsis Definitions Conference

General parameters

Fever (core temperature >38.3°C)

Hypothermia (core temperature <36°C)

Heart rate greater than 90 beats per minute (bpm) or greater than 2 SD above the normal value for age

Tachypnea: greater than 30 bpm

Altered mental status

Significant edema or positive fluid balance (>20 mL/kg over 24 hours)

Hyperglycemia (plasma glucose >110 mg/dL or 7.7 mM/L) in the absence of diabetes

Inflammatory parameters

Leukocytosis (white blood cell count >12,000/μl)

Leukopenia (white blood cell count <4,000/μl)

Normal white blood cell count with greater than 10% immature forms

Plasma C reactive protein greater than 2 SD above the normal value

Plasma procalcitonin greater than 2 SD above the normal value

Hemodynamic parameters

Arterial hypotension (systolic blood pressure <90 mmHg, mean arterial pressure <70, or a systolic blood pressure decrease >40 mmHg)

Mixed venous oxygen saturation greater than 70%

Cardiac index greater than 3.5 l/min/m^2

Organ dysfunction parameters

Arterial hypoxemia (Pao$_2$/Fio$_2$ <300)

Acute oliguria (urine output <0.5 mL kg−1 h−1 or 45 mM/L for at least 2 hours)

Creatinine increase greater than or equal to 0.5 mg/dL

Coagulation abnormalities (international normalized ratio >1.5 or activated partial thromboplastin time >60 seconds)

Ileus (absent bowel sounds)

Thrombocytopenia (platelet count <100,000/μl)

Hyperbilirubinemia (plasma total bilirubin >4 mg/dL or 70 mmol/L)

Tissue perfusion parameters

Hyperlactatemia (>3 mmol/L)

Decreased capillary refill or mottling.

Bacteremia, the presence of viable bacteria in the blood, is found only in about 50% of cases of severe sepsis and septic shock, and no microbial cause of infection is found in 20% to 30% of patients.[1,3]
Diagnosing sepsis early and identifying the origin of the infection, together with appropriate management and monitoring of the disease, can help reduce the high mortality associated with sepsis.[4]

Other parameters that can be monitored on a continuous basis in patients with sepsis include body temperature, heart rate, respiratory rate, cardiac output, systemic vascular resistance, oxygen saturation, mixed venous oxygen saturation, right atrial venous oxygen saturation, urine output, and right ventricular filling pressure or volume.[10–12]

EARLY TREATMENT OF SEPSIS

Early diagnosis of sepsis allows prompt treatment, and several recently published studies have demonstrated that early administration of treatments can decrease mortality among patients with sepsis. Early appropriate antibiotic therapy,[13,14] early goal-directed therapy,[12] corticosteroids,[15] drotrecogin alfa (activated),[16] tight glucose control,[17] and lung protective ventilation strategies[18] have all been associated with survival benefits. These and other therapeutic advances led to the development of the Surviving Sepsis Campaign (SSC) Guidelines[19] as part of a plan to reduce severe sepsis mortality. To improve the care for patients with sepsis, the SSC and the Institute for Healthcare Improvement recommend implementing two sepsis bundles: one marking goals to be achieved within the first 6 hours (resuscitation bundle) and the other within the first 24 hours of presentation (treatment bundle) of patients with severe sepsis or septic shock. Implementation of the bundles is associated to lower mortality.[20–22]

Because successful implementation of the bundles hinges largely on the early detection of sepsis, monitoring of physiologic parameters plays an important role in sepsis management. Early recognition of sepsis is especially important in the most severe patients. Delays in the identification of the most severe patients can be avoided by using easily measured bedside parameters to identify at-risk patients and beginning treatment immediately while waiting for additional information.[23]

These bedside parameters are referred to as the 10 signs of vitality (**Table 2**). When considered in combination, the 10 signs of vitality can help ensure patients at risk are identified early. This early identification of physiologic instability expedites basic resuscitation. Nine of the 10 signs of vitality can be assessed within several minutes; the 10th [base deficit, calculated after arterial puncture, or central venous oxygen saturation (ScVO2), obtained from a central venous catheter] requires a 15-minute

Table 2
The 10 signs of vitality

Ten Signs of Vitality	Triggering Parameter
Temperature	$\leq 36°C$
Pulse	<50/min or >100/min
Pain	New or significant increase
Respiratory rate	<6/min or >20/min
SaO_2	<90% and increased FiO_2
Blood pressure	SBP<90 mmHg, MAP <60 mmHg
Level of consciousness	Anxiety or lethargy
Capillary refill	>3s
Urinary output	<30 mL/h × 5 h, excluding renal failure
$ScvO_2$/base deficit	$ScvO_2$<65% or base deficit ≥ 5 or lactic acid >2.0 mmol/L

Abbreviations: MAP, mean arterial pressure; SAP, systolic arterial pressure; $ScvO_2$, central venous oxygen saturation.

turnaround time at many hospitals. In one study of 500 consecutive patients, using a similar approach for activation of a rapid response team, 50% of assisted patients were subsequently determined to be septic.[24]

PHYSIOLOGIC PARAMETERS ASSOCIATED WITH INFECTION

Several studies have used multiple logistic regression techniques to determine the physiologic parameters associated with the diagnosis of sepsis or to the exacerbation of sepsis (**Table 3**).

The SIRS criteria are not specific to sepsis and could be related to noninfectious causes like trauma, pancreatitis, cerebral hemorrhage, or even myocardial infarction.[25] Several studies have assessed the value of each physiologic parameter for the diagnosis of infection.

Peres and colleagues[26] developed a score to predict the probability of infection in critically ill patients based on physiologic parameters like body temperature, respiratory rate, and heart rate, together with other parameters like white blood cell count, C-reactive protein, and Sequential Organ Failure Assessment (SOFA) score by using multiple regression to calculate the relative weight of each parameter in relation to the presence of infection. The significant variables were: body temperature greater than 37.5°C, heart rate greater than 140, and C-reactive protein greater than 6 mg/dL. Among the clinical variables, heart rate was the best predictor of infection, whereas respiratory rate had the poorest predictive value. However, the investigators decided to include all variables in the Infection Probability Score (IPS), assigning points according the relative weight of each parameter in relation to the presence of infection. The IPS ranges from 0 to 26 points (0–2 for temperature, 0–12 for heart rate, 0–1 for respiratory rate, 0–3 for white blood cell count, 0–6 for C-reactive protein, and 0–2 for SOFA score). The best IPS cutoff value for infection was 14 points, with a positive predictive value of 53.6% and a negative predictive value of 89.5%.

Giuliano[27] used the Project IMPACT dataset to assess whether the physiologic parameters heart rate, mean arterial pressure, body temperature, and respiratory rate could be used to distinguish between critically ill adult patients with and without sepsis in the first 24 hours of admission to an ICU. Only two of the predictor variables, mean arterial pressure and high temperature, were independently associated with sepsis. The odds ratio (OR) for having sepsis was 2.126 for patients with a temperature of 38°C or higher, 3.874 for patients with a mean arterial blood pressure of less than 70 mm Hg, and 4.63 for patients who had both of these conditions.

Jaimes and colleagues[28] developed a clinical prediction rule to detect bacteremia at the bedside. They included in the analysis several physiologic parameters like heart rate, systolic blood pressure, and temperature, together with other simple clinical and biologic parameters. In the final stepwise logistic regression, the significant predictors of bacteremia were age greater than or equal to 30 years (OR, 2.07; 95% CI, 1.19–3.60), heart rate $\geq$90 beats/min (OR, 1.90; 95% CI, 1.13–3.17), temperature greater than or equal to 37.8°C (OR, 2.42; 95% CI, 1.41–4.14), leukocyte count greater than or equal to 12,000 cells/mL (OR, 2.40; 95% CI, 1.41–4.10), use of a central venous catheter (OR, 1.89; 95% CI, 1.02–3.50), and length of hospitalization of greater than or equal to 10 days (OR, 2.02; 95% CI, 1.25–3.24).

A Spanish group constructed a simple score based entirely on epidemiologic and clinical variables to detect bacteremia in patients with community-acquired pneumonia.[29] In the multivariate analysis, only six of the potential predictive factors remained significantly associated with bacteremia and were included in the score: liver disease, pleuritic pain, tachycardia, tachypnea, systolic hypotension, and absence of

Table 3
Studies that evaluate physiologic parameters in sepsis

Study	Risk Evaluated	Independent Parameters
Infection probability score[26]	Infection in ICU	HR >140 beats/min BT >37°C
IMPACT[27]	Sepsis in ICU	BT ≥38°C MAP <70 mmHg
Jaimes et al[28]	Bacteremia in hospitalized patients	HR ≥90 beats/min BT ≥37.8°C
Falguera et al[29]	Bacteremia in community-acquired pneumonia	HR ≥125 beats/min RR >30 cycles/min SAP <90 mmHg
RISSC, European Sepsis Database[41]	Severe sepsis or shock in septic patients	HR ≥120 beats/min SAP <110 mmHg BT ≥38.2°C
MEDS score[42]	Mortality in patients with infection in the ED	SAP <90 mmHg RR >20 cycles/min or pulse oximetry <90% or the need for O_2 supplementation
Varela et al[47]	Mortality in patients with multiorgan failure	BT entropy

Abbreviations: BT, body temperature; HR, heart rate; RR, respiratory rate; SAP, systolic arterial pressure.

prior antibiotic treatment. According to the regression coefficients, one point was assigned to each independent parameter. The score was internally and externally validated. Surprisingly, fever was not identified in the univariate analysis as associated with bacteremia.

Measurement of body temperature is one of the oldest clinical tools available, and fever has been considered a sign of infection for centuries; however, a large spectrum of febrile noninfectious disease must be differentiated from infection.[25] Conversely, infection can be present without fever, especially in elderly and debilitated patients.[30] Moreover, a normal or low body temperature can reflect failure of the host defense against infection.[31] In a series of 300 medical patients, Bossink and colleagues[32] found that only peak body temperature and peak white blood cell count appeared predictive of microbial infection. Body temperature greater than or equal to 38.5°C is related to infection in approximately 50% of patients,[25,26] the risk of sepsis is more than double in patients with temperature greater than 38°C during the first 24 hours in the ICU,[27] and temperature greater than or equal to 37.8°C has been described as an independent predictor of bacteremia in a general hospitalized population[28] but not in community-acquired pneumonia.[29]

Tachycardia is another important sign of infection. As mentioned above, heart rate was the best predictor for infection in the IPS study.[26] The investigators specified two cutoff values, at 80 and 140 beats per minute (bpm). The maximum level of probability for infection (heart rate >140) scored 12 points, whereas heart rates between 81 to 140 were assigned a score of 8. Heart rate greater than or equal to 90 bpm in a general hospitalized population[28] and heart rate greater than 125 bpm in patients with community-acquired pneumonia[29] have also been reported to be independent predictors of bacteremia.

Hypotension is another physiologic marker of infection. In septic shock, the loss of normal sympathetic responsiveness results in decreased vasomotor tone. In the nonresuscitated subject, this presents as hypovolemic shock, but fluid resuscitation does not usually increase blood pressure despite an increase in cardiac output.[33] Hypotension during the first 24 hours in the ICU is highly suggestive of infection.[27] Hypotension (defined as systolic blood pressure <90 mmHg) was found to be an independent predictor of bacteremia in patients with community-acquired pneumonia[29] but not in a general hospitalized population.[28]

Tachypnea has been recognized as a sign of sepsis for many years. The ACCP/SCCM Consensus Conference proposed a respiratory rate greater than 20 breaths per minute (breaths/min) as a cutoff value for infection.[1] In the IPS study, a respiratory rate greater than 25 breaths/min was a better cutoff value for infection, although the predictive value of respiratory rate for sepsis was poor. Tachypnea can develop in ICU patients for many reasons, and the frequent use of mechanical ventilation can influence respiratory rate in many ways. Respiratory rate greater than 30 breaths/min was an independent predictor of bacteremia in patients with community-acquired pneumonia.[29]

Leukocytes are typically increased in sepsis, although leukopenia can also occur and may be associated with a worse prognosis.[34] Using cutoffs of less than 1,000/mm^3 or greater than 15,000/mm^3 and greater than 12,000/mm^3, respectively, Bates and colleagues[35] and Jaimes and colleagues[28] found that leukocyte count was predictive of bacteremia. Stone and colleagues[36] showed that hyperleukocytosis was a predictor of persistent or recurrent sepsis. Another study in 300 hospitalized medical patients found that the peak white blood cell count was predictive of microbial infection.[32] Mellors and colleagues[37] used white blood cell count less than 5000/mm^3 or greater than 10,000/mm^3 together with fever and blood urea nitrogen to develop an index that predicted infection in patients undergoing abdominal surgery. White blood cell count alterations have been reported to be predictive of bacteremia in young febrile patients,[38] in elderly patients,[39] and in septic patients with Gram-negative bacteremia.[40] However, the discriminant value of the leukocyte count is much lower in critically ill patients, as hyperleukocytosis can occur in all stressful situations. In the IPS study,[26] two cutoff values were obtained for leukocyte count, 5,000/mm^3 and 12,000/mm^3. Leukocytosis was scored at only one point, but a higher score was assigned for neutropenia.

PHYSIOLOGIC PARAMETERS ASSOCIATED WITH EVOLUTION FROM SEPSIS TO SEVERE SEPSIS OR SEPTIC SHOCK

Sepsis has been graded in three groups of increasing severity: sepsis, severe sepsis, and septic shock (see **Table 1**), which are viewed as a continuum of risk.[1] One of the main purposes of identifying SIRS and sepsis—the lower severity group—is to help identify patients at risk of progression to a more severe stage to enable early therapeutic intervention. Alberti and colleagues[41] used the European Sepsis Database to estimate the probability of progression from the early stage of sepsis to a more severe one during the ICU stay. Analyzing variables recorded during the first day of infection associated with progression of sepsis to severe sepsis or shock by multivariate analysis, they derived the Risk of Infection to Severe Sepsis and Shock Score (RISSC). Approximately one of four patients presenting with sepsis worsened to a more severe stage during the 30-day follow-up period. Twelve variables were retained in the final multivariate model, including three physiologic variables (temperature, heart rate, and systolic blood pressure), three biologic variables (platelet count, serum sodium, and bilirubin), as well as mechanical ventilation (used in place of respiratory rate in patients on a ventilator), three infection sites (pneumonia, peritonitis, and primary bacteremia), and two categories of microorganisms (gram-positive cocci and aerobic gram-negative bacilli). For the physiologic variables, the cutoff points were defined as follows: temperature greater than 38.2°C, heart rate higher than 120 bpm, and systolic arterial blood pressure less than 110 mm Hg. Interestingly, the cutoff for heart rate associated with sepsis progression was higher (120 bpm) than that empirically selected by the ACCP/SCCM conference (90 bpm). Conversely, a relatively high cutoff was determined for systolic blood pressure (110 mmHg), suggesting that patients having marginally low blood pressure in the context of infection might need close monitoring. Of note, leukocytosis was not retained in the final model. The score derived from the regression coefficient of each variable retained in the final model ranges from 0 to 49, with the highest weights assigned to hyperthermia, primary bacteremia, and mechanical ventilation. It can be concluded from this study that the presence of fever, tachycardia, and hypotension are physiologic risk factors for sepsis worsening.

PHYSIOLOGIC PARAMETERS ASSOCIATED TO MORTALITY

Shapiro and colleagues[42] analyzed the risk factors for mortality in patients with suspected infection in the ED. Vital sign data included temperature, blood pressure, heart rate, respiratory rate, oxygen saturation, and oxygen delivery method. Abnormal temperature was defined as greater than 38°C or less than 35.5°C, tachycardia as greater than 90 bpm, and hypotension as systolic blood pressure less than 90 mmHg. Since arterial blood gases were obtained only in a minority of patients, respiratory difficulty was defined as the presence of any of the following: tachypnea (respiratory rate >20), hypoxemia (pulse oximetry <90%), or the need for oxygen supplementation to maintain adequate oxygenation. A multiple logistic regression model was constructed and used to assign point values for a clinical decision rule: the Mortality in Emergency Department Sepsis (MEDS) score. The covariates in this model identified the factors present in the ED that were independently correlated with the risk of death. The nine independent correlates of 28-day mortality were fatal disease or metastatic cancer, hypotension, respiratory difficulty, low platelet count, bandemia, age greater than 65 years, suspicion of a lower respiratory infection, nursing home residence, and altered mental status. The score ranges from 0 to 27 points, and 3 points are assigned for shock and 3 points for tachypnea or hypoxia. The MEDS score has been validated internally and externally in a multicenter study in patients with SIRS.[43]

VARIABILITY OF PHYSIOLOGIC PARAMETERS

Nonlinear deterministic behavior has been demonstrated or suggested to be the normal condition for a wide variety of human physiologic functions. The signals of many physiologic parameters are characterized as a time series for which interval variations may be analyzed by a variety of nonlinear measurement techniques. Using time series analysis and the statistical technique approximate entropy (ApEn), Godin and colleagues[44] reported that experimental human endotoxemia increases heart-rate regularity. This observation was reproduced by Rassias and colleagues,[45] who demonstrated, using ApEn, that human endotoxemia leads to decreased physiologic variability (increased regularity) of widely diverse in vivo functions like heart rate, innate immune reactivity assessed by neutrophil phagocytosis, and hormonal responses to inflammation assessed by plasma cortisol.

In the clinical setting, the loss of physiologic variability during systemic inflammation has been evaluated for body temperature and heart rate.

In a prospective observational study using ApEn in 24 successive patients admitted to the ICU with multiorgan failure, Varela and colleagues[46] found a correlation between regularity of body temperature and attributed SOFA score. The regularity of the temperature curve was higher in patients who died than in patients who survived. The prognostic value of temperature entropy was corroborated in a second study by the same group.[47] Body temperature was recorded every 10 minutes throughout the entire ICU stay in 50 successive ICU patients with multiorgan failure. The analysis of the entropy of the temperature curves by two independent methods showed that patients with higher regularity (lower entropy) of the temperature curve had worse clinical status, reflected in higher SOFA scores and higher mortality. Nevertheless, the predictive power of entropy to forecast mortality is not different from that of the SOFA score.

However, entropy measurement offers certain advantages over conventional scoring. It is harmless, does not require invasive analytic tests, and is very low cost. Furthermore, it provides data continuously in real time and does not depend on the results of supplementary tests that can only be performed sporadically. Entropy measurement may be useful for assessing the prognosis of patients with multiple organ failure and consequently may be helpful in making clinical decisions. Entropy measurement is a means of achieving a truly quantitative approach to temperature, thereby overcoming the classic febrile-afebrile dichotomy, and may also become a tool providing relevant information in afebrile patients, for whom thermometry is of no use.

Heart rate variability (HRV) analysis is a noninvasive technique that examines the beat-to-beat variation in heart rhythm, and power spectral analysis of HRV enables assessment of the degree of sympathetic and parasympathetic modulation of the heart over relatively short periods.[48,49] Some studies further reported that depressed sympathetic and sympathovagal modulation, detected as a decrease in HRV, may be early signals of deterioration in septic patients in the ICU[50] and may predict significant morbidity or mortality in septic patients in the ED.[51] HRV has been used in septic patients in the ED before the clinical symptoms and signs of septic shock are evident to predict the occurrence of impending septic shock.[52] Septic patients who deteriorated within the first 6 hours were characterized by increased cardiac vagal activity, decreased sympathetic modulation, and impaired sympathovagal balance. In a recent publication, Ahmad and colleagues[53] evaluated the usefulness of HRV in the diagnosis of sepsis. They studied a group of 21 patients at high risk of sepsis using a panel of HRV metrics computed continuously over time before the diagnosis of sepsis; they found that HRV decreases before the clinical diagnosis and treatment of sepsis. These data merit further investigation as a means of providing early warning of sepsis.

SUMMARY

Although the SIRS criteria are not specific to sepsis, several investigators have analyzed which physiologic parameters are independent factors for the diagnosis or the prognosis of sepsis. These physiologic parameters, together with other clinical variables, have been incorporated into scores for the diagnosis and prognosis of sepsis. The variability of physiologic parameters is reduced in septic patients and has a good correlation with outcome. Measurement of body temperature variability and heart rate variability are harmless, very low cost, and provide information in real time that may be helpful in making certain clinical decisions.

REFERENCES

1. American College of Chest Physicians/Society of Critical Care Medicine Consensus Conference: definitions for sepsis and organ failure and guidelines for the use of innovative therapies in sepsis. Crit Care Med 1992;20:864–74.
2. Levy MM, Fink MP, Marshall JC, et al. 2001 SCCM/ESICM/ACCP/ATS/SIS International Sepsis Definitions Conference. Intensive Care Med 2003;29:530–8.
3. Rangel-Frausto MS, Pittet D, Costigan M, et al. The natural history of the systemic inflammatory response syndrome (SIRS). A prospective study. JAMA 1995;273: 117–23.
4. Angus DC, Linde-Zwirble WT, Lidicker J, et al. Epidemiology of severe sepsis in the United States: analysis of incidence, outcome, and associated costs of care. Crit Care Med 2001;29:1303–10.
5. Brun-Buisson C. The epidemiology of the systemic inflammatory response. Intensive Care Med 2000;26(Suppl 1):S64–74.
6. Sprung CL, Sakr Y, Vincent JL, et al. An evaluation of systemic inflammatory response syndrome signs in the Sepsis Occurrence In Acutely Ill Patients (SOAP) study. Intensive Care Med 2006;32:421–7.
7. Alberti C, Brun-Buisson C, Goodman SV, et al. Influence of systemic inflammatory response syndrome and sepsis on outcome of critically ill infected patients. Am J Respir Crit Care Med 2003;168:77–84.
8. Dremsizov T, Clermont G, Kellum JA, et al. Severe sepsis in community-acquired pneumonia: when does it happen, and do systemic inflammatory response syndrome criteria help predict course? Chest 2006;129:968–78.
9. Practice parameters for hemodynamic support of sepsis in adult patients in sepsis. Task Force of the American College of Critical Care Medicine, Society of Critical Care Medicine. Crit Care Med 1999;27:639–60.
10. Dellinger RP. Cardiovascular management of septic shock. Crit Care Med 2003; 31:946–55.
11. Hollenberg SM, Ahrens TS, Annane D, et al. Practice parameters for hemodynamic support of sepsis in adult patients: 2004 update. Crit Care Med 2004; 32:1928–48.
12. Rivers E, Nguyen B, Havstad S, et al. Early goal-directed therapy in the treatment of severe sepsis and septic shock. N Engl J Med 2001;345:1368–77.
13. Garnacho-Montero J, Garcia-Garmendia JL, Barrero-Almodovar A, et al. Impact of adequate empirical antibiotic therapy on the outcome of patients admitted to the intensive care unit with sepsis. Crit Care Med 2003;31:2742–51.
14. Kumar A, Roberts D, Wood KE, et al. Duration of hypotension before initiation of effective antimicrobial therapy is the critical determinant of survival in human septic shock. Crit Care Med 2006;34:1589–96.
15. Annane D, Sebille V, Charpentier C, et al. Effect of treatment with low doses of hydrocortisone and fludrocortisone on mortality in patients with septic shock. JAMA 2002;288:862–71.
16. Bernard GR, Vincent JL, Laterre PF, et al. Efficacy and safety of recombinant human activated protein C for severe sepsis. N Engl J Med 2001;344: 699–709.
17. van den Berghe G, Wouters P, Weekers F, et al. Intensive insulin therapy in the critically ill patients. N Engl J Med 2001;345:1359–67.
18. Ventilation with lower tidal volumes as compared with traditional tidal volumes for acute lung injury and the acute respiratory distress syndrome. The Acute Respiratory Distress Syndrome Network. N Engl J Med 2000;342:1301–8.

19. Dellinger RP, Carlet JM, Masur H, et al. Surviving Sepsis Campaign guidelines for management of severe sepsis and septic shock. Intensive Care Med 2004;30: 536–55.
20. Barochia AV, Cui X, Vitberg D, et al. Bundled care for septic shock: an analysis of clinical trials. Crit Care Med 2010;38:668–78.
21. Ferrer R, Artigas A, Levy MM, et al. Improvement in process of care and outcome after a multicenter severe sepsis educational program in Spain. JAMA 2008;299: 2294–303.
22. Levy MM, Dellinger RP, Townsend SR, et al. The Surviving Sepsis Campaign: results of an international guideline-based performance improvement program targeting severe sepsis. Intensive Care Med 2010;36:222–31.
23. Funk D, Sebat F, Kumar A. A systems approach to the early recognition and rapid administration of best practice therapy in sepsis and septic shock. Curr Opin Crit Care 2009;15:301–7.
24. Sebat F, Musthafa AA, Johnson D, et al. Effect of a rapid response system for patients in shock on time to treatment and mortality during 5 years. Crit Care Med 2007;35:2568–75.
25. Circiumaru B, Baldock G, Cohen J. A prospective study of fever in the intensive care unit. Intensive Care Med 1999;25:668–73.
26. Peres BD, Melot C, Lopes FF, et al. Infection Probability Score (IPS): a method to help assess the probability of infection in critically ill patients. Crit Care Med 2003; 31:2579–84.
27. Giuliano KK. Physiological monitoring for critically ill patients: testing a predictive model for the early detection of sepsis. Am J Crit Care 2007;16:122–30.
28. Jaimes F, Arango C, Ruiz G, et al. Predicting bacteremia at the bedside. Clin Infect Dis 2004;38:357–62.
29. Falguera M, Trujillano J, Caro S, et al. A prediction rule for estimating the risk of bacteremia in patients with community-acquired pneumonia. Clin Infect Dis 2009; 49:409–16.
30. Gleckman R, Hibert D. Afebrile bacteremia. A phenomenon in geriatric patients. JAMA 1982;248:1478–81.
31. Clemmer TP, Fisher CJ Jr, Bone RC, et al. Hypothermia in the sepsis syndrome and clinical outcome. The Methylprednisolone Severe Sepsis Study Group. Crit Care Med 1992;20:1395–401.
32. Bossink AW, Groeneveld AB, Hack CE, et al. The clinical host response to microbial infection in medical patients with fever. Chest 1999;116:380–90.
33. Pinsky MR. Hemodynamic evaluation and monitoring in the ICU. Chest 2007;132: 2020–9.
34. Georges H, Leroy O, Vandenbussche C, et al. Epidemiological features and prognosis of severe community-acquired pneumococcal pneumonia. Intensive Care Med 1999;25:198–206.
35. Bates DW, Cook EF, Goldman L, et al. Predicting bacteremia in hospitalized patients. A prospectively validated model. Ann Intern Med 1990;113:495–500.
36. Stone HH, Bourneuf AA, Stinson LD. Reliability of criteria for predicting persistent or recurrent sepsis. Arch Surg 1985;120:17–20.
37. Mellors JW, Kelly JJ, Gusberg RJ, et al. A simple index to estimate the likelihood of bacterial infection in patients developing fever after abdominal surgery. Am Surg 1988;54:558–64.
38. Kuppermann N, Fleisher GR, Jaffe DM. Predictors of occult pneumococcal bacteremia in young febrile children. Ann Emerg Med 1998;31:679–87.

39. Fontanarosa PB, Kaeberlein FJ, Gerson LW, et al. Difficulty in predicting bacteremia in elderly emergency patients. Ann Emerg Med 1992;21:842–8.
40. Peduzzi P, Shatney C, Sheagren J, et al. Predictors of bacteremia and gram-negative bacteremia in patients with sepsis. The Veterans Affairs Systemic Sepsis Cooperative Study Group. Arch Intern Med 1992;152:529–35.
41. Alberti C, Brun-Buisson C, Chevret S, et al. Systemic inflammatory response and progression to severe sepsis in critically ill infected patients. Am J Respir Crit Care Med 2005;171:461–8.
42. Shapiro NI, Wolfe RE, Moore RB, et al. Mortality in Emergency Department Sepsis (MEDS) score: a prospectively derived and validated clinical prediction rule. Crit Care Med 2003;31:670–5.
43. Sankoff JD, Goyal M, Gaieski DF, et al. Validation of the Mortality in Emergency Department Sepsis (MEDS) score in patients with the systemic inflammatory response syndrome (SIRS). Crit Care Med 2008;36:421–6.
44. Godin PJ, Fleisher LA, Eidsath A, et al. Experimental human endotoxemia increases cardiac regularity: results from a prospective, randomized, crossover trial. Crit Care Med 1996;24:1117–24.
45. Rassias AJ, Holzberger PT, Givan AL, et al. Decreased physiologic variability as a generalized response to human endotoxemia. Crit Care Med 2005;33:512–9.
46. Varela M, Calvo M, Chana M, et al. Clinical implications of temperature curve complexity in critically ill patients. Crit Care Med 2005;33:2764–71.
47. Varela M, Churruca J, Gonzalez A, et al. Temperature curve complexity predicts survival in critically ill patients. Am J Respir Crit Care Med 2006;174:290–8.
48. Heart rate variability: standards of measurement, physiological interpretation and clinical use. Task Force of the European Society of Cardiology and the North American Society of Pacing and Electrophysiology. Circulation 1996;93:1043–65.
49. Kleiger RE, Stein PK, Bigger JT Jr. Heart rate variability: measurement and clinical utility. Ann Noninvasive Electrocardiol 2005;10:88–101.
50. Pontet J, Contreras P, Curbelo A, et al. Heart rate variability as early marker of multiple organ dysfunction syndrome in septic patients. J Crit Care 2003;18:156–63.
51. Barnaby D, Ferrick K, Kaplan DT, et al. Heart rate variability in emergency department patients with sepsis. Acad Emerg Med 2002;9:661–70.
52. Chen WL, Kuo CD. Characteristics of heart rate variability can predict impending septic shock in emergency department patients with sepsis. Acad Emerg Med 2007;14:392–7.
53. Ahmad S, Ramsay T, Huebsch L, et al. Continuous multi-parameter heart rate variability analysis heralds onset of sepsis in adults. PLoS One 2009;4:e6642.

Biomarkers in the Critically Ill Patient: C-reactive Protein

Jean-Louis Vincent, MD, PhD*, Katia Donadello, MD,
Xavier Schmit, MD

KEYWORDS

- Antibiotic • Cirrhosis • C-reactive protein • Infection
- Organ failure • Outcome • Sepsis

Sepsis is the leading cause of death in patients in the intensive care unit (ICU), and delay in diagnosis retards initiation of appropriate treatment. Yet, diagnosis is not always simple, especially in the often-complex critically ill patient in whom the classical signs of sepsis may not be present or may be associated with multiple other pathologic conditions and in whom microbiological cultures are frequently negative. Biomarkers, biologic molecules that characterize normal or pathogenic processes and can be objectively measured, have been suggested as a means of aiding diagnosis, predicting disease severity and outcome, and monitoring response to therapy. More than 170 such markers have been studied for potential use in septic patients,[1] but perhaps the best known and most widely used marker is the acute phase response protein, the C-reactive protein (CRP).

STRUCTURE AND HISTORY

CRP was first described in 1930, when Tillet and Francis[2] reported that serum from individuals acutely ill with lobar pneumonia was able to precipitate a substance derived from the C polysaccharide of *Streptococcus pneumoniae*, which they called fraction C. Importantly, they noted that when serum was taken from patients when they were acutely ill there was a strong precipitation reaction but the strength of the reaction decreased as the patients recovered. This observation suggested that this reaction could be used as a marker of disease. The investigators also reported that this precipitation reaction was not specific to pneumococcal infection but was also present in patients with bacterial endocarditis and acute rheumatic fever, and Ash[3] noted its presence in patients with gram-negative infections. Abernethy and Avery[4]

The authors have nothing to disclose.

Department of Intensive Care, Erasme Hospital, Université Libre de Bruxelles, 808, route de Lennik, 1070, Brussels, Belgium

* Corresponding author.

E-mail address: jlvincen@ulb.ac.be

Crit Care Clin 27 (2011) 241–251

doi:10.1016/j.ccc.2010.12.010

0749-0704/11/$ – see front matter © 2011 Published by Elsevier Inc.

and MacLeod and Avery[5] later determined that the reactive substance being precipitated by fraction C was a protein. The investigators commented that because this substance was present in many different infections, it could not be derived from the bacteria per se, but from the host "as a result of pathologic changes induced by or associated with acute infection."[4] CRP was the first so-called acute phase protein to be described; other proteins include fibrinogen, ferritin, haptoglobin, complement factors, and serum amyloid A.

It is now known that CRP is a member of the pentraxin (from the Greek "penta" meaning 5 and "ragos" meaning berries) family of calcium-dependent ligand-binding plasma proteins. The other member of this family present in humans is serum amyloid P component. The human CRP molecule is composed of 5 identical nonglycosylated polypeptide subunits, each containing 206 amino acid residues, forming an annular configuration.[6] CRP is synthesized principally by hepatocytes in response to stimulation by cytokines, notably interleukin (IL) 6. The plasma half-life of CRP is about 19 hours. In healthy young adults, the normal plasma concentration of CRP is about 0.8 mg/L.[7,8] During infection or acute inflammation, these values can increase by some 10,000-fold.[9] The plasma clearance of CRP is similar in healthy individuals and in those with disease, and the synthesis rate is the only significant determinant of its plasma level, making measurement of CRP levels a useful objective index of the acute phase response.[10]

PHYSIOLOGIC ACTIVITIES

The pentraxin family is highly conserved in evolution, suggesting that members have an important physiologic role. This theory is supported by the fact that there are no known deficiencies of CRP in humans. It has been suggested that CRP may act in a proinflammatory or in an antiinflammatory capacity to aid host defense. In vitro, CRP has been shown to increase release of the antiinflammatory cytokine IL-10[11] and decrease synthesis of several proinflammatory cytokines including IL-12, tumor necrosis factor and interferon-γ.[11,12] CRP also activates complement, enhances phagocytosis,[13,14] inhibits activated neutrophils,[15] increases nitric oxide synthesis,[16] and induces tissue factor[17] and adhesion molecule expressions.[18] Several in vivo models support an effect on host defense. For example, CRP transgenic mice infected with *Streptococcus pneumoniae*[19] or *Salmonella enterica* ser Typhimurium[20] have increased survival rates when compared with wild-type mice. In critically ill patients, the authors have shown a significant correlation between plasma fibrinolytic capacity and serum CRP levels, again supporting a link between CRP and the inflammatory response.[21] Nevertheless, the precise biologic properties of CRP remain somewhat controversial[22] and the variations in form and function among species make it difficult to extrapolate data from animal studies to humans.

CRP AS A BIOMARKER OF DISEASE

CRP is an acute phase protein and as such plasma levels are increased in most forms of acute and chronic inflammatory diseases. CRP is a recognized and widely used marker in rheumatology, with levels elevated in patients with rheumatoid arthritis, ankylosing spondylitis, psoriatic arthritis, polymyalgia rheumatica, to mention just a few. In such patients, CRP levels, especially when using new high-sensitivity CRP assays, can be used to assess the effectiveness of treatment and to monitor periods of disease exacerbation.[23,24] Similarly, CRP is used in gastroenterology, with high levels present in patients with acute relapses of Crohn disease.[25] Increased serum CRP concentrations are also considered a severity marker in pancreatitis.[26,27] CRP has been suggested as a potential marker of severity of asthma[28] and of development of chronic obstructive pulmonary disease (COPD)[29,30] and may be useful for guiding antibiotic therapy in patients with acute exacerbations of respiratory disease.[31]

There has been considerable interest in CRP as a prognostic and predictive marker in acute cardiovascular disease. As early as 1943, it was noted that a substance, later identified as CRP, was present in the sera of patients with acute myocardial infarction,[32] and later studies suggested that persistently elevated CRP levels were predictive of poor outcome after acute myocardial infarction.[33] CRP is, however, not only a marker of the presence of cardiovascular disease but also a biomarker of risk of subsequent cardiovascular disease or stroke.[34–36] Most recently, studies have reported that CRP levels may be used to identify patients who could benefit from preventive therapy.[37] In the Justification for the Use of Statins in Prevention: an Intervention Trial Evaluating Rosuvastatin (JUPITER) study, apparently healthy adults with low concentrations of low-density lipoprotein cholesterol but increased high-sensitivity CRP levels (>2 mg/L) who were randomized to therapy with rosuvastatin had a 54% reduction in myocardial infarction, a 48% reduction in stroke, and a 20% reduction in all-cause mortality when compared with those who received placebo.[37]

CRP AS A BIOMARKER OF INFECTION

A useful biomarker of infection, or rather the host response to infection, should provide additional information to the clinical picture in the fields of diagnosis, disease severity stratification and prognosis, and therapeutic guidance.[38] CRP has been investigated in all these 3 areas.

For Diagnosis

Accurate and rapid diagnosis of infection is important so that appropriate treatment can be initiated early.[39] However, because of prior or current antibiotic therapy, cultures often yield negative results, and multiple comorbidities can complicate diagnosis. The diagnosis of sepsis is thus largely based on clinical suspicion supported by the presence of several signs of sepsis, including elevated white blood cell count, fever, and tachycardia.[40] Laboratory markers of sepsis, similar to the troponins for myocardial disease, would represent a key advance in diagnosis and monitoring disease severity and recovery. However, although many agents have been proposed as sepsis biomarkers, none of them is sufficiently specific or sensitive to be used routinely for diagnosis.[1]

CRP is perhaps the most widely used biomarker of infection in critically ill patients and has been studied in adults[41 42] and children.[43] In 100 adult patients in the ICU, Ugarte and colleagues[41] reported a sensitivity of 67.6% and specificity of 61.3% for diagnosis of infection using a cutoff value of 7.9 mg/dL. In 112 patients in the ICU, Povoa and colleagues[42] reported that a serum CRP concentration greater than 8.7 mg/dL was associated with a diagnosis of infection with a sensitivity of 93.4% and a specificity of 86.1%. The combination of CRP concentration greater than 8.7 mg/dL and temperature greater than 38.2°C increased the specificity for infection diagnosis to 100%. Sierra and colleagues[44] reported a sensitivity of 94.3% and specificity of 87.3% using a cutoff of 8 mg/dL and noted that median CRP levels were significantly higher in patients with sepsis (18.9 mg/dL; 95% confidence interval [CI], 17.1–21.8) than in healthy subjects (0.21 mg/dL; 95% CI, 0.21–0.4), in patients with acute myocardial infarction (2.2 mg/dL; 95% CI, 2.1–4.9), and in noninfected patients with systemic inflammatory response syndrome (1.7 mg/dL; 95% CI, 2.4–5.5). Peres Bota and colleagues[45] suggested that the combination of several signs of sepsis (temperature, heart rate, respiratory rate, white blood cell count) with the CRP concentration and the Sequential Organ Failure Assessment (SOFA) score could provide a useful score to indicate the likelihood of infection. A score less than 14 was associated with a less than 10% chance of having an infection. This infection probability score was shown to be higher in patients with definite or probable infection than in those with unlikely or no infection and had a positive predictive value of 80% and a negative predictive value of 86% for infection.[46]

Importantly, absolute CRP values are in general not helpful. There is a large overlap in CRP levels between infected and noninfected patients, perhaps particularly in patients in the ICU in whom other causes of inflammation may be present. In addition, many patients, perhaps particularly the more elderly,[47] will already have elevated baseline CRP levels before ICU admission because of the presence of comorbidities associated with inflammatory processes. Therefore, although a single high CRP level adds evidence to a strong clinical suspicion of infection, following the pattern of CRP levels over time may provide a clearer picture, with an increasing CRP level suggesting that infection is developing or worsening. In an observational cohort study in which CRP levels were measured daily in patients in the ICU, Povoa and colleagues[48] noted that a maximum daily CRP variation greater than 4.1 mg/dL was a good marker for the prediction of nosocomial infection (sensitivity 92.1%, specificity 71.4%) and that in combination with a CRP concentration greater than 8.7 mg/dL, the discriminative power increased even further (sensitivity 92.1%, specificity 82.1%).

Importantly, although CRP levels are still useful indicators of sepsis in patients with cirrhosis,[49] in patients with fulminant liver failure, CRP levels do not always increase in the presence of sepsis. Therefore, CRP should not be used as a marker of infection in such patients.[50]

In addition to aiding with diagnosis of infection versus other causes of inflammation, attempts have been made to use biomarker levels to distinguish between different types of infection. However, although serum CRP concentrations are generally higher in bacterial infections than in infections of other causes,[51–54] it is unclear whether this is a reliable means of clearly distinguishing among bacterial, fungal, or viral infections in clinical practice. In children hospitalized with community-acquired pneumonia, the CRP level in patients with bacterial infection was higher than that in patients with viral infection (median 9.6 vs 5.4 mg/dL, $P = .008$), but the investigators commented that there was considerable overlapping of values in the 2 groups.[52] In 130 patients with sepsis in the surgical ICU, Martini and colleagues[55] reported that CRP levels in patients with bacterial sepsis were higher than those in patients with candidal sepsis (median [interquartile range] 19.0 [115–316] mg/dL vs 9.4 [66–129] mg/dL, $P = .002$). The best cutoff value for CRP levels to distinguish between bacterial sepsis and candidal sepsis was 10.0 mg/dL, with a sensitivity of 82% and a specificity of 53%. However, no clear cutoff value to distinguish between bacterial and candidal sepsis could be identified from analysis of receiver operating characteristic curves. In a retrospective study of patients with nosocomial bacteremia, serum CRP levels were reported as being substantially higher in patients with gram-negative bacteremia than in those with gram-positive bacteremia.[56] Gram-negative bacteremia was associated with an increase in CRP concentrations from 2 days before diagnosis to 1 day after diagnosis, whereas CRP levels remained unchanged in patients with gram-positive bacteremia.

For Prognosis

As for diagnosis, single CRP values are of less use for prognostication than trends in CRP over time. In 158 patients with sepsis, Silvestre and colleagues[57] reported no correlation between concentrations of CRP measured on the day of sepsis diagnosis and severity of sepsis. However, in a prospective cohort study, Lobo and colleagues[58] reported that at ICU admission patients with serum CRP levels greater than 10 mg/dL when compared with patients with CRP levels less than 1 mg/dL had a significantly higher incidence of respiratory (65% vs 28.8%, $P<.05$), renal (16.6% vs 3.6%, $P<.05$), and coagulation (6.4% vs 0.9%, $P<.05$) failures and higher mortality rates (36% vs 21%, $P<.05$). Moreover, patients who had a CRP concentration greater than 10 mg/dL at ICU admission and in whom the CRP level decreased after 48 hours had mortality rates of 15%, whereas those in whom the CRP level increased had mortality rates of 61% (relative risk, 0.25; 95% CI, 0.07–0.91; $P<.05$).[58] Ho and colleagues[59] reported that a high CRP concentration at ICU discharge was associated with an increased risk of ICU readmission and was an independent predictor of in-hospital mortality after ICU discharge.[60] Similarly, in patients in the nonsurgical ICU, maximum CRP levels during the ICU stay and CRP levels at ICU discharge were independently associated with post-ICU mortality.[61] However, in a mixed medical-surgical ICU, Al-Subaie and colleagues[62] were unable to find a significant difference in the CRP concentration on the day of discharge between patients who required ICU readmission or died in the hospital after ICU discharge and those who did not. Finally, Menendez and colleagues[63] reported that a CRP value greater than or equal to 21.9 mg/dL on admission for community-acquired pneumonia was independently associated with treatment failure (relative risk, 2.6).

For Therapeutic Guidance

The optimal duration of antimicrobial therapy in critically ill patients with sepsis is uncertain, and therefore, the ability to assess ongoing needs for antibiotics using biomarkers is appealing because it may help reduce adverse effects, reduce costs, and potentially reduce the development of antimicrobial resistance. The rationale for using CRP levels to guide antibiotic therapy is supported by several studies suggesting that CRP levels decrease as sepsis resolves. In a retrospective analysis, a decrease in CRP by 25% or more from the previous day's level was reported to be a good indicator of resolution of sepsis, with a sensitivity of 97%, specificity of 95%, and predictive value of 97%.[64] However, data actually linking CRP levels to antibiotic therapy are limited and are mainly from studies in the neonates. In neonates with suspected bacterial infection, Ehl and colleagues[65] stopped antibiotics when CRP levels decreased below 10 mg/L. CRP levels correctly identified 120 of 121 infants as not needing further antibiotics, corresponding to a negative predictive value with respect to further treatment of 99% (95% CI, 95.4%–99.9%). Similarly, Bomela and colleagues[66] reported that repeat CRP estimation correctly identified 99 of 100 infants in their study of neonates with suspected bacterial infection as not requiring further antibiotic therapy (negative predictive value, 99%; 95% CI, 95.6%–99.97%). Recently, in 50 adults with sepsis in the ICU, Schmit and Vincent[67] reported that CRP concentrations decreased more rapidly and more markedly in those with a favorable response to empirical antibiotics than in those who required a change in antibiotic therapy (**Fig. 1**). An increase in CRP of at least 2.2 mg/dL in the first 48 hours was associated with ineffective initial antibiotic therapy with a sensitivity of 77% and a specificity of 67%.[67] In patients with ventilator-acquired pneumonia, mean serum CRP levels 96 hours after diagnosis were significantly lower in patients with appropriate antibiotic treatment than in those with inappropriate empirical treatment (10.3 ± 10 mg/dL vs 19.2 ± 14 mg/dL, $P<.05$). A CRP ratio of 0.8 at 96 hours was a useful indicator of appropriateness of antibiotic therapy (sensitivity 77%, specificity 87%).[68] In patients with community-acquired pneumonia, a less than 60% decrease in CRP levels by

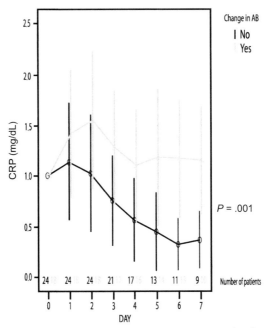

Fig. 1. Time course of the mean CRP concentration in patients with a favorable response to initial antibiotics (AB) (*black line*) and in patients who required a change in antibiotic therapy (*gray line*). Differences, P = .001. (*From* Schmit X, Vincent JL. The time course of blood C-reactive protein concentrations in relation to the response to initial antimicrobial therapy in patients with sepsis. Infection 2008;36:217; with permission.)

3 days after admission (odds ratio [OR], 6.98; 95% CI, 1.56–31.33) or a less than 90% decrease in CRP levels by 7 days (OR, 3.74; 95% CI, 1.12–13.77) were both associated with an increased risk of having received inappropriate empirical antibiotic treatment.[69] Venkatesh and colleagues[70] reported that antibiotic therapy for proven or presumed infection was associated with declining serum CRP levels in critically ill septic patients but that the marked variability made it difficult to define a nadir plasma concentration at which one could recommend discontinuation of antibiotic therapy.

CRP VERSUS PROCALCITONIN

Several studies have suggested that procalcitonin (PCT) is a more reliable marker of sepsis than CRP,[71–75] but not all studies support this.[31,76,77] Luzzani and colleagues[72] reported that PCT levels predicted infection and severity of disease more reliably than CRP levels in 70 critically ill patients, and 2 meta-analyses concluded that PCT was a better diagnostic indicator than CRP.[73,75] Castelli and colleagues[74] reported that PCT reacts faster than CRP, thus allowing an earlier prediction of infection. However, in patients with acute exacerbations of COPD, Daniels and colleagues[31] recently reported that CRP levels were higher in patients with sputum positive for bacteria than in those without, whereas PCT levels were the same in the 2 groups. Also, in patients with suspected community-acquired pneumonia and sepsis, Gaini and colleagues[76] reported that CRP was better than PCT as a diagnostic marker for infection and sepsis, whereas PCT was a better severity marker. A recent literature review of 18 studies in critically ill patients also concluded that PCT could not reliably differentiate sepsis from other inflammatory conditions.[77]

SUMMARY

There is an indisputable need for better techniques to diagnose sepsis, to characterize patients with sepsis, and to monitor therapeutic effectiveness. Use of biomarkers has been suggested as a means of achieving these aims. CRP is one of the many biomarkers that have been proposed for use in patients with sepsis and has been widely studied. The main advantages of serum CRP levels as a biomarker are the availability, ease of use, and low cost of assays. The key disadvantages are that CRP is not specific for sepsis and that its levels may be increased in other inflammatory conditions. Certainly, CRP is not the perfect biomarker for sepsis, but no other biomarkers have clearly and consistently been demonstrated to be better. No biomarker is entirely specific for infection because the body response to infection is not very specific; after all, sepsis is itself an inflammatory marker. There will, therefore, never be a perfect marker to answer the question "Is this patient infected?" In the future, panels of biomarkers are likely to be used to aid diagnosis and guide therapy.

In conclusion, when considering the use of serum CRP levels in critically ill patients, 3 key principles should be remembered:

1. CRP levels, as with other sepsis biomarkers, are more useful to rule out than to rule in sepsis: An elevated value does not necessarily mean that sepsis is present, but a completely normal value makes a diagnosis of sepsis unlikely.
2. Time course is more important that a single value. An increasing CRP level suggests that infection is developing or worsening, whereas a decreasing CRP level during treatment is reassuring in terms of the adequacy of therapy.
3. Serum CRP levels should always be interpreted in the clinical context. CRP levels alone can never be diagnostic, but should be used to support other clinical signs and symptoms.

REFERENCES

1. Pierrakos C, Vincent JL. Sepsis biomarkers: a review. Crit Care 2010;14:R15.
2. Tillett WS, Francis T. Serological reactions in pneumonia with a non-protein somatic fraction of pneumococcus. J Exp Med 1930;52:561–71.
3. Ash R. Nonspecific precipitins for pneumococcic fraction C in acute infections. J Infect Dis 1933;53:89–97.
4. Abernethy TJ, Avery OT. The occurrence during acute infections of a protein not normally present in the blood: I. Distribution of the reactive protein in patients' sera and the effect of calcium on the flocculation reaction with C polysaccharide of pneumococcus. J Exp Med 1941;73:173–02.
5. Macleod CM, Avery OT. The occurrence during acute infections of a protein not normally present in the blood: II. Isolation and proerties of the reactive protein. J Exp Med 1941;73:183–90.
6. Thompson D, Pepys MB, Wood SP. The physiological structure of human C-reactive protein and its complex with phosphocholine. Structure 1999;7: 169–77.
7. Shine B, De Beer FC, Pepys MB. Solid phase radioimmunoassays for human C-reactive protein. Clin Chim Acta 1981;117:13–23.
8. Raitakari M, Mansikkaniemi K, Marniemi J, et al. Distribution and determinants of serum high-sensitive C-reactive protein in a population of young adults: the cardiovascular risk in young Finns study. J Intern Med 2005;258:428–34.
9. Pepys MB, Hirschfield GM. C-reactive protein: a critical update. J Clin Invest 2003;111:1805–12.

10. Vigushin DM, Pepys MB, Hawkins PN. Metabolic and scintigraphic studies of radioiodinated human C-reactive protein in health and disease. J Clin Invest 1993;91:1351–7.
11. Mold C, Rodriguez W, Rodic-Polic B, et al. C-reactive protein mediates protection from lipopolysaccharide through interactions with Fc gamma R. J Immunol 2002; 169:7019–25.
12. Szalai AJ, Nataf S, Hu XZ, et al. Experimental allergic encephalomyelitis is inhibited in transgenic mice expressing human C-reactive protein. J Immunol 2002;168:5792–7.
13. Mold C, Gewurz H, Du Clos TW. Regulation of complement activation by C-reactive protein. Immunopharmacology 1999;42:23–30.
14. Casey R, Newcombe J, McFadden J, et al. The acute-phase reactant C-reactive protein binds to phosphorylcholine-expressing Neisseria meningitidis and increases uptake by human phagocytes. Infect Immun 2008;76:1298–304.
15. Shephard EG, Beer SM, Anderson R, et al. Generation of biologically active C-reactive protein peptides by a neutral protease on the membrane of phorbol myristate acetate-stimulated neutrophils. J Immunol 1989;143:2974–81.
16. Clapp BR, Hirschfield GM, Storry C, et al. Inflammation and endothelial function: direct vascular effects of human C-reactive protein on nitric oxide bioavailability. Circulation 2005;111:1530–6.
17. Nakagomi A, Freedman SB, Geczy CL. Interferon-gamma and lipopolysaccharide potentiate monocyte tissue factor induction by C-reactive protein: relationship with age, sex, and hormone replacement treatment. Circulation 2000;101: 1785–91.
18. Pasceri V, Willerson JT, Yeh ET. Direct proinflammatory effect of C-reactive protein on human endothelial cells. Circulation 2000;102:2165–8.
19. Szalai AJ, Agrawal A, Greenhough TJ, et al. C-reactive protein: structural biology and host defense function. Clin Chem Lab Med 1999;37:265–70.
20. Szalai AJ, VanCott JL, McGhee JR, et al. Human C-reactive protein is protective against fatal Salmonella enterica serovar typhimurium infection in transgenic mice. Infect Immun 2000;68:5652–6.
21. Zouaoui Boudjeltia K, Piagnerelli M, Brohee D, et al. Relationship between CRP and hypofibrinolysis: Is this a possible mechanism to explain the association between CRP and outcome in critically ill patients? Thromb J 2004;2:7.
22. Black S, Kushner I, Samols D. C-reactive protein. J Biol Chem 2004;279:48487–90.
23. Dessein PH, Joffe BI, Stanwix AE. High sensitivity C-reactive protein as a disease activity marker in rheumatoid arthritis. J Rheumatol 2004;31:1095–7.
24. Benhamou M, Gossec L, Dougados M. Clinical relevance of C-reactive protein in ankylosing spondylitis and evaluation of the NSAIDs/coxibs' treatment effect on C-reactive protein. Rheumatology (Oxford) 2010;49:536–41.
25. Mendoza JL, Abreu MT. Biological markers in inflammatory bowel disease: practical consideration for clinicians. Gastroenterol Clin Biol 2009;33(Suppl 3): S158–73.
26. Imamura T, Tanaka S, Yoshida H, et al. Significance of measurement of high-sensitivity C-reactive protein in acute pancreatitis. J Gastroenterol 2002;37: 935–8.
27. Pongprasobchai S, Jianjaroonwong V, Charatcharoenwitthaya P, et al. Erythrocyte sedimentation rate and C-reactive protein for the prediction of severity of acute pancreatitis. Pancreas 2010;39(8):1226–30.
28. Qian FH, Zhang Q, Zhou LF, et al. High-sensitivity C-reactive protein: a predicative marker in severe asthma. Respirology 2008;13:664–9.

29. Dahl M. Genetic and biochemical markers of obstructive lung disease in the general population. Clin Respir J 2009;3:121–2.
30. Kalhan R, Tran BT, Colangelo LA, et al. Systemic inflammation in young adults is associated with abnormal lung function in middle age. PLoS One 2010;5: e11431.
31. Daniels JM, Schoorl M, Snijders D, et al. Procalcitonin versus C-reactive protein as predictive markers of response to antibiotic therapy in acute exacerbations of COPD. Chest 2010;138(5):1108–15.
32. Lofstrom G. Non-specific capsular swelling in pneumococci. Acta Med Scand 1942;110:49–55.
33. De Beer FC, Hind CR, Fox KM, et al. Measurement of serum C-reactive protein concentration in myocardial ischaemia and infarction. Br Heart J 1982;47:239–43.
34. Ridker PM, Cushman M, Stampfer MJ, et al. Inflammation, aspirin, and the risk of cardiovascular disease in apparently healthy men. N Engl J Med 1997;336: 973–9.
35. Ridker PM, Buring JE, Shih J, et al. Prospective study of C-reactive protein and the risk of future cardiovascular events among apparently healthy women. Circulation 1998;98:731–3.
36. Cushman M, Arnold AM, Psaty BM, et al. C-reactive protein and the 10-year incidence of coronary heart disease in older men and women: the cardiovascular health study. Circulation 2005;112:25–31.
37. Ridker PM, Danielson E, Fonseca FA, et al. Rosuvastatin to prevent vascular events in men and women with elevated C-reactive protein. N Engl J Med 2008;359:2195–207.
38. Marshall JC, Reinhart K. Biomarkers of sepsis. Crit Care Med 2009;37:2290–8.
39. Kumar A, Roberts D, Wood KE, et al. Duration of hypotension before initiation of effective antimicrobial therapy is the critical determinant of survival in human septic shock. Crit Care Med 2006;34:1589–96.
40. Levy MM, Fink MP, Marshall JC, et al. 2001 SCCM/ESICM/ACCP/ATS/SIS international sepsis definitions conference. Crit Care Med 2003;31:1250–6.
41. Ugarte H, Silva E, Mercan D, et al. Procalcitonin used as a marker of infection in the intensive care unit. Crit Care Med 1999;27:498–504.
42. Povoa P, Coelho L, Almeida E, et al. C-reactive protein as a marker of infection in critically ill patients. Clin Microbiol Infect 2005;11:101–8.
43. Pulliam PN, Attia MW, Cronan KM. C-reactive protein in febrile children 1 to 36 months of age with clinically undetectable serious bacterial infection. Pediatrics 2001;108:1275–9.
44. Sierra R, Rello J, Bailen MA, et al. C-reactive protein used as an early indicator of infection in patients with systemic inflammatory response syndrome. Intensive Care Med 2004;30:2038–45.
45. Peres Bota D, Melot C, Lopes FF, et al. Infection probability score (IPS): a method to help assess the probability of infection in critically ill patients. Crit Care Med 2003;31:2579–84.
46. Martini A, Gottin L, Melot C, et al. A prospective evaluation of the Infection Probability Score (IPS) in the intensive care unit. J Infect 2008;56:313–8.
47. Lannergard A, Friman G, Ewald U, et al. Serum amyloid A (SAA) protein and high-sensitivity C-reactive protein (hsCRP) in healthy newborn infants and healthy young through elderly adults. Acta Paediatr 2005;94:1198–202.
48. Povoa P, Coelho L, Almeida E, et al. Early identification of intensive care unit-acquired infections with daily monitoring of C-reactive protein: a prospective observational study. Crit Care 2006;10:R63.

49. Bota DP, Van Nuffelen M, Zakariah AN, et al. Serum levels of C-reactive protein and procalcitonin in critically ill patients with cirrhosis of the liver. J Lab Clin Med 2005;146:347–51.

50. Silvestre JP, Coelho LM, Povoa PM. Impact of fulminant hepatic failure in C-reactive protein? J Crit Care 2010;25(4):657, e7–12.

51. Timonen TT, Koistinen P. C-reactive protein for detection and follow-up of bacterial and fungal infections in severely neutropenic patients with acute leukaemia. Eur J Cancer Clin Oncol 1985;21:557–62.

52. Toikka P, Irjala K, Juven T, et al. Serum procalcitonin, C-reactive protein and interleukin-6 for distinguishing bacterial and viral pneumonia in children. Pediatr Infect Dis J 2000;19:598–602.

53. Flood RG, Badik J, Aronoff SC. The utility of serum C-reactive protein in differentiating bacterial from nonbacterial pneumonia in children: a meta-analysis of 1230 children. Pediatr Infect Dis J 2008;27:95–9.

54. Almirall J, Bolibar I, Toran P, et al. Contribution of C-reactive protein to the diagnosis and assessment of severity of community-acquired pneumonia. Chest 2004;125:1335–42.

55. Martini A, Gottin L, Menestrina N, et al. Procalcitonin levels in surgical patients at risk of candidemia. J Infect 2010;60:425–30.

56. Vandijck DM, Hoste EA, Blot SI, et al. Dynamics of C-reactive protein and white blood cell count in critically ill patients with nosocomial Gram positive vs. Gram negative bacteremia: a historical cohort study. BMC Infect Dis 2007;7:106.

57. Silvestre J, Povoa P, Coelho L, et al. Is C-reactive protein a good prognostic marker in septic patients? Intensive Care Med 2009;35:909–13.

58. Lobo SM, Lobo FR, Bota DP, et al. C-reactive protein levels correlate with mortality and organ failure in critically ill patients. Chest 2003;123:2043–9.

59. Ho KM, Dobb GJ, Lee KY, et al. C-reactive protein concentration as a predictor of intensive care unit readmission: a nested case-control study. J Crit Care 2006;21: 259–65.

60. Ho KM, Lee KY, Dobb GJ, et al. C-reactive protein concentration as a predictor of in-hospital mortality after ICU discharge: a prospective cohort study. Intensive Care Med 2008;34:481–7.

61. Grander W, Dunser M, Stollenwerk B, et al. CRP levels and post-intensive care unit mortality in non-surgical intensive care patients. Chest 2010;138(4): 856–62.

62. Al-Subaie N, Reynolds T, Myers A, et al. C-reactive protein as a predictor of outcome after discharge from the intensive care: a prospective observational study. Br J Anaesth 2010;105:318–25.

63. Menendez R, Cavalcanti M, Reyes S, et al. Markers of treatment failure in hospitalised community acquired pneumonia. Thorax 2008;63:447–52.

64. Yentis SM, Soni N, Sheldon J. C-reactive protein as an indicator of resolution of sepsis in the intensive care unit. Intensive Care Med 1995;21:602–5.

65. Ehl S, Gering B, Bartmann P, et al. C-reactive protein is a useful marker for guiding duration of antibiotic therapy in suspected neonatal bacterial infection. Pediatrics 1997;99:216–21.

66. Bomela HN, Ballot DE, Cory BJ, et al. Use of C-reactive protein to guide duration of empiric antibiotic therapy in suspected early neonatal sepsis. Pediatr Infect Dis J 2000;19:531–5.

67. Schmit X, Vincent JL. The time course of blood C-reactive protein concentrations in relation to the response to initial antimicrobial therapy in patients with sepsis. Infection 2008;36:213–9.

68. Lisboa T, Seligman R, Diaz E, et al. C-reactive protein correlates with bacterial load and appropriate antibiotic therapy in suspected ventilator-associated pneumonia. Crit Care Med 2008;36:166–71.
69. Bruns AH, Oosterheert JJ, Hak E, et al. Usefulness of consecutive C-reactive protein measurements in follow-up of severe community-acquired pneumonia. Eur Respir J 2008;32:726–32.
70. Venkatesh B, Kennedy P, Kruger PS, et al. Changes in serum procalcitonin and C-reactive protein following antimicrobial therapy as a guide to antibiotic duration in the critically ill: a prospective evaluation. Anaesth Intensive Care 2009;37:20–6.
71. Muller B, Becker KL, Schachinger H, et al. Calcitonin precursors are reliable markers of sepsis in a medical intensive care unit. Crit Care Med 2000;28:977–83.
72. Luzzani A, Polati E, Dorizzi R, et al. Comparison of procalcitonin and C-reactive protein as markers of sepsis. Crit Care Med 2003;31:1737–41.
73. Uzzan B, Cohen R, Nicolas P, et al. Procalcitonin as a diagnostic test for sepsis in critically ill adults and after surgery or trauma: a systematic review and meta-analysis. Crit Care Med 2006;34:1996–2003.
74. Castelli GP, Pognani C, Cita M, et al. Procalcitonin as a prognostic and diagnostic tool for septic complications after major trauma. Crit Care Med 2009;37:1845–9.
75. Simon L, Gauvin F, Amre DK, et al. Serum procalcitonin and C-reactive protein levels as markers of bacterial infection: a systematic review and meta-analysis. Clin Infect Dis 2004;39:206–17.
76. Gaini S, Koldkjaer OG, Pedersen C, et al. Procalcitonin, lipopolysaccharide-binding protein, interleukin-6 and C-reactive protein in community-acquired infections and sepsis: a prospective study. Crit Care 2006;10:R53.
77. Tang BM, Eslick GD, Craig JC, et al. Accuracy of procalcitonin for sepsis diagnosis in critically ill patients: systematic review and meta-analysis. Lancet Infect Dis 2007;7:210–7.

Biomarkers in the Critically Ill Patient: Procalcitonin

Konrad Reinhart, Dr Med[a], Michael Meisner, Dr Med Habil[b],*

KEYWORDS

• Procalcitonin • Biomarker • Sepsis • Antibiotic

USE OF PCT IN CRITICALLY ILL PATIENTS

PCT differs from other propsed sepsis markers such as cytokines, C-reactive protein (CRP), or lipopolysaccharide-binding protein (LBP) primarily by the fact that it better reflects the severity of the systemic inflammatory response to infection, and it has some potential to differentiate between the infectious and sterile causes of systemic inflammation. Because the level of PCT is related to the severity of the systemic inflammatory response, PCT values have some prognostic value as well. In critically ill patients, PCT is used to confirm or exclude the diagnosis of sepsis, severe sepsis, and septic shock. This use has various consequences, for example, to initiate or stop sepsis-related treatment, to search for an area of focus or follow up the course of the disease, and to estimate the success of therapy. Recently, measurements that are highly sensitive in a low range became possible. Because the negative predictive value to exclude sepsis and severe bacterial infections is high, PCT has successfully been evaluated to guide antibiotic therapy in various types of patients, such as outpatients with suspected lower respiratory tract infections (LRTIs) and critically ill patients with sepsis, severe sepsis, and septic shock. PCT-guided antibiotic stewardship resulted in a reduction of antibiotic exposure between 20% and 70% without a negative effect on patient outcomes. Besides prevention of antibiotic overuse, the rapid diagnosis of infection and sepsis is of outstanding significance because an hour delay in appropriate antimicrobial therapy increases the mortality by 5% to 10%. As a result, antibiotic therapy is started, without a definitive microbiological test result, based on clinical signs and routine laboratory parameters such as white blood cell count and CRP levels, which have high sensitivity but lack specificity. Diagnostic uncertainty is compensated for by the liberal use of broad-spectrum antibiotics. The resulting increase in antibiotic resistance has become an increasing public health problem.

[a] Clinic of Anaesthesiology and Intensive Care Medicine, Friedrich-Schiller-University Jena, Erlanger Allee 101, 07740 Jena, Germany
[b] Clinic of Anaesthesiology and Intensive Care Medicine, Staedtisches Krankenhaus Dresden-Neustadt, Industriestr, 40, 01229 Dresden, Germany
* Corresponding author.
E-mail address: Michael.meisner@khdn.de

Crit Care Clin 27 (2011) 253–263
doi:10.1016/j.ccc.2011.01.002
0749-0704/11/$ – see front matter © 2011 Published by Elsevier Inc.

criticalcare.theclinics.com

BIOCHEMISTRY AND INDUCTION

PCT is the prohormone of the hormone calcitonin. Induction of the prohormone is differentially regulated during sepsis and infection as for hormonal activities of the mature hormone.[2] PCT levels, start to increase upon an infectious stimulus somewhat slowly after 2 hours and peak at 24 hours, provided no second infectious hit occurs. This response is considerably faster than that of CRP, whose levels increase slowly and only peak at 48 hours. PCT has various immunologic functions, modulating the immune response during sepsis, infection, and inflammation. Among those functions are chemotactic functions, modulation of inducible nitric oxide synthase, and cytokine induction, and the protein interferes with receptor binding of other peptide hormones involved in modulating intravascular fluid and vascular tone (calcitonin gene–related peptide, adrenomedullin).[3,4] Induction of the protein is strictly regulated and depends on cell-cell interactions. Circulating blood cells produce cytokines, but no PCT. Migration of adherent monocytic cells into the tissue obviously plays a major role in PCT induction because only adherent monocytic cells produce PCT in a time-dependent manner and contact of such cells with adipocytes, for example, triggers a major and sustained PCT response in vitro.[5]

STUDY FINDINGS ON PCT MEASUREMENT IN CRITICALLY ILL PATIENTS

Table 1 summarizes the findings of studies that assessed the potential of PCT in several clinical settings, such as presence and severity of a systemic inflammatory response caused by infection, differential diagnosis between infectious and noninfectious causes, and the effectiveness of measures of source control.

DIAGNOSIS OF SEPSIS, SEVERE SEPSIS, AND SEPTIC SHOCK

In patients with sepsis, severe sepsis, or septic shock compared with infected patients without signs of systemic inflammation or patients with sterile systemic inflammation, PCT levels are significantly elevated. The odds ratio for increased PCT levels (>0.5 ng/mL) in a meta-analysis was around 15.7 as compared with 5.4 for CRP levels.[14] High PCT levels have been reported especially in patients with septic shock. As depicted in **Table 2**, the cutoffs may also vary.[6,7,10,48,56,57] There are several other conditions, such as autoimmune disorders (Kawasaki syndrome), that may result in elevated PCT levels without signs of infection.[58,59] Basically, for all diagnostic tests, the diagnostic accuracy can be increased if further clinical data are implemented into decision making.

DIAGNOSIS OF INFECTION AND SEPSIS

In the absence of other factors that may induce an increase in PCT levels, a PCT value of 0.25 to 0.5 ng/mL suggests the presence of a bacterial infection that requires antimicrobial treatment. If PCT levels are less than 0.25 ng/mL, severe bacterial infection and sepsis are very unlikely; however, local infection may be present. The clinical relevance of the potential of PCT to differentiate between infectious and noninfectious causes of inflammation has been questioned by Tang and colleagues.[60] However, in most studies included in this meta-analysis, this question was not the primary aim of the study. Despite the limitations of PCT, to date, there is no other biomarker that differentiates better between the infectious and noninfectious causes and severity of inflammation in patients with a systemic inflammatory response. This is especially true in comparison with CRP, LBP, and interleukin 6. **Table 3** depicts the average

Table 1
Potential benefits of the measurement of PCT levels

Aim of the Study	Findings	References
PCT levels in patients with sepsis, severe sepsis, and septic shock	PCT is significantly elevated in patients with sepsis, severe sepsis, and septic shock. Especially high concentrations were found in patients with severe stages of the disease (severe sepsis, septic shock)	6–13
PCT in severe bacterial infection	PCT levels were significantly higher in patients with bacterial infection than in those with viral and fungal infections and sepsis	14–18
PCT as a marker for effectiveness of source control and prognosis	PCT levels decline by successful measures of source control, and sustained elevated PCT levels are associated with poor prognosis. This finding was demonstrated in adult and pediatric patients with sepsis, VAP, and CAP	6,19–25
Usefulness of PCT for antibiotic stewardship	PCT-guided antibiotic therapy may result in a 20%–70% decrease in antibiotic exposure without a negative effect on patient outcome	26–29
PCT in specific indications (see also **Table 3**)	Pancreatitis: low PCT levels were found in patients with sterile less-severe pancreatitis. High levels (>0.5 ng/mL) were reported in patients with infected necrosis and in those with severe pancreatitis Fungal infection: elevated PCT levels were reported in patients with fungal infection; however, there are reports on invasive fungal infections without major increase in PCT levels. Any PCT level increase, especially if it does not respond to antibiotic therapy, may indicate invasive or systemic fungal infection Bacteremia: it is more likely in patients with high PCT levels, but low PCT level does not exclude bacteremia Transplantation: in transplant patients, PCT is superior to conventional infection markers to differentiate between acute ejection and infectious complications	30–35 36–40 18,41–47 48–53

Abbreviations: CAP, community-acquired pneumonia; VAP, ventilator-associated pneumonia.

PCT levels that differentiated between infectious and noninfectious agents in various disease entities in published studies.

NONINFECTIOUS CAUSES OF PCT INDUCTION

Various causes of nonbacterial systemic inflammation and/or organ dysfunction have been reported, including

Major surgery and trauma
Severe burns

Table 2
PCT levels in patients with bacterial infection and different severities of systemic inflammation

| SIRS | | | | | | |
Median (Range)	Mean (SD)	Sepsis	Severe Sepsis	Septic Shock	Number of Patients (n)	References
—	—	2.4 ± 0.5 (mean, SD)	37 ± 16	45 ± 22	145	12
—	0.6 ± 2.2	6.6 ± 22.5	—	35 ± 68	337	13,54
—	1.3 ± 0.2	2.0 ± 0	8.7 ± 2.5	39 ± 5.9	100	55
<0.5 ng/mL	—	0.8 ng/mL	—	4.3 ng/mL	190	7
—	3.8 ± 6.9	1.3 ± 2.7	9.1 ± 18.2	38 ± 59	101	8
3.0 (0.7–29.5)	—	—	19.1 (2.8–351)	16.8 (0.9–351) All septic patients	33	9
—	0.5 ± 0.2 (approx)	2.0 ± 2.0 (approx)	18.0 ± 10.0 (approx)	20 ± 10 (approx)	101	6
0.38 (0.16–0.93 quartiles)	—	3.0 (1.48–15)	5.58 (1.84–33)	13.1 (6.1–42)	101	11
0.6 (0–5.3)	—	3.5 (0.4–6.7)	6.2 (2.2–85)	21.3 (1.2–654)	78	10

Abbreviations: approx, approximately; SIRS, systemic inflammatory response syndrome.

Table 3
Cutoff values for the differentiation between infectious and noninfectious causes of inflammation

Diagnosis	Cutoff (PCT)	Sensitivity/Specificity (%)	PCT (ng/mL)	Number of Patients	References
Acute meningitis Viral vs bacterial infection (children)	>0.5 µg/L	94/100	(Mean, range) 0.32 (0–1.7) vs 54.5 (4.8–110)	41 vs 18	61
Autoimmune disorders No infection vs bacterial infection	>0.5 g/L	100/84	(Mean, SD) <0.5 vs 1.9 ± 1.19	42 vs 16	62
Renal transplantation Diagnosis of acute rejection vs infection	>0.5 µg/L	87/70	—	13 vs 17	63
Pneumonia Bacterial vs atypical agents	—	—	(Median, range) 1.41 (0.05–65) vs 0.05 (0.05–7.5)	27 vs 9	64
Pneumonia Bacterial vs viral agents	2 ng/mL	63/96	(Mean, range) 2.7 (0.6–91) vs 0.63 (0.01–4.38)	43 vs 29	65
Invasive vs local infection in children	0.9 ng/mL	93/78	(Mean, SD) 27.5 ± 70 vs 0.32 ± 0.32	64 vs 27	66
Pancreatitis/edematous vs sterile necrosis vs infected necrosis	>1.8 µg/L	94/91	—	18 vs 14 vs 18	67
Patients in the ICU No infection vs infection	>0.6 µg/L	67/61	0.5 (median) vs 2.5 (median)	79 vs 111	7

Cardiogenic shock, birth stress in newborns

Heat shock

Different types of immune therapy, such as granulocyte transfusions, administration of antilymphocyte globulin, anti-CD3, or therapy with cytokines or related antibodies (alemtuzumab, interleukin 2, tumor necrosis factor α) and patients with acute graft-versus-host disease.

Likewise some autoimmune diseases (Kawasaki disease, different types of vasculitis) and paraneoplastic syndromes may be associated with elevated PCT levels.[68,69]

ANTIBIOTIC STEWARDSHIP WITH PCT

To date, several randomized controlled trials (RCTs) have demonstrated that an individual patient-adapted antibiotic therapy can be given with the support of the measurement of PCT levels. More recently, the use of this therapy was also demonstrated in the intensive care unit (ICU) setting. However, the concept of PCT-guided antibiotic stewardship and the studies that support it still face several criticisms. The main concern is that these studies aimed to demonstrate noninferiority within a rather large range of 7.5% to 10% difference in mortality between PCT-guided therapy and control groups. Such high cutoffs have been questioned because no study in an ICU setting has ever shown such a dramatic difference in mortality. Furthermore, Bouadma and colleagues[70] found a 3.8% higher 28- and 60-day mortality rates in the PCT-guided group, which was not statistically significant, but the design and the power of the trial imply that a negative effect on mortality attributable to the PCT strategy cannot be definitively excluded. Excluding a true excess mortality of 4%, similar to that seen in the trial, would require about 4220 patients; a study to exclude an excess mortality of 2% would need to be powered for 16,500 patients.[71,72] In a recent review, Schuetz and colleagues[73] summarized the results of 11 RCTs on PCT-guided antibiotic therapy, which were performed in adult patients. A total of 3691 patients were enrolled; 166 patients died in the control arm and 159 in the PCT arm. Although there remains some uncertainty on the safety of PCT-guided antibiotic therapy, the evidence in favor of this concept is increasing. But several open questions remain. Most of the higher-quality studies were performed in patients with pneumonia and LRTIs. There is only 1 smaller study in patients with severe sepsis. Studies in patients in the postsurgical ICU and immunocompromised patients are also warranted because it is well known that PCT is far from being an ideal infection marker. The user has to know that surgical trauma and other conditions may result in increases in PCT levels without concomitant infection. Likewise, there are several other noninfectious causes that may induce elevated PCT serum levels. It has also been argued that less-expensive biomarkers, such as CRP, have shown test characteristics similar to PCT when assessed in an outpatient population.[74,75]

SUMMARY

Among the numerous sepsis and infection markers that have been proposed, PCT is by far the most widely evaluated marker. This marker may help to make diagnosis earlier, to differentiate infectious from sterile causes of severe systemic inflammation, and to assess the severity of systemic inflammation caused by bacterial infection. PCT's potential to prevent unnecessary antibiotic use was assessed in 11 RCTs, and ongoing trials assess its clinical utility and safety as a guide for antibiotic therapy in settings such as severe sepsis.

REFERENCES

1. Bohoun C, Petitjean S, Assicot M. Blood procalcitonin is a new biological marker of the human septic response. New data on the specificity. Clin Intens Care 1994; 5(Suppl 2):88.
2. Becker K, Müller B, Nylen E, et al. Calcitonin gene family of peptides. In: Becker K, editor. Principles and practice of endocrinology and metabolism. 3rd edition. Philadelphia: J.B. Lippincott Co; 2001. p. 520–34.
3. Sexton PM, Christopoulous G, Christopoulous A, et al. Procalcitonin has bioactivity at calcitonin receptor family complexes: potential mediator implications in sepsis. Crit Care Med 2008;36:1637–40.
4. Hoffmann G, Totzke G, Seibel M, et al. In vitro modulation of inducible nitric oxide synthase gene expression and nitric oxide synthesis by procalcitonin. Crit Care Med 2001;29:112–6.
5. Linscheid P, Seboek D, Schaer JD, et al. Expression and secretion of procalcitonin and calcitonin gene-related peptide by adherent monocytes and macrophage-activated adipocytes. Crit Care Med 2004;32:1715–21.
6. Müller B, Becker KL, Schächinger H, et al. Calcitonin precursors are reliable markers of sepsis in a medical intensive care unit. Crit Care Med 2000;28(4): 977–83.
7. Ugarte H, Silva E, Mercan D, et al. Procalcitonin used as a marker of infection in the intensive care unit. Crit Care Med 1999;27:498–504.
8. Suprin K, Camus C, Gacoucin A, et al. Procalcitonin: a valuable indicator of infection in a medical ICU? Intensive Care Med 2000;26:1232–8.
9. Selberg O, Hecker H, Martin M, et al. Discrimination of sepsis and systemic inflammatory response syndrome by determination of circulating plasma concentrations of procalcitonin, protein complement 3a, and interleukin-6. Crit Care Med 2000;28:2793–8.
10. Harbarth S, Holeckova K, Froidevaux C, et al. Diagnostic value of procalcitonin, interleukin-6 and interleukin-8 in critically ill patients admitted with suspected sepsis. Am J Respir Crit Care Med 2001;164:396–402.
11. Castelli GP, Pognani C, Meisner M, et al. Procalcitonin and C-reactive protein during systemic inflammatory response syndrome, sepsis and organ dysfunction. Crit Care 2004;8:R234 40.
12. Zeni F, Viallon A, Assicot M, et al. Procalcitonin serum concentrations and severity of sepsis. Clin Intens Care 1994;5(Suppl 2):89–98.
13. Al-Nawas B, Krammer I, Shah PM. Procalcitonin in diagnosis of severe infections. Eur J Med Res 1996;1:331–3.
14. Uzzan B, Cohen R, Nicolas P, et al. Procalcitonin as a diagnostic test for sepsis in critically ill adults and after surgery or trauma: a systematic review and meta-analysis. Crit Care Med 2006;34(7):1–8.
15. Bohoun C, Assicot M, Raymond J, et al. Procalcitonin, a marker of bacterial meningitis in children in childhood. Bull Acad Natl Med 1998;182:1469–75.
16. Prat C, Dominguez J, Rodrigo C, et al. Use of quantitative and semiquantitative procalcitonin measurements to identify children with sepsis and meningitis. Eur J Clin Microbiol Infect Dis 2004;23:136–8.

17. Mueller C, Huber P, Laifer G, et al. Procalcitonin and the early diagnosis of infective endocarditis. Circulation 2004;109:1707–10.
18. Gras-le-Guen C, Delmas C, Launay E, et al. Contribution of procalcitonin to occult bacteremia detection in children. Scand J Infect Dis 2007;39:157–9.
19. Wanner GA, Keel M, Steckholzer U, et al. Relationship between procalcitonin plasma levels and severity of injury, sepsis, organ failure, and mortality in injured patients. Crit Care Med 2000;28:950–7.
20. Schröder J, Staubach KH, Zabel P, et al. Procalcitonin as a marker of severity in septic shock. Langenbecks' Arch Surg 1999;384:33–8.
21. Seligman R, Meisner M, Lisboa TC, et al. Decreases in procalcitonin and C-reactive protein are strong predictors of survival in ventilator-associated pneumonia. Crit Care 2006;10:R125.
22. Luyt CE, Guerin V, Combes A, et al. Procalcitonin kinetics as a prognostic marker of ventilator-associated pneumonia. Am J Respir Crit Care Med 2005;171:48–53.
23. Chastre J, Luyt CE, Trouillet JL, et al. New diagnostic and prognostic markers of ventilator-associated pneumonia. Curr Opin Crit Care 2006;124:446–51.
24. Jensen JU, Heslet L, Jensen TH, et al. Procalcitonin increase in early identification of critically ill patients at high risk of mortality. Crit Care Med 2006;34: 2596–602.
25. Hatherill M, Shane MT, Turner C, et al. Procalcitonin and cytokine levels: relationship to organ failure and mortality in pediatric septic shock. Crit Care Med 2000; 28:2591–4.
26. Christ-Crain M, Jaccard-Stolz D, Bingisser R, et al. Effect of procalcitonin-guided treatment on antibiotic use and outcome in lower respiratory tract infections: cluster randomised, single-blinded intervention trial. Lancet 2004;363:6000–7.
27. Briel M, Schuetz P, Mueller B, et al. Procalcitonin-guided antibiotic use vs a standard approach for acute respiratory tract infections in primary care. Arch Intern Med 2008;168:2000–7.
28. Stolz D, Christ-Crain M, Bingisser R, et al. Antibiotic treatment of exacerbations of COPD: a randomized, controlled trial comparing procalcitonin-guidance with standard therapy. Chest 2007;131:9–19.
29. Schuetz P, Christ-Crain M, Thomann R, et al. Effect of procalcitonin-based guidelines vs standard guidelines on antibiotic use in lower respiratory tract infections. JAMA 2009;302:1059–66.
30. Kylänpää-Bäck ML, Takala A, Kamppainen EA, et al. Procalcitonin, soluble interleukin-2 receptor, and soluble E-selectin in predicting the severity of acute pancreatitis. Crit Care Med 2001;29:63–9.
31. Kylänpää-Bäck ML, Takala A, Kemppainen E, et al. Procalcitonin strip test in the early detection of severe acute pancreatitis. Br J Surg 2000;88:1–6.
32. Bülbüller N, Doğru O, Ayten R, et al. Procalcitonin is a predictive marker for severe acute pancreatitis. Ulus Travma Acil Cerrahi Derg 2006;12(2):115–20.
33. Rau B, Kemppainen EA, Gumps AA, et al. Early assessment of pancreatic infections and overall prognosis in severe acute pancreatitis by procalcitonin (PCT). Ann Surg 2007;245:745–54.
34. Riche FC, Cholley BP, Laisne MJC, et al. Inflammatory cytokines, C reactive protein, and procalcitonin as early predictors of necrosis infection in acute necrotizing pancreatitis. Surgery 2003;133:257–62.
35. Purkayastha S, Chow A, Athanasiou T, et al. Does serum procalcitonin have a role in evaluating the severity of acute pancreatitis? A question revisited. World J Surg 2006;30:1713–21.

36. Distefano G, Curreri R, Betta P, et al. Procalcitonin serum levels in perinatal bacterial and fungal infection of preterm infants. Acta Paediatr 2004;93:216–9.
37. Christofilopoulou S, Charvalos E, Petrikkos G. Could procalcitonin be a predictive biological marker in systemic fungal infections? Eur J Intern Med 2002;13: 493–5.
38. Jemli B, Aouni Z, Lebben I, et al. [Procalcitonine et candidoses invasives en milieu de reanimation]. Ann Biol Clin (Paris) 2007;65:169–73 [in French].
39. Han YY, Doughty LA, Kofos D, et al. Procalcitonin is persistently increased among children with poor outcome from bacterial sepsis. Pediatr Crit Care Med 2003;4: 21–5.
40. Gerard Y, Hober D, Petitjean S, et al. High serum procalcitonin level in a 4-year old liver transplant recipient with disseminated candidiasis [letter]. Infection 1995;23:310–1.
41. Bell K, Wattie M, Byth K, et al. Procalcitonin: a marker of bacteraemia and SIRS. Anaesth Intensive Care 2003;31:629–36.
42. Chan YL, Tseng CP, Tsay PK, et al. Procalcitonin as a marker of bacterial infection in the emergency department: an observational study. Crit Care 2004;8(1): R12–20.
43. Caterino JM, Scheatzle MD, Forbes ML, et al. Bacteremic elder emergency department patients: procalcitonin and white count. Acad Emerg Med 2004; 11(4):393–6.
44. Liaudat S, Dayer E, Praz G, et al. Usefulness of procalcitonin serum level for the diagnosis of bacteremia. Eur J Clin Microbiol Infect Dis 2001;20:524–7.
45. Chirouze C, Schuhmacher H, Rabaud C, et al. Low serum procalcitonin level accurately predicts the absence of bacteremia in adult patient with acute fever. Clin Infect Dis 2002;35:156–61.
46. Persson L, Engervall P, Magnuson A, et al. Use of inflammatory markers for early detection of bacteremia in patients with febrile neutropenia. Scand J Infect Dis 2004;36:365–71.
47. Jimeno A, Garcia-Valasco A, Del Val O, et al. Assessment of procalcitonin as a diagnostic and prognostic marker in patients with solid tumors and febrile neutropenia. Cancer 2004;100:2462–9.
48. Hammer S, Meisner F, Dirschedl P, et al. Procalcitonin: a new marker for diagnosis of acute rejection and bacterial infection in patients after heart and lung transplantation. Transpl Immunol 1998;6:235–41.
49. Hammer S, Meisner F, Dirschedl P, et al. Procalcitonin: a new marker for diagnosis of acute rejection and becterial infection in patients after heart and lung transplantation. Transpl Immunol 2006;6:235–41.
50. Fazakas J, Gondos T, Varga M, et al. Analysis of systemic and regional procalcitonin serum levels during liver transplantation. Transpl Int 2003;16(7):465–70.
51. Kuse ER, Langefeld I, Jaeger K, et al. Procalcitonin in fever of unknown origin (FUO) following liver transplantation - a parameter to differentiate acute rejection from infection. Intensive Care Med 2000;(Suppl 2):S187–92.
52. Qedra N, Wagner F, Jonitz B, et al. Procalcitonin (PCT) is a new biological marker for the diagnosis of non-viral infections after transplantation of intrathoracic organs. J Heart Lung Transplant 2001;20(2):239.
53. Wagner FD, Jonitz B, Potapov E, et al. Procalcitonin: a donor-specific predictor of early graft failure-related mortality after heart transplantation [abstract]. J Heart Lung Transplant 2001;2:206.
54. Al-Nawas B, Shah PM. Procalcitonin in patients with and without immunosuppression and sepsis. Infection 1996;24:434–6.

55. Oberhoffer M, Bitterlich A, Hentschel T, et al. Procalcitonin (ProCT) correlates better with the ACCP/SCCM consensus conference definitions than other specific markers of the inflammatory response. Clin Intens Care 1996;7(Suppl 1):46.

56. De Talance N, Burlet C, Claudel C. La procalcitonine (PCT) est-elle le marqueur specifique du choc septique? Immunoanalyse et Biologie Specialisee 2003;18: 120–2 [in French].

57. Brunkhorst FM, Wegscheider K, Forycki ZF, et al. Procalcitonin for early diagnosis and differentiation of SIRS, sepsis, severe sepsis, and septic shock. Intensive Care Med 2000;26(Suppl):S148–52.

58. Okada Y, Minakami H, Tomomasa T, et al. Serum procalcitonin concentrations in patients with Kawasaki disease. J Infect 2003;48:199–205.

59. Ciaccio M, Fugardi G, Titone L, et al. Procalcitonin levels in plasma in oncohae-matological patients with and without bacterial infections. Clin Chim Acta 2004; 340:149–52.

60. Tang BM, Eslick GD, Craig JC, et al. Accuracy of procalcitonin for sepsis diagnosis in critically ill patients: systematic review and meta-analysis. Lancet Infect Dis 2007;7:210–7.

61. Gendrel D, Raymond J, Assicot M, et al. Measurement of procalcitonin levels in children with bacterial and viral meningitis. Clin Infect Dis 1997;24:1240–2.

62. Eberhard OK, Haubitz M, Brunkhorst FM, et al. Usefulness of procalcitonin for differentiation between activity of systemic autoimmune disease (systemic lupus erythematosus/systemic antineutrophil cytoplasmatic antibody-associated vasculitis) and invasive bacterial infection. Arthritis Rheum 1997;40:1250–6.

63. Eberhard OK, Langefeld I, Kuse E, et al. Procalcitonin in the early phase after renal transplantation – will it add to diagnostic accuracy? Clin Transplant 1998; 12:206–11.

64. Hedlund J, Hansson LO. Procalcitonin and C-reactive protein levels in community-acquired pneumonia: correlation with etiology and prognosis. Infection 2000;28:68–73.

65. Moulin F, Raymond J, Lorrot M, et al. Procalcitonin in children admitted to hospital with community acquired pneumonia. Arch Dis Child 2001;84:332–6.

66. Lacour AG, Gervaix A, Zamora SA, et al. Procalcitonin, IL-6, IL-8, IL-1 receptor antagonist and C-reactive protein as identificators of serious bacterial infections in children with fever without localising signs. Eur J Pediatr 2001;160:95–100.

67. Rau B, Steinbach G, Baumgart K, et al. The clinical value of procalcitonin in the prediction of infected necrosis in acute pancreatitis. Intensive Care Med 2000;26: S159–64.

68. Ilhan N, Ilhan N, Ilhan Y, et al. C-reactive protein, procalcitonin, interleukin-6, vascular endothelial growth factor and oxidative metabolites in diagnosis of infection and staging in patients with gastric cancer. World J Gastroenterol 2004;10(8): 1115–20.

69. Matzaraki V, Alexandraki K, Venetsanou K, et al. Evaluation of serum procalcitonin and interleukin-6 levels as markers of liver metastasis. Clin Biochem 2007;40: 336–42.

70. Bouadma L, Luyt CE, Tubach F, et al; PRORATA trial group. Use of procalcitonin to reduce patients' exposure to antibiotics in intensive care units (PRORATA trial): a multicentre randomised controlled trial. Lancet 2010;375(9713):463–74.

71. Gibot S. Procalcitonin in intensive care units: the PRORATA trial. Lancet 2010; 375:1605–6.

72. Tarnow-Mordi W, Gebski V. Procalcitonin in intensive care units: the PRORATA trial. Lancet 2010;375:1605.

73. Schuetz P, Albrich W, Christ-Crain M, et al. Procalcitonin for guidance of antibiotic therapy. Expert Rev Anti Infect Ther 2010;8:575–87.
74. Holm A, Pedersen SS, Nexoe J, et al. Procalcitonin versus C-reactive protein for predicting pneumonia in adults with lower respiratory tract infection in primary care. Br J Gen Pract 2007;57:555–60.
75. Cals JW, Butler CC, Hopstaken RM, et al. Effect of point-of-care testing for C-reactive protein and training in communication skills on antibiotic use in lower respiratory tract infections: cluster randomised trial. BMJ 2009;338:1374.

Triggering Receptor Expressed on Myeloid Cell 1

Damien Barraud, MD, Sébastien Gibot, MD, PhD*

KEYWORDS

- Sepsis • Infection • Innate immunity • TREM-1
- Soluble TREM-1

Sepsis is a common cause of morbidity and mortality in intensive care units (ICUs). Clinical and laboratory signs of systemic inflammation, including changes in body temperature, tachycardia, or leukocytosis, are neither sensitive nor specific enough for the diagnosis of sepsis and can often be misleading. Trauma, burns, pancreatitis, major surgery, and many other conditions may elicit clinical signs of a systemic inflammatory response syndrome (SIRS) in the absence of microbial infection. There is no gold standard for diagnosing sepsis because culture results may be negative especially in cases of antibiotic pretreatment or inadequate sampling. Indeed, more than 30% of infected patients remain without a clear microbial documentation. Moreover, results of microbiological studies are not immediately available. Clinicians often feel uncomfortable about the diagnosis and may administer unneeded antibiotics awaiting laboratory results. However, the empirical use of broad-spectrum antibiotics in patients without infection is potentially harmful, facilitating colonization and superinfection with multiresistant bacteria. Thus, there is a so far unsatisfied need for clinical or laboratory tools allowing to distinguish between SIRS and sepsis. Among the potentially useful markers of sepsis, procalcitonin (PCT) has been suggested to be the most promising marker. However, several investigators have questioned the diagnostic and prognostic accuracy of routine PCT measurements, reporting inconsistent and variable results depending on the severity of illness and infection in the patient population studied.[1]

A vast amount of research, from intuitive approaches to highly sophisticated genomic or proteomic studies, has centered on the discovery of the ideal biomarker of sepsis, which would allow for the early recognition of infection and may guide the treatment from antibiotics to immunomodulating agents.

The authors declare no conflict of interest.
Medical ICU, University Hospital of Nancy, Avenue de Lattre de Tassigny, 54000 Nancy, France
* Corresponding author.
E-mail address: s.gibot@chu-nancy.fr

doi:10.1016/j.ccc.2010.12.006
criticalcare.theclinics.com

THE TRIGGERING RECEPTOR EXPRESSED ON MYELOID CELLS 1

Recently, a new family of receptors expressed on myeloid cells, distantly related to NKp44, has been described: the triggering receptor expressed on myeloid cells (TREMs) family. The TREM isoforms share low sequence homology with each other or with other immunoglobulin superfamily members and are characterized by having only 1 immunoglobulinlike domain. Five *trem* genes have been identified, with 4 genes encoding putative functional type I transmembrane glycoproteins. The *trem* genes are clustered on human chromosome 6 (and mouse chromosome 17). All TREMs associate with the adaptor DAP12 for signaling.[2]

Among this family, TREM-1 has been identified on both human and murine polymorphonuclear cells and mature monocytes. Its expression by these effector cells is dramatically increased in skin, biologic fluids, and tissues infected by grampositive or gram-negative bacteria and by fungi.[3,4] By contrast, TREM-1 is not upregulated in samples from patients with noninfectious inflammatory disorders such as psoriasis, ulcerative colitis, or vasculitis caused by immune complexes.[4] In mice, the engagement of TREM-1 with agonist monoclonal antibodies has been shown to stimulate the production of proinflammatory cytokines and chemokines, such as interleukin (IL) 8, monocyte chemoattractant proteins 1 and 3, and macrophage inflammatory protein 1α, along with rapid neutrophil degranulation and oxidative burst.[5,6] The activation of TREM-1 in the presence of toll-like receptor (TLR) 2 or TLR4 ligands amplifies the production of proinflammatory cytokines (tumor necrosis factor α, IL-1β, granulocyte-macrophage colony stimulating factor), together with the inhibition of IL-10 release.[7] In addition, activation of these TLRs upregulates TREM-1 expression.[6] Thus, TREM-1 and TLRs seem to cooperate in producing an inflammatory response.

The role of TREM-1 as an amplifier of the inflammatory response has been confirmed in a mouse model of septic shock, in which blocking signaling through TREM-1 partially protected animals from death.[4,8] Both in vitro and in vivo, synthetic peptides mimicking short highly interspecies-conserved domains of TREM-1 attenuated the cytokine production of human monocytes and protected septic animals from hyperresponsiveness and death.[9] These peptides were efficient in not only preventing but also downmodulating the deleterious effects of proinflammatory cytokines.[8]

Besides its membrane-bound form, a soluble form of TREM-1 is liberated by the cleavage of its extracellular domain.[10] Soluble TREM-1 (sTREM-1) acts as a decoy receptor, sequestering TREM-1 ligand, which may exist in soluble form in the sera of septic patients,[11] and dampening TREM-1 activation.[4,12] To counteract excessive inflammatory reaction, several mechanisms exist, 1 of which involves another TREM family member. Hamerman and colleagues[13] suggested that 1 or more DAP12-associated receptors could negatively regulate TLRs signaling. One of these receptors could be TREM-2. When TREM-2 is expressed on monocytes/macrophages, its activation downregulates TLRs signaling through DAP12.[14] These data suggest that immune cells are able to integrate the sum of different signals through sensor receptors, such as TREM-1 and TREM-2, to induce a balanced inflammatory response.

TREM-1 is also implicated in the platelet/neutrophil dialog. Indeed, a TREM-1 ligand is constitutively expressed on platelets and megacaryocytes.[12] Although the interaction of the TREM-1 ligand (expressed on platelets) with the TREM-1 receptor (expressed on neutrophils) is not responsible for platelet-neutrophil complex formation, it mediates platelet-induced activation of neutrophils.

STREM-1 AS A DIAGNOSTIC MARKER OF INFECTION

Considering the modest reliability of traditional biomarkers, such as C-reactive protein (CRP) and PCT, and the a priori specific involvement of TREM-1 during infections, the usefulness of sTREM-1 in diagnosing sepsis has been the focus of several studies during the recent 5 years.

TREM-1 and the Diagnosis of Sepsis

Studies reporting on the performance of sTREM-1 in diagnosing sepsis are summarized in **Tables 1** and **2**.

Objective analysis of the published literature on this subject is tricky because of a huge heterogeneity between studies: many did not take into account the Bayes theory, the case mix is highly variable (eg, immunodepression, previous antibiotics), the selected cutoffs range from picograms to nanograms per mL, and so on. Most importantly, the techniques used to measure the sTREM-1 concentrations are not always comparable with large variations both during the preanalytical (such as technique of sampling, conservation) and the analytical periods (dilutions, homemade or commercial kits, some of which have been withdrawn from the market during the fall of 2008 due to unreliable results).

sTREM-1 and Systemic Sepsis

In order to distinguish between sepsis and SIRS in critically ill patients, 3 studies determined the usefulness of measuring plasma sTREM-1 concentrations in adults and 2 in pediatric patients (see **Table 1**). In a cohort of 76 patients admitted to an adult medical ICU with a suspicion of infection, Gibot and colleagues[15] determined that plasma concentrations of CRP, PCT, and sTREM-1 were higher in infected patients than in those with noninfectious SIRS. sTREM-1 performed better than other markers in diagnosing infection, with sensitivity, specificity, positive predictive value, and negative predictive value at 96%, 89%, 94%, and 93%, respectively. These initial encouraging results were not confirmed in 2 subsequent studies by Latour-Perez and colleagues[16] and Barati and colleagues,[17] involving a total of 246 critically ill patients, in which the sensitivity ranged from 49% to 70% and the specificity from 60% to 79%. In these studies, sTREM-1 was inferior than CRP or PCT. In the emergency room, the measurement of sTREM-1 concentrations alone also proved disappointing with an area under the receiver operating characteristic (ROC) curve at 0.61. Interestingly, the combined determination of sTREM-1 and 3 or 6 other marker levels performed far better than each marker taken alone.[18]

A similar discordance is found in pediatric patients. In 44 neonates, Chen and colleagues[19] found that sTREM-1 was superior to CRP or immature to total neutrophil ratio in diagnosing severe bacterial infections, whereas Sarafidis and colleagues[20] determined that in a neonatal ICU setting, sTREM-1 performed lower than IL-6, with 71% sensitivity and 78% specificity.

Finally, How and colleagues[21] determined *Trem-1* mRNA expression in 127 patients in the ICU and found that it was not better than determining CRP levels to diagnose infection.

Therefore, the measurement of plasma sTREM-1 concentrations does not seem to hold its initial promises in diagnosing systemic infections. Indeed, it now seems that many inflammatory conditions may be responsible for an elevation of plasma sTREM-1 concentrations (see later discussion). Whether determination of plasma sTREM-1 concentrations in association with other markers could prove useful remains to be studied.

Table 1
Soluble TREM-1 and systemic sepsis

	Patients	Confirmed Sepsis	Kits	Sample	Comparator	Sensibility (%)	Specificity (%)	PPV (%)	NPV (%)	Cutoff	AUC of ROC Curve (95% CI)	LR+ (95% CI)	LR− (95% CI)
Gibot et al[15]	Prospective, 76 consecutive adults, medical ICU	62	ELISA Original antibody	Plasma	CRP, PCT	96	89	94	93	60 ng/mL	0.97 (0.94–1)	8.6 (3.8–21.5)	0.04 (0.01–0.2)
Latour-Perez et al[16]	114 adults, ICU	63	ELISA Quantikine[a]	Plasma	CRP, PCT	49	79	80	47	463 pg/mL	0.62 (0.51–0.72)	3.47 (1.45–8.28)	—
Barati et al[17]	132 adults, ICU	39	ELISA Quantikine[a]	Plasma	ESR, CRP	70	60	67	65	725 pg/mL	0.65 (0.53–0.76)	—	—
Kofoed et al[18]	Prospective, 151 adults, emergency room	77	ELISA Luminex multiple assay	Plasma	CRP, PCT, MIF, sUPAR, combinations	82	40	71	56	3.5 ng/mL	0.61 (0.52–0.71)	—	—
Chen et al[19]	44 consecutive children younger than 3 mo	52	ELISA Quantikine[a]	Plasma	CRP, IT ratio	87	51	83	85	24 ng/mL	0.88 (0.78–0.99)	4.6 (1.6–11.2)	0.2 (0.1–0.4)
Sarafidis et al[20]	52 newborns	59	ELISA Quantikine[a]	Plasma	IL-6	70	71	78	62	143 pg/mL	0.73 (0.58–0.88)	—	—

Abbreviations: AUC, area under the curve; CI, confidence interval; ELISA, enzyme-linked immunosorbent assay; ESR, erythrocyte sedimentation rate; IT, immature to total neutrophil; LR+, positive likelihood ratio; LR−, negative likelihood ratio; MIF, macrophage inhibition factor; NPV, negative predictive value; PPV, positive predictive value; ROC, receiver operating characteristic; sUPAR, soluble urokinase plasminogen activator receptor.
[a] R&D Systems Inc, Minneapolis, MN, USA.

sTREM-1 and Localized Infections

Since the initial publication by Gibot and colleagues,[22] many studies have dealt with the local measurement of sTREM-1 concentrations during a variety of localized infections, from nosocomial pneumonia to peritonitis (see **Table 2**).

Pleuropulmonary infections constitute the core of research on TREM-1 diagnostic performance. The first study was published in 2004 by Richeldi and colleagues.[23] It showed that the expression of TREM-1 at the surface of alveolar neutrophils and macrophages (determined by flow cytometry) was increased during bacterial pneumonia as compared with levels found in patients with noninfectious interstitial lung diseases. Gibot and colleagues[22] investigated alveolar sTREM-1 as a marker of infectious pneumonia in 148 consecutive patients under mechanical ventilation. In this study, alveolar sTREM-1 concentrations were highly predictive of lung infection and performed better than any other clinical or biologic finding (including CRP and PCT) in both community-acquired pneumonia (CAP) and ventilator-associated pneumonia (VAP), with a diagnostic odds ratio of 41.5. Several other studies then confirmed these preliminary results. Huh and colleagues[24] found that sTREM-1 concentrations were useful during bacterial or fungal pneumonias, while sTREM-1 concentrations remained low in case of viral infection. The study by Determann and colleagues[25] focusing on VAP added kinetics data; alveolar sTREM-1 concentrations increased a few days before the clinical diagnosis of VAP, and the investigators concluded that the combination of more than 200 pg/mL of sTREM-1 with an increase of more than 100 pg/mL as compared with the value obtained 2 days earlier was highly predictive of the presence of VAP. Finally, El Solh and colleagues[26] showed that alveolar sTREM-1 allowed for the discrimination between aspiration pneumonia and pneumonitis.

However, several other studies, although confirming the elevation of alveolar sTREM-1 concentrations during lung infections, reported a lower discriminative value of measurement of sTREM-1concentrations. During VAP, alveolar sTREM-1 performed lower than the usual clinical pulmonary infection score, and clearly, plasma concentration measurement was not interesting.[27,28]

There is much less controversy over the diagnosis of pleural effusions. Indeed, 5 different studies including about 350 patients showed the role of pleural sTREM-1 in discriminating between infectious (due to empyema, parapneumonia) and noninfectious pleural effusions (due to cardiac insufficiency, cancer), with sensitivity ranging from 71% to 94% and specificity from 74% to 93%.[29–33]

Identifying the bacterial cause of meningitis can also be challenging, especially when patients have already received antibiotics. Two different studies showed that the increase in sTREM-1 concentrations in the cerebrospinal fluid was able to discriminate between infectious and viral meningitis. Of note, sTREM-1 concentrations were similar during pneumococcal and meningococcal infections.[34,35]

Only 1 study investigated sTREM-1 concentrations in urine for the diagnosis of lower urinary tract infections, and the results were inconclusive.[36]

The usefulness of peritoneal sTREM-1 in the diagnosis of peritonitis has also been investigated.[37] Determann and colleagues[37] showed in a cohort of 83 patients operated for secondary peritonitis that the peritoneal concentration of sTREM-1 progressively decreased in the patients of good outcome but remained persistently elevated and even increased in case of patients with residual sepsis and tertiary peritonitis. Thus, persistent elevation of peritoneal sTREM-1 concentrations could prompt the clinician to a new and urgent evaluation of the patient.

Finally, elevated sTREM-1 concentrations were also found in the synovial fluid of patients with septic arthritis.[38]

Table 2
Soluble TREM-1 and localized infections

		Population	Confirmed Sepsis	Kits	Sample	Sensibility (%)	Specificity (%)	PPV (%)	NPV (%)	Cutoff	AUC of ROC Curve (95% CI)	LR+	LR−
Pneumonia	Gibot et al[22]	Prospective, 148 consecutive patients, medical ICU, pneumonia suspected	31% VAP	Immunoblot	Mini-BAL	98	90	93	96	5 pg/mL	—	—	—
	El Solh et al[26]	Prospective, 75 consecutive patients in the ICU, inhalational pneumonia	51%	ELISA DuoSet[a]	Plasma	—	—	—	—	250 pg/mL	0.51 (0.39–0.62)	—	—
					BAL	66	92	89	72		0.87 (0.78–0.94)		
	Huh et al[24]	Prospective, 80 patients, medical ICU, pneumonia suspected	36%	ELISA DuoSet[a]	BAL	86	90	83	92	184 pg/mL	0.91 (0.83–0.98)	8.79	0.11
	Phua et al[27]	Prospective, 150 patients, respiratory unit, CAP, COPD, asthma	48%	Immunoblot	Plasma	81 / 70	65 / 77	62 / 68	83 / 79	163 ng/mL / 219 ng/mL	0.77 (0.70–0.84)	—	—
	Horonenko et al[66]	Prospective, 23 patients, medical ICU, VAP suspected	63%	ELISA DuoSet[a]	BAL / EVC	100 / 78	11 / 89	64 / 92	100 / 73	—	—	—	—
	Anand et al[67]	Prospective, 105 patients, medical ICU, pneumonia suspected	18% (53 indetermined)	ELISA Quantikine[a]	BAL	42	75	27	85.5	200 pg/mL	0.55 (0.40–0.70)	—	—
	Oudhuis et al[68]	Retrospective, 207 patients in the ICU, VAP suspected	40%	ELISA Quantikine[a]	BAL	—	—	—	—	—	0.58 (0.50–0.65)	—	—
	Determann et al[25]	Prospective, 28 consecutive patients in the ICU, VAP suspected	32%	ELISA DuoSet[a]	Plasma / BAL	— / 88	— / 84	— / 70	— / 94	200 pg/mL	0.83 (0.65–1.00)	—	—

Category	Study	Population	Method	Sample	Sens	Spec	PPV	NPV	Cutoff	AUC	CI	LR+	LR−
Pleural Effusion	Chan et al[29]	Prospective, 67 patients in the ICU, pleural effusion	ELISA	Pleural fluid	88	90	—	—	114 pg/mL	0.84	(0.70–0.93)	8.46	0.14
		57% (32% empyema, 42% TB, 26% parapneumonia)			94	91	—	—	374 pg/mL	0.93	(0.80–0.99)	10.31	0.07
	Huang et al[30]	Prospective, 109 patients in respiratory unit, pleural effusion	Expression TREM-1 cytometry	Plasma	—	—	—	—	—	—		12.6	—
		48% (60% TB)	ELISA[a]	Pleural fluid	86	93	75	96	768 pg/mL	0.93	(0.86–0.99)		
	Bishara et al[31]	89 consecutive patients, pleural effusion	ELISA DuoSet[a]	Pleural fluid	94	93	70	98	114 pg/mL	0.97	(0.90–1.00)	—	—
		76% (71% empyema, 29% parapneumonia)											
	Determann et al[32]	36 consecutive patients in the ICU, pleural effusion	ELISA DuoSet[a]	Pleural fluid	93	86	—	—	50 pg/mL	0.93	(0.84–1.00)	—	—
		36%											
	Kim et al[33]	48 consecutive patients, pleural effusion	ELISA	Pleural fluid	71	74	60	82	55 pg/mL	—		—	—
		35%											
CNS Infections	Determann et al[34]	Prospective, 100 patients, meningitis	ELISA DuoSet[a]	CSF	73	77	94	34	20 pg/mL	0.82	(0.74–0.90)	3.1	—
		92% bacterial											
	Bishara et al[35]	Prospective, 21 patients, meningitis	ELISA DuoSet[a]	CSF	77	100	100	86	128 pg/mL	0.89	(0.72–1.00)	—	—
		43%											
UTIs	Determann et al[36]	89 consecutive patients, UTI	ELISA DuoSet[a]	Urine	19	89	93	12	—	—		—	—
		79%											
Intra-abdominal Infections	Determann et al[37]	83 consecutive surgical patients, postoperative peritonitis, suspected ongoing infection	ELISA DuoSet[a]	Plasma, ascites					160 pg/mL				
		44%		H48	88	67	70	86		0.76	(0.63–0.90)	2.63	0.19
				H72	86	63	66	85		0.79	(0.66–0.92)	2.33	0.22

Abbreviations: AUC, area under the curve; BAL, bronchoalveolar lavage; CAP, community-acquired pneumonia; CI, confidence interval; CNS, central nervous system; COPD, chronic obstructive pulmonary disease; CSF, cerebrospinal fluid; ELISA, enzyme-linked immunosorbent assay; EVC, exhaled ventilator condensate; LR+, positive likelihood ratio; LR−, negative likelihood ratio; NPV, negative predictive value; PPV, positive predictive value; TB, tuberculosis; UTI, urinary tract infection; VAP, ventilator-associated pneumonia; H48, 48 hours post-operative; H72, 72 hours post-operative.
[a] R&D Systems Inc, Minneapolis, MN, USA.

Nearly all the above-discussed studies thus suggest that the determination of sTREM-1 concentrations at the site of the presumed infection may be useful in clinical practice, but obviously, more research is necessary before implementing this assay into practical algorithms.

A recent meta-analysis from Jiyong and colleagues[39] reviewed 13 studies (1032 patients, 605 patients with bacterial infection and 427 with nonbacterial infection). The global sensitivity was 0.82 (95% confidence interval [CI], 0.69–0.91), specificity was 0.84 (95% CI, 0.75–0.90), positive likelihood ratio was 5.01 (95% CI, 3.07–8.18), negative likelihood ratio was 0.21 (95% CI, 0.11–0.40), diagnostic odds ratio was 23.41 (95% CI, 8.95–61.22), and area under the curve of summary ROC was 0.90 (95% CI, 0.87–0.92).

These encouraging data must now be translated into interventional studies, with the demonstration that measurement of sTREM-1 concentrations can safely guide and reduce the use of antibiotics by analogy to what is suggested for PCT.

STREM-1 BEYOND THE DIAGNOSIS OF INFECTION

A recent growing body of evidence suggests that sTREM-1 concentrations could increase in biologic fluids even in the absence of infection. Indeed, TREM-1 expression depends on the activation of several TLRs or NOD-like receptors, and it has become clear that many danger-associated molecular motifs (or alarmins, such as high mobility group box nuclear protein 1, heat shock proteins, free cyclic AMP) that activate these receptors may be produced during noninfectious inflammatory disorders. It is, therefore, not surprising that TREM-1 is also involved in the pathogenesis of many inflammatory conditions such as hemorrhagic shock (HS), ischemia-reperfusion, and inflammatory intestinal diseases.

Three different studies dealt with acute pancreatitis. Yasuda and colleagues[40] (48 patients), Ferat-Osorio and colleagues[41] (29 patients, among them 11 were critically ill), and Wang and colleagues[42] (18 patients, 8 were critically ill) showed an elevation of plasma sTREM-1 concentrations and an increase in the expression of monocytic TREM-1 and/or *Trem-1* mRNA during acute pancreatitis as compared with control patients and healthy subjects. Plasma sTREM-1 concentrations were also shown to correlate to the severity, the risk of developing remote organ failure, and the presence of infected necrosis.

In the surgical patient, the diagnostic usefulness of sTREM-1 has been explored in digestive or cardiac surgery and polytrauma. During the postoperative period of a cardiac surgery under extracorporeal assistance, Adib-Conquy and colleagues[43] (76 patients) showed an early increase of plasma sTREM-1 concentrations, although at a lower level than those encountered during severe sepsis. These concentrations correlated neither with the length of aorta clamping nor with the length of extracorporeal circulation. Similar findings were observed by Ferat-Osorio and colleagues[44] in patients who underwent a major abdominal surgery. The patients presented an upregulation of TREM-1 expression that did not correlate with the presence of an ongoing sepsis. Importantly, concentrations of sTREM-1 were not determined in this study.

Studying a cohort of 54 patients resuscitated from a cardiac arrest, Adib-Conquy and colleagues[43] were able to demonstrate that 60% of the patients presented with elevated plasma sTREM-1 concentrations. Such an elevation was especially present among patients who had multiorgan failure.

Physiologically, TREM-1 is not expressed by the macrophages infiltrating the lamina propria of the digestive tract. This phenomenon could be explained by the presence of IL-10 and transforming growth factor β that refrain TREM-1 expression and oppose to an excessive immune activation in response to the intestinal flora.[45] The development of chronic inflammatory bowel disease (IBD) may be the result of aberrations of the innate intestinal immune response to endogenous intestinal flora.[46] Indeed, Schenk and colleagues[45] demonstrated that TREM-1 was overexpressed on the surface of intestinal macrophages in patients with IBD. This upregulation was responsible for a huge production of proinflammatory cytokines and correlated to the disease severity. This finding has recently been confirmed by Tzivras and colleagues[46] and Park and colleagues,[47] who showed in 39 and 53 patients with IBD, respectively, that plasma sTREM-1 concentrations were increased and correlated with the disease activity.

The TREM-1 involvement in gastric ulcer has been pointed out by Koussoulas and colleagues.[48] This group found that sTREM-1 concentrations were elevated in the gastric juice of patients with peptic ulcer, independently of the presence of *Helicobacter pylori* infection, and that this increase correlated with the histologic score. These data suggested that TREM-1 could be implicated in the pathogenesis of gastric ulcer.

TREM-1 has also been investigated in chronic obstructive pulmonary disease (COPD) and bronchopulmonary cancer. In 12 patients with stable COPD, plasma sTREM-1 concentrations were mildly elevated and inversely correlated to the severity of the disease.[49] Clinical data suggest that enhanced innate immunity is a significant factor influencing malignant outcome, and thus, manipulation of the immune system could constitute an approach for antitumor therapy.[50] Ho and colleagues[50] showed that in humans, sTREM-1 concentrations were elevated in malignant pleural effusions and correlated with poor outcomes, making sTREM-1 an independent predictor of patient survival. Also, TREM-1 expression was upregulated in tumor-associated macrophages (TAMs) but not in cancer cells. Coculture of blood monocytes and lung cancer cells leads to monocytic TREM-1 upregulation both at the gene and the protein levels. Finally, TREM-1 engagement by αTREM-1 facilitated metastasis, whereas TAMs *Trem-1* silencing resulted in the loss of invasiveness of cancer cells. These data underline the potential therapeutic interest of the TREM-1 modulation in lung cancer to prevent cancer progression.

Finally, and despite the initial thought that TREM-1 was not involved in vasculitis, several recent studies reported on the role of TREM-1 in pure inflammatory disorders such as vasculitis and autoimmune diseases. Retrospective data published by Daikeler and colleagues[51] showed elevated concentrations of plasma sTREM-1 in patients with antineutrophil cytoplasmic autoantibody (ANCA)-associated vasculitis. More recently, serum sTREM-1 concentrations were found elevated among 41 patients with active myeloperoxidase (MPO)-ANCA–associated vasculitis and inactive MPO-ANCA–associated vasculitis but with a concomitant infection as compared with patients with inactive disease at the time of sampling. Of note, the serum sTREM-1/creatinine ratio was higher in patients with inactive vasculitis with infectious complications than that in those with active vasculitis and in those with inactive vasculitis without infection but not significantly different from that in patients with acute pyelonephritis. On ROC curve analysis, a lower-limit value of 9.40 ng/mg for this ratio had a sensitivity of 84.6% and a specificity of 90.8% in differentiating patients with infection from those without infection.[52] Finally, sTREM-1 concentrations have been shown to be elevated in the synovial fluid of patients with rheumatoid arthritis.[38]

STREM-1 TO PREDICT OUTCOME

Beyond the use of sTREM-1 as a diagnostic marker, the determination of its concentration may also be of some help to prognosticate the outcome of a septic patient.

Gibot and colleagues[53] sequentially measured plasma sTREM-1 concentrations and monocytic TREM-1 expression in 63 consecutive septic patients. The baseline (at admission) value of monocytic TREM-1 expression was unable to discriminate between survivors and nonsurvivors. By contrast, the baseline plasma sTREM-1 concentration was higher in survivors and was found to be an independent factor associated with outcome. The patterns of evolution were also different according to the outcome, with a progressive decrease in sTREM-1 concentrations in survivors, whereas concentrations remained high in nonsurvivors. Giamarellos-Bourboulis and colleagues,[54] Tejera and colleagues,[55] and Adib-Conquy and colleagues[43] confirmed the prognostic value of sTREM-1 in pneumonia (VAP and CAP) and cardiac arrest, respectively.

Two recent studies lead to a different conclusion. Studying patients with CAP who are admitted to an emergency room, Muller and colleagues[28] did not find any relationship between plasma sTREM-1 concentrations and severity or outcome. In a surgical setting, Bopp and colleagues[56] found that plasma sTREM-1 was useless to predict outcome in SIRS, sepsis, or severe sepsis.

THERAPEUTIC MANIPULATION OF THE TREM-1 PATHWAY

A relevant biomarker should provide diagnostic, or prognostic, information and should be of physiologic relevance. The therapeutic modulation of the TREM-1 pathway has been the subject of many experimental studies.

Acute Inflammatory Disorders

Sepsis

Implication of TREM-1 as an amplifier of the host immune response to microbial infection was first described by Bouchon and colleagues.[4] In this study, infected tissues were infiltrated by neutrophils and macrophages that express high levels of TREM-1. In vitro, polymorphonuclear cells and monocytes stimulated with lipopolysaccharide (LPS) and αTREM-1, a monoclonal antibody against TREM-1 that is used as a specific agonist, were overactivated when compared with LPS challenge only. TREM-1 blockade by a chimeric protein composed of an Fc fragment and the extracellular portion of murine TREM-1 (mTREM-1/IgG1) protected septic mice from death.

LP17, a TREM-1 peptide antagonist, administration to septic mice resulted in a decreased plasma concentration of several proinflammatory cytokines. LP17-treated animals were also protected against organ failure, hemodynamic disorders, and finally, against death.[8,57] Moreover, data (Damien Barraud, MD, and Sébastien Gibot, MD, PhD, unpublished data, 2010) recently obtained the authors' laboratory confirm that TREM-1 modulation confers cardiovascular protection during polymicrobial sepsis.

In a rat model of *Pseudomonas aeruginosa*–induced pneumonia as well as in melioidosis, LP17 treatment was associated with hemodynamic improvement, as well as with dampening of the tissue and systemic inflammatory responses and a decrease of coagulation activation. In fine, LP17 treatment improved survival.[58,59]

HS, ischemia-reperfusion, pancreatitis

Severe HS and ischemia-reperfusion lead to an exaggerated production of inflammatory mediators, such as cytokines and chemokines, which may play a significant role in the development of multiorgan failure, especially during the reperfusion phase. In a rat model of HS, the TREM-1 modulation by LP17 attenuated the hemodynamic compromise and the development of lactic acidosis, prevented cytokine production and organ dysfunction, and improved survival.[60]

Gibot and colleagues[61] showed that modulation of TREM-1 during ischemia-reperfusion in rats was beneficial in terms of systemic inflammation, lactatemia, hemodynamic deterioration, activation of hepatic NF-κB, bacterial translocation, and mortality. These results have recently been comforted by Pamuk and colleagues[62] who demonstrated that inhibition of spleen tyrosine kinase (Syk), involved in TREM-1/DAP12 pathway, provides similar protective effects.

Finally, in a mouse model of acute pancreatitis, Kamei and colleagues[63] were able to demonstrate a salutary effect of TREM-1 modulation with an LP17-associated organ dysfunction improvement.

Chronic Inflammatory Disorders

The TREM-1 pathway modulation was also showed to be interesting in several chronic inflammatory conditions such as IBDs,[45] inflammatory rheumatoid disorders,[64] and even lung cancer.[65]

SUMMARY

TREM-1 is a recently described cell-surface receptor on neutrophils and macrophages. Now recognized to be a crucial actor of the complex network of innate immunity, TREM-1 acts as an amplifier of inflammatory responses, especially against bacterial infections. Nevertheless, a growing body of evidence suggests new roles for TREM-1 in other inflammatory diseases or even cancer.

sTREM-1 seems to be a reliable marker of bacterial infection and has already been tested with success in various clinical situations at the bedside. Whether this marker could guide antibiotic strategy warrants additional studies.

The therapeutic modulation of the TREM-1 signaling pathway, with peptides like LP17, presents the great advantage by not totally abrogating the inflammatory response but allowing a fine-tuning. The modulation of TREM-1 at the bench seems promising and paves the way for new immunomodulatory strategies not only in infectious diseases but also during aseptic inflammatory conditions.

REFERENCES

1. Tang BM, Eslick GD, Craig JC, et al. Accuracy of procalcitonin for sepsis diagnosis in critically ill patients: systematic review and meta-analysis. Lancet Infect Dis 2007;7(3):210–7.
2. Ford JW, McVicar DW. TREM and TREM-like receptors in inflammation and disease. Curr Opin Immunol 2009;21(1):38–46.
3. Colonna M, Facchetti F. TREM-1 (triggering receptor expressed on myeloid cells): a new player in acute inflammatory responses. J Infect Dis 2003;187(Suppl 2):S397–401.
4. Bouchon A, Facchetti F, Weigand MA, et al. TREM-1 amplifies inflammation and is a crucial mediator of septic shock. Nature 2001;410(6832):1103–7.
5. Radsak MP, Salih HR, Rammensee HG, et al. Triggering receptor expressed on myeloid cells-1 in neutrophil inflammatory responses: differential regulation of activation and survival. J Immunol 2004;172(8):4956–63.
6. Bouchon A, Dietrich J, Colonna M. Cutting edge: inflammatory responses can be triggered by TREM-1, a novel receptor expressed on neutrophils and monocytes. J Immunol 2000;164(10):4991–5.
7. Bleharski JR, Kiessler V, Buonsanti C, et al. A role for triggering receptor expressed on myeloid cells-1 in host defense during the early-induced and adaptive phases of the immune response. J Immunol 2003;170(7):3812–8.

8. Gibot S, Kolopp-Sarda MN, Bene MC, et al. A soluble form of the triggering receptor expressed on myeloid cells-1 modulates the inflammatory response in murine sepsis. J Exp Med 2004;200(11):1419–26.

9. Lanier LL, Bakker AB. The ITAM-bearing transmembrane adaptor DAP12 in lymphoid and myeloid cell function. Immunol Today 2000;21(12):611–4.

10. Gomez-Pina V, Soares-Schanoski A, Rodriguez-Rojas A, et al. Metalloproteinases shed TREM-1 ectodomain from lipopolysaccharide-stimulated human monocytes. J Immunol 2007;179(6):4065–73.

11. Wong-Baeza I, Gonzalez-Roldan N, Ferat-Osorio E, et al. Triggering receptor expressed on myeloid cells (TREM-1) is regulated post-transcriptionally and its ligand is present in the sera of some septic patients. Clin Exp Immunol 2006; 145(3):448–55.

12. Haselmayer P, Grosse-Hovest L, von Landenberg P, et al. TREM-1 ligand expression on platelets enhances neutrophil activation. Blood 2007;110(3):1029–35.

13. Hamerman JA, Tchao NK, Lowell CA, et al. Enhanced Toll-like receptor responses in the absence of signaling adaptor DAP12. Nat Immunol 2005;6(6):579–86.

14. Hamerman JA, Ogasawara K, Lanier LL. Cutting edge: toll-like receptor signaling in macrophages induces ligands for the NKG2D receptor. J Immunol 2004; 172(4):2001–5.

15. Gibot S, Kolopp-Sarda MN, Bene MC, et al. Plasma level of a triggering receptor expressed on myeloid cells-1: its diagnostic accuracy in patients with suspected sepsis. Ann Intern Med 2004;141(1):9–15.

16. Latour-Perez J, Alcala-Lopez A, Garcia-Garcia MA, et al. Diagnostic accuracy of sTREM-1 to identify infection in critically ill patients with systemic inflammatory response syndrome. Clin Biochem 2010;43(9):720–4.

17. Barati M, Bashar FR, Shahrami R, et al. Soluble triggering receptor expressed on myeloid cells 1 and the diagnosis of sepsis. J Crit Care 2010;25(2):362, e1–6.

18. Kofoed K, Andersen O, Kronborg G, et al. Use of plasma C-reactive protein, procalcitonin, neutrophils, macrophage migration inhibitory factor, soluble urokinase-type plasminogen activator receptor, and soluble triggering receptor expressed on myeloid cells-1 in combination to diagnose infections: a prospective study. Crit Care 2007;11(2):R38.

19. Chen HL, Hung CH, Tseng HI, et al. Soluble form of triggering receptor expressed on myeloid cells-1 (sTREM-1) as a diagnostic marker of serious bacterial infection in febrile infants less than three months of age. Jpn J Infect Dis 2008;61(1):31–5.

20. Sarafidis K, Soubasi-Griva V, Piretzi K, et al. Diagnostic utility of elevated serum soluble triggering receptor expressed on myeloid cells (sTREM)-1 in infected neonates. Intensive Care Med 2010;36(5):864–8.

21. How CK, Chern CH, Wu MF, et al. Expression of the triggering receptor expressed on myeloid cells-1 mRNA in a heterogeneous infected population. Int J Clin Pract 2009;63(1):126–33.

22. Gibot S, Cravoisy A, Levy B, et al. Soluble triggering receptor expressed on myeloid cells and the diagnosis of pneumonia. N Engl J Med 2004;350(5):451–8.

23. Richeldi L, Mariani M, Losi M, et al. Triggering receptor expressed on myeloid cells: role in the diagnosis of lung infections. Eur Respir J 2004;24(2):247–50.

24. Huh JW, Lim CM, Koh Y, et al. Diagnostic utility of the soluble triggering receptor expressed on myeloid cells-1 in bronchoalveolar lavage fluid from patients with bilateral lung infiltrates. Crit Care 2008;12(1):R6.

25. Determann RM, Millo JL, Gibot S, et al. Serial changes in soluble triggering receptor expressed on myeloid cells in the lung during development of ventilator-associated pneumonia. Intensive Care Med 2005;31(11):1495–500.

26. El Solh AA, Akinnusi ME, Peter M, et al. Triggering receptors expressed on myeloid cells in pulmonary aspiration syndromes. Intensive Care Med 2008;34(6):1012–9.

27. Phua J, Koay ES, Zhang D, et al. Soluble triggering receptor expressed on myeloid cells-1 in acute respiratory infections. Eur Respir J 2006;28(4):695–702.

28. Muller B, Gencay MM, Gibot S, et al. Circulating levels of soluble triggering receptor expressed on myeloid cells (sTREM)-1 in community-acquired pneumonia. Crit Care Med 2007;35(3):990–1.

29. Chan MC, Chang KM, Chao WC, et al. Evaluation of a new inflammatory molecule (triggering receptor expressed on myeloid cells-1) in the diagnosis of pleural effusion. Respirology 2007;12(3):333–8.

30. Huang LY, Shi HZ, Liang QL, et al. Expression of soluble triggering receptor expression on myeloid cells-1 in pleural effusion. Chin Med J (Engl) 2008; 121(17):1656–61.

31. Bishara J, Goldberg E, Ashkenazi S, et al. Soluble triggering receptor expressed on myeloid cells-1 for diagnosing empyema. Ann Thorac Surg 2009;87(1):251–4.

32. Determann RM, Achouiti AA, El Solh AA, et al. Infectious pleural effusions can be identified by sTREM-1 levels. Respir Med 2010;104(2):310–5.

33. Kim JH, Park EI, Kim WH, et al. Soluble triggering receptor expressed on myeloid cells-1: role in diagnosis of pleural effusions. Tuberc Respir Dis 2007;62:290–8.

34. Determann RM, Weisfelt M, de Gans J, et al. Soluble triggering receptor expressed on myeloid cells 1: a biomarker for bacterial meningitis. Intensive Care Med 2006;32(8):1243–7.

35. Bishara J, Hadari N, Shalita-Chesner M, et al. Soluble triggering receptor expressed on myeloid cells-1 for distinguishing bacterial from aseptic meningitis in adults. Eur J Clin Microbiol Infect Dis 2007;26(9):647–50.

36. Determann RM, Schultz MJ, Geerlings SE. Soluble triggering receptor expressed on myeloid cells-1 is not a sufficient biological marker for infection of the urinary tract. J Infect 2007;54(6):e249–50.

37. Determann RM, van Till JW, van Ruler O, et al. sTREM-1 is a potential useful biomarker for exclusion of ongoing infection in patients with secondary peritonitis. Cytokine 2009;46(1):36–42.

38. Collins CE, La DT, Yang HT, et al. Elevated synovial expression of triggering receptor expressed on myeloid cells 1 in patients with septic arthritis or rheumatoid arthritis. Ann Rheum Dis 2009;68(11):1768–74.

39. Jiyong J, Tiancha H, Wei C, et al. Diagnostic value of the soluble triggering receptor expressed on myeloid cells-1 in bacterial infection: a meta-analysis. Intensive Care Med 2009;35(4):587–95.

40. Yasuda T, Takeyama Y, Ueda T, et al. Increased levels of soluble triggering receptor expressed on myeloid cells-1 in patients with acute pancreatitis. Crit Care Med 2008;36(7):2048–53.

41. Ferat-Osorio E, Wong-Baeza I, Esquivel-Callejas N, et al. Triggering receptor expressed on myeloid cells-1 expression on monocytes is associated with inflammation but not with infection in acute pancreatitis. Crit Care 2009;13(3):R69.

42. Wang DY, Qin RY, Liu ZR, et al. Expression of TREM-1 mRNA in acute pancreatitis. World J Gastroenterol 2004;10(18):2744–6.

43. Adib-Conquy M, Monchi M, Goulenok C, et al. Increased plasma levels of soluble triggering receptor expressed on myeloid cells 1 and procalcitonin after cardiac surgery and cardiac arrest without infection. Shock 2007;28(4):406–10.

44. Ferat-Osorio E, Esquivel-Callejas N, Wong-Baeza I, et al. The increased expression of TREM-1 on monocytes is associated with infectious and noninfectious inflammatory processes. J Surg Res 2008;150(1):110–7.

45. Schenk M, Bouchon A, Seibold F, et al. TREM-1–expressing intestinal macrophages crucially amplify chronic inflammation in experimental colitis and inflammatory bowel diseases. J Clin Invest 2007;117(10):3097–106.
46. Tzivras M, Koussoulas V, Giamarellos-Bourboulis EJ, et al. Role of soluble triggering receptor expressed on myeloid cells in inflammatory bowel disease. World J Gastroenterol 2006;12(21):3416–9.
47. Park JJ, Cheon JH, Kim BY, et al. Correlation of serum-soluble triggering receptor expressed on myeloid cells-1 with clinical disease activity in inflammatory bowel disease. Dig Dis Sci 2009;54(7):1525–31.
48. Koussoulas V, Tzivras M, Giamarellos-Bourboulis EJ, et al. Can soluble triggering receptor expressed on myeloid cells (sTREM-1) be considered an anti-inflammatory mediator in the pathogenesis of peptic ulcer disease? Dig Dis Sci 2007;52(9):2166–9.
49. Radsak MP, Taube C, Haselmayer P, et al. Soluble triggering receptor expressed on myeloid cells 1 is released in patients with stable chronic obstructive pulmonary disease. Clin Dev Immunol 2007;2007:52040.
50. Ho CC, Liao WY, Wang CY, et al. TREM-1 expression in tumor-associated macrophages and clinical outcome in lung cancer. Am J Respir Crit Care Med 2008; 177(7):763–70.
51. Daikeler T, Regenass S, Tyndall A, et al. Increased serum levels of soluble triggering receptor expressed on myeloid cells-1 in antineutrophil cytoplasmic antibody-associated vasculitis. Ann Rheum Dis 2008;67(5):723–4.
52. Hirayama K, Nagai M, Ebihara I, et al. Serum ratio of soluble triggering receptor expressed on myeloid cells-1 to creatinine is a useful marker of infectious complications in myeloperoxidase-antineutrophil cytoplasmic antibody-associated renal vasculitis. Nephrol Dial Transplant 2011;26(3):868–74.
53. Gibot S, Cravoisy A, Kolopp-Sarda MN, et al. Time-course of sTREM (soluble triggering receptor expressed on myeloid cells)-1, procalcitonin, and C-reactive protein plasma concentrations during sepsis. Crit Care Med 2005;33(4):792–6.
54. Giamarellos-Bourboulis EJ, Zakynthinos S, Baziaka F, et al. Soluble triggering receptor expressed on myeloid cells 1 as an anti-inflammatory mediator in sepsis. Intensive Care Med 2006;32(2):237–43.
55. Tejera A, Santolaria F, Diez ML, et al. Prognosis of community acquired pneumonia (CAP): value of triggering receptor expressed on myeloid cells-1 (TREM-1) and other mediators of the inflammatory response. Cytokine 2007; 38(3):117–23.
56. Bopp C, Hofer S, Bouchon A, et al. Soluble TREM-1 is not suitable for distinguishing between systemic inflammatory response syndrome and sepsis survivors and nonsurvivors in the early stage of acute inflammation. Eur J Anaesthesiol 2009; 26(6):504–7.
57. Gibot S, Buonsanti C, Massin F, et al. Modulation of the triggering receptor expressed on the myeloid cell type 1 pathway in murine septic shock. Infect Immun 2006;74(5):2823–30.
58. Gibot S, Alauzet C, Massin F, et al. Modulation of the triggering receptor expressed on myeloid cells-1 pathway during pneumonia in rats. J Infect Dis 2006;194(7):975–83.
59. Wiersinga WJ, Veer CT, Wieland CW, et al. Expression profile and function of triggering receptor expressed on myeloid cells-1 during melioidosis. J Infect Dis 2007;196(11):1707–16.
60. Gibot S, Massin F, Alauzet C, et al. Effects of the TREM 1 pathway modulation during hemorrhagic shock in rats. Shock 2009;32(6):633–7.

61. Gibot S, Massin F, Alauzet C, et al. Effects of the TREM-1 pathway modulation during mesenteric ischemia-reperfusion in rats. Crit Care Med 2008;36(2): 504–10.
62. Pamuk ON, Lapchak PH, Rani P, et al. Spleen tyrosine kinase inhibition prevents tissue damage after ischemia reperfusion injury. Am J Physiol Gastrointest Liver Physiol 2010;299(2):G391–9.
63. Kamei K, Yasuda T, Ueda T, et al. Role of triggering receptor expressed on myeloid cells-1 in experimental severe acute pancreatitis. J Hepatobiliary Pancreat Sci 2010;17(3):305–12.
64. Murakami Y, Akahoshi T, Aoki N, et al. Intervention of an inflammation amplifier, triggering receptor expressed on myeloid cells 1, for treatment of autoimmune arthritis. Arthritis Rheum 2009;60(6):1615–23.
65. Johansson M, Tan T, de Visser KE, et al. Immune cells as anti-cancer therapeutic targets and tools. J Cell Biochem 2007;101(4):918–26.
66. Horonenko G, Hoyt JC, Robbins RA, et al. Soluble triggering receptor expressed on myeloid cell-1 is increased in patients with ventilator-associated pneumonia: a preliminary report. Chest 2007;132(1):58–63.
67. Anand NJ, Zuick S, Klesney-Tait J, et al. Diagnostic implications of soluble triggering receptor expressed on myeloid cells-1 in BAL fluid of patients with pulmonary infiltrates in the ICU. Chest 2009;135(3):641–7, 68.
68. Oudhuis GJ, Beuving J, Bergmans D, et al. Soluble triggering receptor expressed on myeloid cells-1 in bronchoalveolar lavage fluid is not predictive for ventilator-associated pneumonia. Intensive Care Med 2009;35(7):1265–70.

Coagulation Biomarkers in Critically Ill Patients

Marcel Levi, MD[a],*, Marcus Schultz, MD[b], Tom van der Poll, MD[c,d]

KEYWORDS

- Coagulation • Fibrinolysis • Platelets • Critically ill patients
- Intensive care

In critically ill patients, coagulation abnormalities are commonly found.[1] A variety of altered coagulation parameters may be detectable, such as thrombocytopenia, prolonged global coagulation times, reduced levels of coagulation inhibitors, or high levels of fibrin split products. In addition, more sophisticated tests for activation of individual factors or pathways of coagulation may point to specific involvement of these components in the pathogenesis of the underlying disease in critically ill patients. Both conventional markers and sensitive molecular markers may be used to specifically determine the nature of the coagulopathy, but also as predictors of an adverse clinical course. Moreover, coagulation biomarkers can be helpful to guide in the selection of patients that require specific, often expensive, interventions in the coagulation system.

RELEVANCE OF ABNORMAL COAGULATION BIOMARKERS

There is ample evidence that activation of coagulation in concert with inflammatory activation can result in microvascular thrombosis and thereby contributes to multiple organ failure in patients with critical illness and systemic inflammatory states.[2] First, extensive data has been reported on postmortem findings of patients with coagulation abnormalities in patients with severe infectious diseases.[3,4] These autopsy findings include diffuse bleeding at various sites, hemorrhagic necrosis of tissue, microthrombi in small blood vessels, and thrombi in midsize and larger arteries and veins. The

All three authors have nothing to disclose.

[a] Department of Vascular Medicine and Internal Medicine, Academic Medical Centre F-4, Meibergdreef 9, 1105 AZ Amsterdam, The Netherlands

[b] Department of Intensive Care Medicine, Academic Medical Centre F-4, University of Amsterdam, Meibergdreef 9, 1105 AZ Amsterdam, The Netherlands

[c] Laboratory for Experimental and Molecular Medicine, Academic Medical Centre F-4, University of Amsterdam, Meibergdreef 9, 1105 AZ Amsterdam, The Netherlands

[d] Center for Infection and Immunity Amsterdam, Academic Medical Center F-4, University of Amsterdam, Meibergdreef 9, 1105 AZ Amsterdam, The Netherlands

* Corresponding author.

E-mail address: m.m.levi@amc.uva.nl

Crit Care Clin 27 (2011) 281–297
doi:10.1016/j.ccc.2010.12.009
0749-0704/11/$ – see front matter © 2011 Elsevier Inc. All rights reserved.

criticalcare.theclinics.com

demonstration of ischemia and necrosis was invariably due to fibrin deposition in small and midsize vessels of various organs.[5] Importantly, the presence of these intravascular thrombi appears to be clearly and specifically related to the clinical dysfunction of the organ. Secondly, experimental animal studies of disseminated intravascular coagulation (DIC) show fibrin deposition in various organs. Experimental bacteremia or endotoxemia causes intra- and extravascular fibrin deposition in kidneys, lungs, liver, brain, and various other organs. Amelioration of the hemostatic defect by various interventions in these experimental models appears to improve organ failure and, in some but not all cases, mortality.[6–9] Interestingly, some studies indicate that amelioration of the systemic coagulation activation will have a profound beneficial effect on resolution of local fibrin deposition and improvement of organ failure.[10,11] Finally, clinical studies support the notion of coagulation as an important denominator of clinical outcome. Hypercoagulability has shown to be an independent predictor of organ failure and mortality in patients with sepsis.[12,13]

Apart from microvascular thrombosis and organ dysfunction, coagulation abnormalities may also have other harmful consequences. The relevance of thrombocytopenia in patients with sepsis is in the first place related to an increased risk of bleeding. Indeed, in particular critically ill patients with a platelet count of less than 50×10^9/l have a four- to fivefold higher risk for bleeding as compared to patients with a higher platelet count.[14,15] The risk of intracerebral bleeding in patients with sepsis during intensive care admission is relatively low (0.3%–0.5%), but in 88% of patients with this complication the platelet count is less than 100×10^9/l.[16] Regardless of the cause, thrombocytopenia is an independent predictor of intensive care unit (ICU) mortality in multivariate analyses with a relative risk of 1.9 to 4.2 in various studies.[14,15,17] In particular, a sustained thrombocytopenia during more than 4 days after ICU admission or a drop in platelet count of greater than 50% during ICU stay is related to a four to sixfold increase in mortality.[14,18] The platelet count was shown to be a stronger predictor for ICU mortality than composite scoring systems, such as the Acute Physiology and Chronic Evaluation (APACHE) II score or the Multiple Organ Dysfunction Score (MODS). Also low levels of coagulation factors in patients with sepsis, as reflected by prolonged global coagulation times, may be a risk factor for bleeding and mortality. A prothrombin time (PT) or activated partial thromboplastin time (aPTT) ratio greater than 1.5 in critically ill patients was found to predict excessive bleeding and increased mortality.[19,20]

THROMBOCYTOPENIA AND ABNORMAL ROUTINE CLOTTING TIMES

The incidence of thrombocytopenia (platelet count $<150 \times 10^9$/l) in critically ill medical patients is 35% to 44%.[14,15,21] A platelet count of less than 100×10^9/l is seen in 20% to 25% of patients, whereas 12% to 15% of patients have a platelet count less than 50×10^9/l. In surgical and trauma patients the incidence of thrombocytopenia is higher with 35% to 41% of patients having less than 100×10^9/l platelets.[17,22] Typically, the platelet count decreases during the first 4 days on the intensive care unit.[18] **Fig. 1** shows that the number of platelets in critically ill patients is inversely related to survival. In particular, sustained thrombocytopenia over more than 4 days after ICU admission or a drop in platelet count of greater than 50% during ICU stay is related to a four to sixfold increase in mortality.[14,18] A platelet count of less than 100×10^9/l is also related to a longer ICU stay but not the total duration of hospital admission.[15]

A prolonged global coagulation time (such as PT or aPTT) occurs in 14% to 28% of ICU patients.[19,20] In particular, trauma patients seem to have a high incidence of

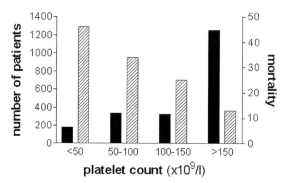

Fig. 1. Number of patients within strata of platelet counts (black bars) and mortality (striped bars) in a pooled analysis of for clinical studies of consecutive groups of patients admitted to the ICU. (*Data from* Refs.[1,3,4,6])

coagulation time prolongation. A PT or aPTT ratio greater than 1.5 was found to predict excessive bleeding.[19] In a prospective study of trauma patients a prolonged PT or aPTT were strong and independent predictors of mortality.[20]

It is important to emphasize that global coagulation tests, such as the PT and the aPTT, poorly reflect in vivo hemostasis. However, these tests are a convenient method to quickly estimate the concentration of one or at times multiple coagulation factors for which each test is sensitive.[23] In general, coagulation tests will prolong if the level of coagulation factors are below 50%. This is relevant since the levels of coagulation factors, that are needed for adequate hemostasis, are somewhere between 25% and 50%.[24] The normal values and the sensitivity of these tests for deficiencies of coagulation factors may vary markedly between tests, dependent on the reagents used. Therefore, an increasing number of laboratories use the International Normalized Ratio (INR) instead of the PT. Although this may carry the advantage of increased standardization between centers, it should be mentioned that the INR has only been validated for control of the intensity of vitamin K antagonist therapy and has never been developed for the use as a screening test for coagulation abnormalities.[25]

MOLECULAR MARKERS FOR ABNORMAL COAGULATION IN CRITICALLY ILL PATIENTS

Other coagulation test abnormalities frequently observed in ICU patients include elevated fibrin split products and reduced levels of coagulation inhibitors. Fibrin split products are detectable in 42% of a consecutive series of ICU patients, in 80% of trauma patients and in 99% of patients with sepsis.[26–28] Fibrin degradation products (FDPs) may be detected by specific enzyme-linked immunosorbent assays (ELISAs), or by latex agglutination assays, allowing rapid and bedside determination in emergency cases.[29] None of the available assays for FDP discriminates between degradation products of cross-linked fibrin and fibrinogen degradation, which may cause spuriously high results.[30] The specificity of high levels of FDP is therefore limited and many other conditions, such as trauma, recent surgery, inflammation, or venous thromboembolism, are associated with elevated FDPs. Because FDPs are metabolized by the liver and secreted by the kidneys, FDP levels are influenced by liver and kidney function.[31] Other tests are specifically aimed at the detection of neoantigens on degraded cross-linked fibrin. One of these tests detects an epitope related to plasmin-degraded cross-linked γ-chain, resulting in fragment D-dimer. These tests better differentiate degradation of cross-linked fibrin from fibrinogen or FDPs.[26]

D-dimer levels are high in patients with DIC, but also poorly distinguish patients with DIC from patients with venous thromboembolism, recent surgery, or inflammatory conditions.

The dynamics of the coagulopathy in critically ill patients can be judged by measuring activation markers that are released upon the conversion of a coagulation factor zymogen to an active protease. Examples of such markers are prothrombin activation fragment F1+2 (F1+2), and the activation peptides of factors IX and X.[30,32] Indeed, these markers are markedly elevated in critically ill patients. Elevated plasma concentrations of thrombin-antithrombin complexes may well reflect the increased generation of thrombin and thrombin-mediated fibrinogen to fibrin conversion can be monitored by increased levels of fibrinogen activation peptide fibrinopeptide-A.[33] All these markers are increased in patients with critical illness and their high sensitivity may be helpful in detecting even low-grade activation of coagulation. The specificity of high levels of markers for coagulation factor activation is probably limited, since many other conditions may lead to elevated plasma levels. Another drawback may be that these assays are very much dependent on optimal venous puncture, which may be difficult in sick patients and during routine (intensive) care. The most important disadvantage of these tests may be that their use is limited to specialized coagulation laboratories and that they are not available for routine use in most clinical centers. Thus, although these tests are very relevant for research in critically ill patients and the effect of specific interventions in the coagulation cascade, their practical use in clinical medicine is very limited so far.

NATURAL COAGULATION INHIBITORS IN CRITICALLY ILL PATIENTS

Low levels of coagulation inhibitors, such as antithrombin and protein C, are found in 40% to 60% of trauma patients and 90% of sepsis patients.[28,34] Antithrombin is a serine protease inhibitor and the main inhibitor of thrombin and factor Xa. During severe inflammatory responses, antithrombin levels are markedly decreased due to consumption (as a result of ongoing thrombin generation), impaired synthesis (as a result of a negative acute phase response) and degradation by elastase from activated neutrophils.[35,36] A reduction in glycosaminoglycan availability at the endothelial surface (due to the influence of proinflammatory cytokines on endothelial synthesis) will also contribute to reduced antithrombin function, since glycosaminoglycans act as physiological heparin-like cofactors of antithrombin. Binding of glycosaminoglycans to antithrombin induces a conformational change at the reactive center of the antithrombin molecule, thereby rendering this protease inhibitor from a slow to a very efficient inhibitor of thrombin and other active coagulation factors.[37] Prospective clinical studies in patients at high risk for sepsis have shown that a marked decrease in levels of antithrombin precedes the clinical manifestation of the infection, which may indicate that antithrombin is involved in the early stages of coagulation activation during sepsis.[38]

Endothelial dysfunction is even more important in the impairment of the protein C system during inflammation. Under physiologic conditions protein C is activated by thrombin bound to the endothelial cell membrane-associated thrombomodulin. Thrombomodulin is a membrane protein with several domains, including a lectin-like domain, six epidermal growth factor (EGF)-like repeats, a transmembrane domain and a short cytoplasmic tail.[39] The binding of thrombin to thrombomodulin occurs at the site of the EGF-repeats.[40] This binding not only results in an about 100-fold increase in the activation of protein C, but also blocks the thrombin-mediated conversion of fibrinogen into fibrin and inhibits the binding of thrombin to other cellular

receptors on platelets and inflammatory cells. In addition, thrombomodulin acceler-
ates the activation of the plasma carboxypeptidase thrombin-activatable fibrinolysis
inhibitor, an important inhibitor of fibrinolysis.[41] Activated protein C regulates coagulation activation by proteolytic cleavage of the essential cofactors Va and VIIIa.
Binding of protein C to the endothelial protein C receptor results in a fivefold augmen-
tation of the activation of protein C by the thrombomodulin-thrombin complex.[42]
However, during severe inflammation, such as occurs in sepsis, in addition to low
levels of protein C due to impaired synthesis[35] and degradation by neutrophil elastase
(which has been described at least in vitro),[43] the protein C system is defective due to
downregulation of thrombomodulin at the endothelial surface, mediated by the proinflammatory cytokines tumor necrosis factor-α (TNF-α) and IL-1β.[44] Observations in
patients with severe gram-negative septicemia indeed confirmed the downregulation
of thrombomodulin in vivo and impaired activation of protein C.[45] In this study, histo-
logical analysis of skin biopsies from patients with meningococcal sepsis showed
decreased endothelial expression of thrombomodulin, both in vessels with and
without thrombosis. Low levels of free protein S (the cofactor of activated protein C)
may further compromise an adequate function of the protein C system. In plasma,
60% of protein S is complexed to a complement regulatory protein, C4b binding
protein (C4bBP). Increased plasma levels of C4bBP as a consequence of the acute
phase reaction in inflammatory diseases may result in a relative free protein S deficiency. Although it has been shown that the β-chain of C4bBP (which mainly governs
the binding to protein S) is not very much affected during the acute phase response,[46]
support from this hypothesis comes from studies showing that infusion of C4bBP
increases organ dysfunction and mortality in septic baboons.[47] Animal experiments
of severe inflammation-induced coagulation activation convincingly show that
compromising the protein C system results in increased morbidity and mortality,
whereas restoring an adequate function of activated protein C improves survival
and organ failure.[48] Interestingly, experiments in mice with a one-allele targeted dele-
tion of the protein C gene (resulting in heterozygous protein C deficiency) have more
severe DIC and organ dysfunction and a higher mortality than wild-type littermates.[49]

A third inhibitory mechanism of thrombin generation involves tissue factor pathway
inhibitor (TFPI), the main inhibitor of the tissue factor-factor VIIa complex. TFPI is
a complex multidomain Kunitz-type protease inhibitor, which binds to the tissue
factor-factor VIIa complex and factor Xa.[50] The TFPI-factor Xa complex may bind to
negatively charged membrane surfaces, which may increase the local concentration
of TFPI at cellular sites and facilitate inhibition of membrane-bound tissue factor-
factor VIIa complex. The role of TFPI in the regulation of inflammation-induced coagulation activation is not completely clear. Experiments showing that administration of
recombinant TFPI (and thereby achieving higher than physiological plasma concentrations of TFPI) blocks inflammation-induced thrombin generation in humans and the
observation that pharmacological doses of TFPI are capable of preventing mortality
during systemic infection and inflammation suggest that high concentrations of TFPI
are capable of importantly modulating tissue factor mediated coagulation.[6,51]
However, the endogenous concentration of TFPI is presumably insufficiently capable
of regulating coagulation activation and downstream consequences during systemic
inflammation, as has been confirmed in a clinical study of patients with sepsis.[52,53]

THE CONTACT ACTIVATION PATHWAY IN CRITICALLY ILL PATIENTS

In critically ill patients activation of the contact system is detectable with sensitive
assays for complexes between activated contact system factors and their inhibitors.[54]

However, the contribution of the contact system to the activation of blood coagulation associated with severe infection or sepsis was shown not to be of importance. It was elegantly shown that blocking contact activation by means of a monoclonal antibody to factor XIIa did not affect *Escherichia coli*-induced coagulation abnormalities in baboons.[55] Recent experiments in a murine model of streptococcal necrotizing fasciitis showed no coagulopathy or bleeding, despite dramatically reduced factor XII and prekallikrein levels.[56] In endotoxemic humans, activation of factor XI did not result in contact system activation.[57] Hence, activation of the contact system may not be relevant for activation of coagulation, but there is emerging evidence that the contact system plays an important role in other physiologic and pathophysiologic mechanisms, most importantly on the occurrence of shock in sepsis.[58,59] In clinical and experimental studies contact system activation was associated with more severe hypotension.[58,60,61] Also, it was demonstrated that blocking contact system activation in experimental bacteremia in baboons prevented irreversible hypotension.[55] The mechanism by which the contact system affects blood pressure regulation is most likely dependent on the formation and release of bradykinin and other kinins upon contact system activation. There is also emerging evidence that the contact system plays a role in fibrinolysis and complement activation in septic conditions.[62]

FIBRINOLYSIS IN CRITICAL ILLNESS

The acute fibrinolytic response in critical illness is the release of plasminogen activators, in particular tissue-type plasminogen activator and urokinase-type plasminogen activator, from storage sites in vascular endothelial cells. However, this increase in plasminogen activation and subsequent plasmin generation, is counteracted by a delayed but sustained increase in plasminogen activator inhibitor, type 1 (PAI-1).[63,64] The resulting effect on fibrinolysis is a complete inhibition and, as a consequence, inadequate fibrin removal, thereby contributing to microvascular thrombosis. Experiments in mice with targeted disruptions of genes encoding components of the plasminogen-plasmin system confirm that fibrinolysis plays a major role in inflammation-induced coagulation. Mice with a deficiency of plasminogen activators have more extensive fibrin deposition in organs when challenged with endotoxin, whereas PAI-1 knockout mice, in contrast to wild-type controls, have no microvascular thrombosis upon endotoxin.[65,66] Of interest, studies have shown that a functional mutation in the PAI-1 gene, the 4G/5G polymorphism, not only influenced the plasma levels of PAI-1, but was also linked to clinical outcome of meningococcal septicemia. Patients with the 4G/4G genotype had significantly higher PAI-1 concentrations in plasma and an increased risk of death.[67] Further investigations demonstrated that the PAI-1 polymorphism did not influence the risk of contracting meningitis as such, but probably increased the likelihood of developing septic shock from meningococcal infection.[68]

LOCALIZED COAGULATION ABNORMALITIES IN CRITICALLY ILL PATIENTS

Although the mechanisms mentioned above have been demonstrated to occur in vivo as a general response in critical illness, it is likely that marked differences in the procoagulant response as well as the underlying pathogenetic pathway may exist between cells and tissues.[69] This may be caused by differences in cell-specific gene expression, environmental factors, and organ specific differences. First, localization of coagulation activity may relate to a cell specific gene expression. For example, inflammatory mediators enhance PAI-1 gene expression in a complex and tissue-specific way.[70] Recent studies have demonstrated that the von Willebrand factor promoter contains cell-specific elements, and similar response elements may be involved in protein synthesis in cells in general.[71] Second, the tissue environment may determine whether specific gene transcription occurs.[72] It is not completely clear why specific sites and organs are at greater risk of developing microvascular thrombosis and also local differences in the consequences of (micro)thrombosis are still poorly understood. Environmental factors underlying the inflammatory response are thought to play a role in this differential coagulative response as well. In mice with disturbances in the plasminogen-plasmin system subjected to hypoxia, the formation of fibrin is induced and is particularly evident in the lungs.[65] In contrast, these same mice respond to endotoxemia with fibrin deposition in the microvasculature of the kidney in particular. Similarly, mice with a functional thrombomodulin deficiency had a marked increase in pulmonary fibrin deposition after hypoxic challenge.[73] In addition, when mice with a functional defect in the thrombomodulin gene were challenged with endotoxin in sublethal amounts, fibrin formation was apparent in the lungs, but not in any other organ studied. In the latter model, fibrin was only temporarily present, and had disappeared after 24 hours.[74] These models illustrate the assumption that fibrin formation is a localized phenomenon, rather than a generalized process.

Finally, various organ systems may markedly differ in their endothelial cell response towards inflammation and injury. In general, endothelial cells play a central role in the coagulation response upon systemic inflammation.[75] The endothelium plays a central role in all major pathways involved in the pathogenesis of hemostatic derangement during severe inflammation. Endothelial cells appear to be directly involved in the initiation and regulation of thrombin generation and the inhibition of fibrin removal. Endothelial cells may express tissue factor, which is the main initiator of coagulation. In addition, physiological anticoagulant pathways, such as antithrombin, the protein C system, or TFPI, are mostly located on endothelial cells and endothelial cell dysfunction is directly related to impaired regulation of coagulation. Also, endothelial cells are the main storage site of plasminogen activators and inhibitors and can acutely release these factors, thereby importantly mediating fibrinolytic activity or inhibition. Proinflammatory cytokines are crucial in mediating these effects on endothelial cells, which themselves may also express cytokines, thereby amplifying the coagulative response.[76] Although not completely clear, various organs may differ in all these endothelial cell-related factors influencing local coagulation activation and fibrin deposition.

POINT OF CARE TESTS

Thromboelastography (TEG) is a method that has been developed decades ago and provides an overall picture of ex vivo coagulation. Modern techniques, such as rotational thromboelastography (ROTEM) enable bedside performance of this test and has become very popular recently in acute care settings.[77] The theoretical advantage of TEG over conventional coagulation assays is that is provides an idea of platelet function as well as fibrinolytic activity. Hyper- and hypocoagulability as demonstrated with TEG was shown to correlate with clinically relevant morbidity and mortality in several studies,[78,79] although its superiority over conventional tests has not unequivocally been established.[80] Also, TEG seems to be overly sensitive to some interventions in the coagulation system, such as administration of fibrinogen, of which the therapeutic benefit remains to be established.

Another new method that has proved highly sensitive and specific for hypercoagulability in critically ill patients is the aPTT test biphasic waveform analysis.[81,82] This test, which requires specific instrumentation, detects the presence of precipitates of a complex of very-low-density lipoprotein and C-reactive protein that appears very early in DIC. When such complexes first appear in the plasma of individuals with diseases known to predispose to hypercoagulability, they confer a greater than 90% sensitivity and specificity for subsequent development of DIC and fatal outcome.[81]

COMPOSITE SCORING SYSTEMS FOR COAGULATION ABNORMALITIES IN CRITICAL ILLNESS

For the diagnosis of the most extreme form of coagulation activation in critically ill patients, DIC, a simple scoring system has been developed.[83] The score can be calculated based on routinely available laboratory tests, that is, platelet count, PT, a fibrin-related marker (usually D-dimer), and fibrinogen. Tentatively, a score of five or more is compatible with DIC, whereas a score of less than five may be indicative but is not affirmative for non-overt DIC. By using receiver-operating characteristics curves, an optimal cut-off for a quantitative D-dimer assay was determined, thereby optimizing sensitivity and the negative predictive value of the system.[84] Prospective studies show that the sensitivity of the DIC score is 93%, and the specificity is 98%.[85,86] The severity of DIC according to this scoring system is related to the mortality in patients with sepsis.[87] Linking prognostic determinants from critical care measurement scores such as APACHE II to DIC scores is an important means to assess prognosis in critically ill patients. Similar scoring systems have been developed in Japan.[88]

In a prospective study in 840 patients continuation of coagulopathy during the first calendar day correlated with development of new organ failure and 28-day mortality in patients with severe sepsis.[89] Coagulopathy risk points (based on sustained abnormalities in PT and platelet count) were related to progression from single to multiple organ failure, time to resolution of organ failure, and 28-day mortality (p<.001). Adding the scoring system to APACHE. II improved ability to predict which patients may progress from single to multiple organ failure.

DIFFERENTIAL DIAGNOSIS OF COAGULATION ABNORMALITIES IN CRITICALLY ILL PATIENTS

Table 1 summarizes the most frequently occurring diagnoses recognized in intensive care patients with thrombocytopenia. The relative incidence of each of these disorders in ICU patients is provided along with the differential diagnostic approach to distinguish each of these entities.

Sepsis is a clear risk factor for thrombocytopenia in critically ill patients and the severity of sepsis correlates with the decrease in platelet count.[90] The principal factors that contribute to thrombocytopenia in patients with sepsis are impaired platelet production, increased consumption or destruction, or sequestration platelets in the spleen or along the endothelial surface. Impaired production of platelets from within the bone marrow may seem contradictory to the high levels of platelet production-stimulating proinflammatory cytokines, such as TNF-α and IL-6, and high concentration of circulating thrombopoietin in patients with sepsis.[91] These cytokines and growth factors should theoretically stimulate megakaryopoiesis in the bone marrow.[92] However, in a substantial number of patients with sepsis marked hemophagocytosis may occur. This pathologic process consists of active phagocytosis of megakaryocytes and other hematopoietic cells by monocytes and macrophages, hypothetically due to stimulation with high levels of macrophage colony stimulating factor in sepsis.[93] Platelet consumption probably also plays an important role in patients with sepsis, due to ongoing generation of thrombin (which is the most potent activator of platelets in vivo), in its most fulminant form known as disseminated intravascular coagulation.

Table 1		
Differential diagnosis of thrombocytopenia in the ICU		
Differential Diagnosis	**Relative Incidence**	**Additional Diagnostic Clues**
Sepsis	52.4%	Positive (blood) cultures, positive sepsis criteria, hematophagocytosis in bone marrow aspirate
DIC[a]	25.3%	Prolonged aPTT and PT, increased fibrin split products, low levels of physiological anticoagulant factors (antithrombin, protein C)
Massive blood loss	7.5%	Major bleeding, low hemoglobin, prolonged aPTT and PT,
Thrombotic microangiopathy	0.7%	Schistocytes in blood smear, Coombs-negative hemolysis, fever, neurologic symptoms, renal insufficiency
Heparin-induced thrombocytopenia	1.2%	Use of heparin, venous or arterial thrombosis, positive HIT test (usually ELISA for heparin-platelet factor IV antibodies), rebound of platelets after cessation of heparin
Immune thrombocytopenia	3.4%	Antiplatelet antibodies, normal or increased number of megakaryocytes in bone marrow aspirate, thrombopoietin decreased
Drug-induced thrombocytopenia	9.5%	Decreased number of megakaryocytes in bone marrow aspirate or detection of drug-induced anti-platelet antibodies, rebound of platelet count after cessation of drug

Seven major causes of thrombocytopenia (platelet count $<150 \times 10^9/l$) are listed. Relative incidences are based on two studies in consecutive ICU patients.[1,6] Patients with hematological malignancies were excluded.

[a] Patients with sepsis and DIC are classified as DIC.

Platelet activation, consumption, and destruction may also occur at the endothelial site as a result of the extensive endothelial cell-platelet interaction in sepsis, which may vary between different vascular beds in various organs.[94]

In patients with DIC, the platelet count is invariably low or rapidly decreasing.[12] DIC is the most extreme form of systemic coagulation activation, which may complicate a variety of underlying disease processes, including sepsis, trauma, cancer, or obstetrical calamities, such as placental abruption (see later discussion).

The group of thrombotic microangiopathies encompasses syndromes such as thrombotic thrombocytopenic purpura, hemolytic-uremic syndrome, severe malignant hypertension, chemotherapy-induced microangiopathic hemolytic anemia, and the HELLP syndrome.[95] A common pathogenetic feature of these clinical entities appears to be endothelial damage, causing platelet adhesion and aggregation, thrombin formation, and an impaired fibrinolysis. The multiple clinical consequences of this extensive endothelial dysfunction include thrombocytopenia, mechanical fragmentation of red cells with hemolytic anemia, and obstruction of the microvasculature of various organs, such as kidney and brain (leading to renal failure and neurologic dysfunction, respectively). Despite this common final pathway, the various thrombotic microangiopathies have different underlying etiologies. Thrombotic thrombocytopenic purpura is caused by deficiency of von Willebrand factor cleaving protease (ADAMTS-13), resulting in endothelial cell-attached ultra-large von Willebrand multimers, that readily bind to platelet surface glycoprotein Ib and cause platelet adhesion and aggregation.[96] In hemolytic uremic syndrome, a cytotoxin released upon infection with a specific serogroup of gram-negative microorganisms (usually E coli serotype O157:H7) is responsible for endothelial cell and platelet activation. In case of malignant hypertension or chemotherapy-induced thrombotic microangiopathy, presumably direct mechanical or chemical damage to the endothelium is responsible for the enhanced endothelial cell-platelet interaction, respectively. A diagnosis of thrombotic microangiopathy relies upon the combination of thrombocytopenia, Coombs-negative hemolytic anemia, and the presence of schistocytes in the blood smear. Additional information can be achieved by measurement of ADAMTS-13 and autoantibodies towards this metalloprotease and culture (usually from the stool or urine) of microorganisms capable of cytotoxin production.

Heparin-induced thrombocytopenia (HIT) is caused by a heparin-induced antibody that binds to the heparin-platelet factor IV complex on the platelet surface.[94] This may result in massive platelet activation and as a consequence a consumptive thrombocytopenia and arterial and venous thrombosis occurs. The incidence of HIT may be as high as 5% of patients receiving heparin and is dependent on the type and dose of heparin and the duration of its administration (especially when given more than 4 days). A consecutive series of critically ill ICU patients who received heparin revealed an incidence of 1% in this setting.[97] Unfractionated heparin carries a higher risk of HIT than low molecular weight heparin.[98] Thrombosis may occur in 25% to 50% of patients with HIT (with fatal thrombosis in 4%–5%) and may also become manifest after discontinuation of heparin.[98] The diagnosis of HIT is based on the detection of HIT antibodies in combination with the occurrence of thrombocytopenia in a patient receiving heparin, with or without concomitant arterial or venous thrombosis. It should be mentioned that the commonly used ELISA for HIT antibodies has a high negative predictive value (100%) but a very low positive predictive value (10%).[97] A more precise diagnosis may be made with a 14C-serotonin release assay, but this test is not routinely available in most settings.[99] Normalization in the number of platelets in 1 to 3 days after discontinuation of heparin may further support the diagnosis of HIT.

Drug-induced thrombocytopenia is another frequent cause of thrombocytopenia in the ICU setting.[17] Thrombocytopenia may be caused by drug-induced myelosuppression, such as caused by cytostatic agents, or by immune-mediated mechanisms. Examples of drug-induced immune-mediated thrombocytopenia are HIT or quinine-induced thrombocytopenia. A large number of other agents may cause thrombocytopenia by similar mechanisms, including medications that are frequently used in critically ill patients such as antibiotics (including cephalosporins or trimethoprim-sulfamethoxazole), benzodiazepines, or nonsteroidal antiinflammatory agents. Novel inhibitors of platelet aggregation, such as glycoprotein IIb/IIIa antagonists (eg, abciximab) or thienopyridine derivatives (clopidogrel) are increasingly used in the management of patients with acute coronary syndromes and may also cause severe thrombocytopenia.[100] Drug-induced thrombocytopenia is a difficult diagnosis in the ICU setting as these patients are often exposed to multiple agents and have numerous other potential reasons for platelet depletion. Drug-induced thrombocytopenia is often diagnosed based upon the timing of initiation of a new agent in relationship to the development of thrombocytopenia, after exclusion of other causes of thrombocytopenia. The observation of rapid restoration of the platelet count after discontinuation of the suspected agent is highly suggestive of drug-induced thrombocytopenia. In some cases, specific drug-dependent antiplatelet antibodies can be detected.

A prolongation of global coagulation tests may be due to a deficiency of one or more coagulation factors (**Table 2**). In addition, the presence of an inhibiting antibody, which can have major in vivo relevance (such as in acquired hemophilia) but can also be a clinically insignificant laboratory phenomenon, should be considered. The presence of such inhibiting antibody can be confirmed by a simple mixing experiment. As a general rule, if a prolongation of a global coagulation test cannot be corrected by mixing 50% of patient plasma with 50% of normal plasma, then an inhibiting antibody is likely to be present.

In the vast majority of critically ill patients, deficiencies of coagulation factors are acquired and the authors will not discuss the various congenital coagulation defects here. In general, deficiencies in coagulation factors may be due to impaired synthesis, massive loss, or increased turnover (consumption). Impaired synthesis is often due to liver insufficiency or vitamin K deficiency. The PT is most sensitive to both conditions, since this test is highly dependent on the plasma levels of factor VII (a vitamin K-dependent coagulation factor with a shortest half-life of the clotting factors). Liver failure may be differentiated from vitamin K deficiency by measuring factor V, which is not vitamin K dependent. In fact, factor V plays an important role in various scoring systems for severe acute liver failure.[101] Uncompensated loss of coagulation factors may occur after massive bleeding, for example in trauma patients or patients undergoing major surgical procedures. This is particularly common in patients with major blood loss where intravascular volume is rapidly replaced with crystalloids, colloids, and red cells without simultaneous administration of coagulation factors. This resulting depletional form of coagulopathy may persist and exacerbate the bleeding. In hypothermic patients (eg, trauma patients) measurement of the global coagulation tests may underestimate coagulation in vivo, since in the laboratory test-tube assays are standardized and performed at $37°C$ to mimic normal body temperature. Consumption of coagulation factors may occur in the framework of disseminated intravascular coagulation (see later discussion). In complicated cases, various causes for a prolongation of global coagulation times may be present simultaneously and the cause may also change over time. For example, multitrauma patients will often present with a loss of coagulation factors due to severe bleeding but can later develop a consumption

Table 2
Results of global coagulation assays in critically ill patients

Test Result	Cause
PT prolonged, aPTT normal	Factor VII deficiency Mild vitamin K deficiency Mild liver insufficiency Low doses of vitamin K antagonists
PT normal, aPTT prolonged	Factor VIII, IX, or XI deficiency Use of unfractionated heparin Inhibiting antibody or anti-phospholipid antibody Factor XII or prekallikrein deficiency (no relevance for in vivo coagulation)
Both PT and aPTT prolonged	Factor X, V, II or fibrinogen deficiency Severe vitamin K deficiency Use of vitamin K antagonists Global clotting factor deficiency Synthesis: liver failure Loss: massive bleeding Consumption: DIC

coagulopathy due to DIC as a consequence of a systemic inflammatory response. Coagulopathy may subsequently ensue from trauma-induced liver injury and acute hepatic decompensation with resultant impaired coagulation factor synthesis.

Some anticoagulant agents will also prolong global coagulation times. Unfractionated heparin prolongs the aPTT, but confusingly low molecular weight heparins do not (or only very modestly) have such an effect. Warfarin or other vitamin K antagonists causes a reduction in vitamin K dependent coagulation factors, resulting in an initial prolongation the PT followed by elevations of both the PT and aPTT.

SUMMARY

Coagulation abnormalities occur frequently in critically ill patients and may have a major impact on the outcome. An adequate explanation for the cause of the coagulation abnormality is important, since many underlying disorders may require specific treatment. Treatment of coagulation abnormalities in critically ill patients should be directed at the underlying condition, but supportive therapy may be required. Deficiencies in platelets and coagulation factors in bleeding patients or patients at risk for bleeding can be achieved by transfusion of platelet concentrate or plasma products, respectively. In addition, prohemostatic treatment may be beneficial in case of severe bleeding, whereas restoring physiological anticoagulant pathways may be helpful in patients with sepsis and DIC.

REFERENCES

1. Levi M, Opal SM. Coagulation abnormalities in critically ill patients. Crit Care 2006;10(4):222.
2. Levi M, Keller TT, van Gorp E, et al. Infection and inflammation and the coagulation system. Cardiovasc Res 2003;60(1):26–39.
3. Robboy SJ, Major MC, Colman RW, et al. Pathology of disseminated intravascular coagulation (DIC). Analysis of 26 cases. Hum Pathol 1972;3(3):327–43.
4. Shimamura K, Oka K, Nakazawa M, et al. Distribution patterns of microthrombi in disseminated intravascular coagulation. Arch Pathol Lab Med 1983;107(10): 543–7.
5. Coalson JJ. Pathology of sepsis, septic shock, and multiple organ failure. Perspective on sepsis and septic shock. Fullerton (CA): Society of Critical Care Medicine; 1986. p. 27–59.
6. Creasey AA, Chang AC, Feigen L, et al. Tissue factor pathway inhibitor reduces mortality from Escherichia coli septic shock. J Clin Invest 1993;91(6):2850–6.
7. Kessler CM, Tang Z, Jacobs HM, et al. The suprapharmacologic dosing of antithrombin concentrate for Staphylococcus aureus-induced disseminated intravascular coagulation in guinea pigs: substantial reduction in mortality and morbidity. Blood 1997;89(12):4393–401.
8. Taylor FBJ, Chang A, Ruf W, et al. Lethal E. coli septic shock is prevented by blocking tissue factor with monoclonal antibody. Circ Shock 1991;33(3):127–34.
9. Taylor FBJ, Chang AC, Esmon CT, et al. Baboon model of Escherichia coli sepsis: description of its four stages and the role of tumor necrosis factor, tissue factors, and the protein C system in septic shock. Curr Stud Hematol Blood Transfus 1991;58:8–14.
10. Welty-Wolf KE, Carraway MS, Miller DL, et al. Coagulation blockade prevents sepsis-induced respiratory and renal failure in baboons. Am J Respir Crit Care Med 2001;164(10 Pt 1):1988–96.

11. Miller DL, Welty-Wolf K, Carraway MS, et al. Extrinsic coagulation blockade attenuates lung injury and proinflammatory cytokine release after intratracheal lipopolysaccharide. Am J Respir Cell Mol Biol 2002;26(6):650–8.
12. Levi M, ten Cate H. Disseminated intravascular coagulation. N Engl J Med 1999; 341(8):586–92.
13. Fourrier F, Chopin C, Goudemand J, et al. Septic shock, multiple organ failure, and disseminated intravascular coagulation. Compared patterns of antithrombin III, protein C, and protein S deficiencies [see comments]. Chest 1992;101(3): 816–23.
14. Vanderschueren S, De Weerdt A, Malbrain M, et al. Thrombocytopenia and prognosis in intensive care. Crit Care Med 2000;28(6):1871–6.
15. Strauss R, Wehler M, Mehler K, et al. Thrombocytopenia in patients in the medical intensive care unit: bleeding prevalence, transfusion requirements, and outcome. Crit Care Med 2002;30(8):1765–71.
16. Oppenheim-Eden A, Glantz L, Eidelman LA, et al. Spontaneous intracerebral hemorrhage in critically ill patients: incidence over six years and associated factors. Intensive Care Med 1999;25(1):63–7.
17. Stephan F, Hollande J, Richard O, et al. Thrombocytopenia in a surgical ICU. Chest 1999;115(5):1363–70.
18. Akca S, Haji Michael P, de Medonca A, et al. The time course of platelet counts in critically ill patients. Crit Care Med 2002;30:753–6.
19. Chakraverty R, Davidson S, Peggs K, et al. The incidence and cause of coagulopathies in an intensive care population. Br J Haematol 1996;93(2):460–3.
20. MacLeod JB, Lynn M, McKenney MG, et al. Early coagulopathy predicts mortality in trauma. J Trauma 2003;55(1):39–44.
21. Baughman RP, Lower EE, Flessa HC, et al. Thrombocytopenia in the intensive care unit. Chest 1993;104(4):1243–7.
22. Hanes SD, Quarles DA, Boucher BA. Incidence and risk factors of thrombocytopenia in critically ill trauma patients. Ann Pharmacother 1997;31(3):285–9.
23. Greaves M, Preston FE. Approach to the bleeding patient. In: Colman RW, Hirsh J, Marder VJ, et al, editors. Hemostasis and thrombosis. Basic principles and clinical practice. 4th edition. Philadelphia: Lippingcott William & Wilkins; 2001. p. 1031–43.
24. Edmunds LH. Hemostatic problems in surgical patients. In: Colman RW, Hirsh J, Marder VJ, et al, editors. Hemostasis and thrombosis. Basic principles and clinical practice. 4th edition. Philadelphia: Lippingcott William & Wilkins; 2001. p. 1031–43.
25. Kitchen S, Preston FE. Standardization of prothrombin time for laboratory control of oral anticoagulant therapy. Semin Thromb Hemost 1999;25(1):17–25.
26. Shorr AF, Thomas SJ, Alkins SA, et al. D-dimer correlates with proinflammatory cytokine levels and outcomes in critically ill patients. Chest 2002;121(4):1262–8.
27. Owings JT, Gosselin RC, Anderson JT, et al. Practical utility of the D-dimer assay for excluding thromboembolism in severely injured trauma patients. J Trauma 2001;51(3):425–9.
28. Bernard GR, Vincent JL, Laterre PF, et al. Efficacy and safety of recombinant human activated protein C for severe sepsis. N Engl J Med 2001;344(10): 699–709.
29. Levi M, Toh CH, Thachil J, et al. Guidelines for the diagnosis and management of disseminated intravascular coagulation. Br J Haematol 2009;145(1):24–33.
30. Boisclair MD, Ireland H, Lane DA. Assessment of hypercoagulable states by measurement of activation fragments and peptides. Blood Rev 1990;4(1):25–40.

31. Levi M. The coagulant response in sepsis. Clin Chest Med 2008;29(4):627–42, viii.
32. ten Cate H, Bauer KA, Levi M, et al. The activation of factor X and prothrombin by recombinant factor VIIa in vivo is mediated by tissue factor. J Clin Invest 1993;92(3):1207–12.
33. Nossel HL, Yudelman I, Canfield RE, et al. Measurement of fibrinopeptide A in human blood. J Clin Invest 1974;54(1):43–53.
34. Gando S, Nanzaki S, Sasaki S, et al. Significant correlations between tissue factor and thrombin markers in trauma and septic patients with disseminated intravascular coagulation. Thromb Haemost 1998;79(6):1111–5.
35. Vary TC, Kimball SR. Regulation of hepatic protein synthesis in chronic inflammation and sepsis. Am J Physiol 1992;262(2 Pt 1):C445–52.
36. Seitz R, Wolf M, Egbring R, et al. The disturbance of hemostasis in septic shock: role of neutrophil elastase and thrombin, effects of antithrombin III and plasma substitution. Eur J Haematol 1989;43(1):22–8.
37. Opal SM, Kessler CM, Roemisch J, et al. Antithrombin, heparin, and heparan sulfate. Crit Care Med 2002;30(Suppl 5):S325–31.
38. Mesters RM, Mannucci PM, Coppola R, et al. Factor VIIa and antithrombin III activity during severe sepsis and septic shock in neutropenic patients [see comments]. Blood 1996;88(3):881–6.
39. Esmon CT. New mechanisms for vascular control of inflammation mediated by natural anticoagulant proteins. J Exp Med 2002;196(5):561–4.
40. Zushi M, Gomi K, Yamamoto S, et al. The last three consecutive epidermal growth factor-like structures of human thrombomodulin comprise the minimum functional domain for protein C-activating cofactor activity and anticoagulant activity. J Biol Chem 1989;264(18):10351–3.
41. Bajzar L, Morser J, Nesheim M. TAFI, or plasma procarboxypeptidase B, couples the coagulation and fibrinolytic cascades through the thrombin-thrombomodulin complex. J Biol Chem 1996;271(28):16603–8.
42. Taylor FB Jr, Peer GT, Lockhart MS, et al. Endothelial cell protein C receptor plays an important role in protein C activation in vivo. Blood 2001;97(6):1685–8.
43. Eckle I, Seitz R, Egbring R, et al. Protein C degradation in vitro by neutrophil elastase. Biol Chem Hoppe Seyler 1991;372(11):1007–13.
44. Nawroth PP, Stern DM. Modulation of endothelial cell hemostatic properties by tumor necrosis factor. J Exp Med 1986;163(3):740–5.
45. Faust SN, Levin M, Harrison OB, et al. Dysfunction of endothelial protein C activation in severe meningococcal sepsis. N Engl J Med 2001;345(6):408–16.
46. Garcia de Frutos P, Alim RI, Hardig Y, et al. Differential regulation of alpha and beta chains of C4b-binding protein during acute-phase response resulting in stable plasma levels of free anticoagulant protein S. Blood 1994;84(3):815–22.
47. Taylor F, Chang A, Ferrell G, et al. C4b-binding protein exacerbates the host response to Escherichia coli. Blood 1991;78(2):357–63.
48. Taylor FBJ, Dahlback B, Chang AC, et al. Role of free protein S and C4b binding protein in regulating the coagulant response to Escherichia coli. Blood 1995;86(7):2642–52.
49. Levi M, Dorffler-Melly J, Reitsma PH, et al. Aggravation of endotoxin-induced disseminated intravascular coagulation and cytokine activation in heterozygous protein C deficient mice. Blood 2003;101:4823–7.
50. Broze GJ Jr, Girard TJ, Novotny WF. Regulation of coagulation by a multivalent Kunitz-type inhibitor. Biochemistry 1990;29(33):7539–46.

51. de Jonge E, Dekkers PE, Creasey AA, et al. Tissue factor pathway inhibitor (TFPI) dose-dependently inhibits coagulation activtion without influencing the fibrinolytic and cytokine response during human endotoxemia. Blood 2000;95: 1124–9.

52. Gando S, Kameue T, Morimoto Y, et al. Tissue factor production not balanced by tissue factor pathway inhibitor in sepsis promotes poor prognosis. Crit Care Med 2002;30:1729–34.

53. Levi M. The imbalance between tissue factor and tissue factor pathway inhibitor in sepsis. Crit Care Med 2002;30(8):1914–5.

54. Nuijens JH, Huijbregts CC, Eerenberg-Belmer AJ, et al. Quantification of plasma factor XIIa-Cl(-)-inhibitor and kallikrein-Cl(-)-inhibitor complexes in sepsis. Blood 1988;72(6):1841–8.

55. Pixley RA, De LC, Page JD, et al. The contact system contributes to hypotension but not disseminated intravascular coagulation in lethal bacteremia. In vivo use of a monoclonal anti-factor XII antibody to block contact activation in baboons. J Clin Invest 1993;91(1):61–8.

56. Sriskandan S, Kemball-Cook G, Moyes D, et al. Contact activation in shock caused by invasive group A *Streptococcus* pyogenes. Crit Care Med 2000; 28:3684–91.

57. Minnema MC, Pajkrt D, Wuillemin WA, et al. Activation of clotting factor XI without detectable contact activation in experimental human endotoxemia. Blood 1998;92(9):3294–301.

58. Colman RW, Schmaier AH. Contact system: a vascular biology modulator with anticoagulant, profibrinolytic, antiadhesive, and proinflammatory attributes [review]. Blood 1997;90(10):3819–43.

59. Levi M. Keep in contact: the role of the contact system in infection and sepsis. Crit Care Med 2000;28(11):3765–6.

60. O'Donnell TFJ, Clowes GHJ, Talamo RC, et al. Kinin activation in the blood of patients with sepsis. Surg Gynecol Obstet 1976;143(4):539–45.

61. Kaufman N, Page JD, Pixley RA, et al. Alpha 2-macroglobulin-kallikrein complexes detect contact system activation in hereditary angioedema and human sepsis. Blood 1991;77(12):2660–7.

62. Jansen PM, Pixley RA, Brouwer M, et al. Inhibition of factor XII in septic baboons attenuates the activation of complement and fibrinolytic systems and reduces the release of interleukin-6 and neutrophil elastase. Blood 1996;87(6):2337–44.

63. van der Poll T, Levi M, Buller HR, et al. Fibrinolytic response to tumor necrosis factor in healthy subjects. J Exp Med 1991;174(3):729–32.

64. Biemond BJ, Levi M, ten Cate H, et al. Plasminogen activator and plasminogen activator inhibitor I release during experimental endotoxaemia in chimpanzees: effect of interventions in the cytokine and coagulation cascades. Clin Sci (Lond) 1995;88(5):587–94.

65. Yamamoto K, Loskutoff DJ. Fibrin deposition in tissues from endotoxin-treated mice correlates with decreases in the expression of urokinase-type but not tissue-type plasminogen activator. J Clin Invest 1996;97(11):2440–51.

66. Pinsky DJ, Liao H, Lawson CA, et al. Coordinated induction of plasminogen activator inhibitor-1 (PAI-1) and inhibition of plasminogen activator gene expression by hypoxia promotes pulmonary vascular fibrin deposition. J Clin Invest 1998; 102(5):919–28.

67. Hermans PW, Hibberd ML, Booy R, et al. 4G/5G promoter polymorphism in the plasminogen-activator-inhibitor-1 gene and outcome of meningococcal disease. Meningococcal Research Group. Lancet 1999;354(9178):556–60.

68. Westendorp RG, Hottenga JJ, Slagboom PE. Variation in plasminogen-activator-inhibitor-1 gene and risk of meningococcal septic shock. Lancet 1999; 354(9178):561–3.

69. Aird WC. Vascular bed-specific hemostasis: role of endothelium in sepsis pathogenesis. Crit Care Med 2001;29(Suppl 7):S28–34.

70. Sawdey MS, Loskutoff DJ. Regulation of murine type 1 plasminogen activator inhibitor gene expression in vivo. Tissue specificity and induction by lipopolysaccharide, tumor necrosis factor-alpha, and transforming growth factor-beta. J Clin Invest 1991;88(4):1346–53.

71. Rosenberg RD, Aird WC. Vascular-bed–specific hemostasis and hypercoagulable states [review]. N Engl J Med 1999;340(20):1555–64.

72. Aird WC, Edelberg JM, Weiler-Guettler H, et al. Vascular bed-specific expression of an endothelial cell gene is programmed by the tissue microenvironment. J Cell Biol 1997;138(5):1117–24.

73. Healy AM, Hancock WW, Christie PD, et al. Intravascular coagulation activation in a murine model of thrombomodulin deficiency: effects of lesion size, age, and hypoxia on fibrin deposition. Blood 1998;92(11):4188–97.

74. ten Cate H. Pathophysiology of disseminated intravascular coagulation in sepsis. Crit Care Med 2000;28:S9–11.

75. Levi M, van der Poll T, Buller HR. Bidirectional relation between inflammation and coagulation. Circulation 2004;109(22):2698–704.

76. Levi M, van der Poll T, ten Cate H, et al. The cytokine-mediated imbalance between coagulant and anticoagulant mechanisms in sepsis and endotoxaemia. Eur J Clin Invest 1997;27(1):3–9.

77. Dempfle CE, Borggrefe M. Point of care coagulation tests in critically ill patients. Semin Thromb Hemost 2008;34(5):445–50.

78. Johansson PI, Stensballe J, Vindelov N, et al. Hypocoagulability, as evaluated by thrombelastography, at admission to the ICU is associated with increased 30-day mortality. Blood Coagul Fibrinolysis 2010;21(2):168–74.

79. Park MS, Martini WZ, Dubick MA, et al. Thromboelastography as a better indicator of hypercoagulable state after injury than prothrombin time or activated partial thromboplastin time. J Trauma 2009;67(2):266–75.

80. Collins PW, Macchiavello LI, Lewis SJ, et al. Global tests of haemostasis in critically ill patients with severe sepsis syndrome compared to controls. Br J Haematol 2006;135(2):220–7.

81. Toh CH, Samis J, Downey C, et al. Biphasic transmittance waveform in the APTT coagulation assay is due to the formation of a Ca($++$)-dependent complex of C-reactive protein with very-low-density lipoprotein and is a novel marker of impending disseminated intravascular coagulation. Blood 2002;100(7):2522–9.

82. Toh CH. Transmittance waveform of routine coagulation tests is a sensitive and specific method for diagnosing non-overt disseminated intravascular coagulation. Blood Rev 2002;16(Suppl 1):S11–4.

83. Taylor FBJ, Toh CH, Hoots WK, et al. Towards definition, clinical and laboratory criteria, and a scoring system for disseminated intravascular coagulation. Thromb Haemost 2001;86(5):1327–30.

84. Horan JT, Francis CW. Fibrin degradation products, fibrin monomer and soluble fibrin in disseminated intravascular coagulation. Semin Thromb Hemost 2001; 27(6):657–66.

85. Bakhtiari K, Meijers JC, de Jonge E, et al. Prospective validation of the international society of thrombosis and maemostasis scoring system for disseminated intravascular coagulation. Crit Care Med 2004;32:2416–21.

86. Toh CH, Hoots WK. The scoring system of the Scientific and Standardisation Committee on Disseminated Intravascular Coagulation of the International Society on thrombosis and haemostasis: a five year overview. J Thromb Haemost 2007;5:604–6.
87. Dhainaut JF, Yan SB, Joyce DE, et al. Treatment effects of drotrecogin alfa (activated) in patients with severe sepsis with or without overt disseminated intravascular coagulation. J Thromb Haemost 2004;2:1924–33.
88. Levi M. Settling the score for disseminated intravascular coagulation. Crit Care Med 2005;33(10):2417–8.
89. Kinasewitz GT, Zein JG, Lee GL, et al. Prognostic value of a simple evolving DIC score in patients with severe sepsis. Crit Care Med 2005;33:2214–21.
90. Mavrommatis AC, Theodoridis T, Orfanidou A, et al. Coagulation system and platelets are fully activated in uncomplicated sepsis. Crit Care Med 2000; 28(2):451–7.
91. Anas A, Wiersinga WJ, de Vos AF, et al. Recent insights into the pathogenesis of bacterial sepsis. Neth J Med 2010;68:147–52.
92. Folman CC, Linthorst GE, van Mourik J, et al. Platelets release thrombopoietin (Tpo) upon activation: another regulatory loop in thrombocytopoiesis? Thromb Haemost 2000;83(6):923–30.
93. Francois B, Trimoreau F, Vignon P, et al. Thrombocytopenia in the sepsis syndrome: role of hemophagocytosis and macrophage colony-stimulating factor. Am J Med 1997;103(2):114–20.
94. Warkentin TE, Aird WC, Rand JH. Platelet-endothelial interactions: sepsis, HIT, and antiphospholipid syndrome. Hematology Am Soc Hematol Educ Program 2003;497–519.
95. Moake JL. Thrombotic microangiopathies. N Engl J Med 2002;347(8):589–600.
96. Tsai HM. Platelet activation and the formation of the platelet plug: deficiency of ADAMTS13 causes thrombotic thrombocytopenic purpura. Arterioscler Thromb Vasc Biol 2003;23(3):388–96.
97. Verma AK, Levine M, Shalansky SJ, et al. Frequency of heparin-induced thrombocytopenia in critical care patients. Pharmacotherapy 2003;23(6):745–53.
98. Warkentin TE. Heparin-induced thrombocytopenia: pathogenesis and management. Br J Haematol 2003;121(4):535–55.
99. Sheridan D, Carter C, Kelton JG. A diagnostic test for heparin-induced thrombocytopenia. Blood 1986;67(1):27–30.
100. Makoni SN. Acute profound thrombocytopenia following angioplasty: the dilemma in the management and a review of the literature. Heart 2001; 86(6):o18.
101. Bailey B, Amre DK, Gaudreault P. Fulminant hepatic failure secondary to acetaminophen poisoning: a systematic review and meta-analysis of prognostic criteria determining the need for liver transplantation. Crit Care Med 2003; 31(1):299–305.

Lactate: Biomarker and Potential Therapeutic Target

Okorie Nduka Okorie, MD[a,b,*], Phil Dellinger, MD[c,d]

KEYWORDS

• Lactate • Hypoperfusion • Critically ill • Biomarker

Critical illness is characterized by disruptions in homeostasis that result in single- or multiple-organ injury and reversible or irreversible organ dysfunction. To a large extent, the duration of exposure to injurious stimuli/conditions determines the reversibility or irreversibility of organ dysfunction in critical illness. Therefore, it is highly important that organ system dysfunction in critically ill patients is recognized as early as possible and appropriate therapeutic interventions are applied to improve outcomes in these patients. Traditionally, recognition of organ dysfunction in patients has relied on its clinical signs and symptoms (eg, oliguria and/or elevated creatinine levels for the kidney). Historically, recognition of circulatory failure and the likelihood of tissue hypoperfusion relied on the presence of persistent or refractory (to fluid resuscitation) hypotension. This approach is complicated by a relative lack of sensitivity of clinical signs and symptoms to predict the presence or absence of organ injury or tissue hypoperfusion. In addition, some clinical examination techniques lack standardization, for example, the assessment of capillary refill time (CRT) as an index of peripheral hypoperfusion. In one study, it was noted that clinicians used several different methods to assess CRT, including either finger "pulp" or finger "nail" pressure.[1] The same study showed substantial interobserver variability between measurements of CRT when a cutoff value of 2 seconds was used in patients presenting to an emergency department (ED). The cutoff values used to define normal CRT have been variously listed, with values between 2 and 6 seconds.[2,3] Few clinical examination measurements used at present in critically ill patients have been subjected to rigorous standards of validation.

[a] Florida State University School of Medicine, Orlando, FL, USA
[b] Department of Critical Care Medicine, Orlando Regional Medical Center, 86 West Underwood Street, Suite 102, Orlando, FL, USA
[c] University of Medicine and Dentistry of New Jersey, Robert Wood Johnson Medical School, Camden, NJ, USA
[d] Division of Critical Care Medicine, Cooper University Hospital, Camden, NJ, USA
* Corresponding author. Department of Critical Care Medicine, Orlando Regional Medical Center, 86 West Underwood Street, Suite 102, Orlando, FL
E-mail address: Okorie.Okorie@orlandohealth.com

Crit Care Clin 27 (2011) 299–326
doi:10.1016/j.ccc.2010.12.013   criticalcare.theclinics.com

It is against this background that measurements of serum lactate either singly or serially may have a role as a biomarker to estimate the likelihood and extent of tissue hypoperfusion, as well as in the judgment of treatment response and prognosis.

Traditionally, the terms lactate and lactic acid are used interchangeably. Lactic acid is a weak acid, which means that it only partially dissociates in water. Lactic acid dissociates in water resulting in ion lactate and H^+. Depending on the environmental pH, weak acids, such as lactic acid, are present as either acid in their undissociated form at low pH or ion salt at higher pH. The pH at which 50% of the acid is dissociated is called the pKa, which for lactic acid is 3.85. The pKa of lactic acid is much lower than that of cells and the extracellular fluid compartment, and thus, it exists predominantly in the ionized state. This reaction can be illustrated by the Henderson-Hasselbalch equation:

$$pH = pKa + \log [H^+][A^-]/[HA].$$

The ratio of lactate to lactic acid at physiologic pH (7.4) and the lowest limits of pH compatible with life over a protracted period (6.8) can be calculated as follows:

$$7.4 = 3.85 + \log [(lactate)/(lactic\ acid)] = 3548:1$$

$$6.8 = 3.85 + \log [(lactate)/(lactic\ acid)] = 891:1$$

From these equations, it is clear that lactic acid in human subjects exists predominantly in its ionized form even in severely low pH states. Accordingly, measurements are made of blood or plasma lactate, not lactic acid.

This review discusses the role of lactate as a biomarker in diagnosing and assessing the severity of systemic hypoperfusion, as well as the role of serum lactate measurements in guiding clinical care and enabling prognosis in critically ill patients.

HISTORICAL PERSPECTIVE

Lactate was first described in 1780 as a substance in sour milk by the Swedish chemist, Karl Wilhelm Scheele.[4] This discovery was followed by its first description in animals by another Swedish chemist, Jons Jacob Berzelius, in 1807, when he discovered it in the muscle tissue of hunted stags.[5] The Japanese chemist, Trasaburo Araki, demonstrated that in states of oxygen deprivation, no matter how, mammals produced and excreted lactate.[6–9] The findings were replicated in experiments conducted by Hermann Zillessen.[10] The works done by Araki and Zillessen serve as the earliest demonstrations of the relationship between tissue hypoxia and lactate production.

The German chemist and physician, Joseph Scherer,[11] in 1843, first demonstrated the presence of lactate in human blood (post mortem) in a series of case reports involving 7 young women who died of puerperal fever. In 1851, he subsequently reported the same finding in the tissue fluids of a patient who had died of leukemia.[12] This report was followed by demonstration of elevated lactate levels in the blood of a living patient by Carl Folwarczny in 1858.[13] These observations were the basis for the understanding of the significance of elevated lactate levels in critically ill patients.

Essentially, hyperlactatemia was viewed primarily as the result of anaerobic metabolism due to inadequate tissue oxygen delivery.[14] This understanding persisted for most of the last century, and it was only in the later half of the last century that the understanding of the significance of elevated serum lactate levels was modified to include disease states other than tissue hypoxia.[15] Further work on lactate metabolism elucidated the role of hyperlactatemia as a product of metabolic adjustment in critical illness.[16,17]

LACTATE PRODUCTION, METABOLISM, AND EXCRETION

Glycolysis is the first step in the metabolism of glucose (**Fig. 1**), and its end product is pyruvate. Once formed, pyruvate can follow several metabolic pathways. It can cross the mitochondrial membranes into the tricarboxylic acid pathway and produce energy (38 molecules of ATP). It can be converted into lactate by the action of the enzyme lactate dehydrogenase. It can be used as a substrate in gluconeogenesis for the production of glucose, or it can undergo transamination to alanine. The conversion of pyruvate to lactate is reserved primarily for excess pyruvate levels. Conversion of pyruvate to lactate is favored during hypoxic tissue conditions and several other clinically relevant conditions (**Box 1**).

$$Glucose + 2ADP + 2NAD^+ \rightarrow 2Pyruvate + 2ATP + 2NADH$$

$$Pyruvate + NADH + H^+ \leftrightarrow Lactate + NAD^+$$

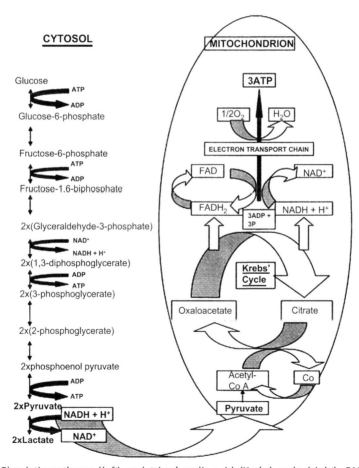

Fig. 1. Glycolytic pathway (*left*) and tricarboxylic acid (Krebs) cycle (*right*). FAD/FADH$_2$, oxidized/reduced flavin cofactors, respectively; CoA, Coenzyme A. (*From* Handy J. Lactate—the bad boy of metabolism, or simply misunderstood? Curr Anaesth Crit Care 2006;17(1/2):73; with permission.)

Box 1
Conditions favoring the conversion of pyruvate to lactate

Systemic hypoperfusion necessitating anaerobic metabolism

Regional hypoperfusion and microcirculatory dysfunction

Increased aerobic glycolysis, with pyruvate production exceeding pyruvate dehydrogenase capacity. This condition may be seen in response to cytokine release, increased circulating catecholamine levels, or the accumulation of leukocytes at the site of inflammation/infection

Mitochondrial dysfunction shunting pyruvate away from the tricarboxylic acid cycle, which may be seen in sepsis and drug toxicity

Impaired activity of pyruvate dehydrogenase, which is essential for the conversion of pyruvate into acetyl coenzyme A, a necessary step in aerobic metabolism. This condition may be seen in excessive alcohol use and cofactor deficiency states (beriberi)

The serum arterial lactate concentration reflects the balance between net lactate production and net lactate consumption/clearance. This concentration is generally less than 2 mmol/L. The daily production of lactate is about 1400 mmol, and although all tissues can produce lactate, physiologic lactate production is primarily from skeletal muscle (25%), skin (25%), brain (20%), intestine (10%), and red blood cells (20%).[18] In pathologic conditions, significant lactate production occurs in other organs.

In the critically ill, lactate is produced in tissues outside the "usual lactate producers," including the lungs, white blood cells, and splanchnic organs. Physiologic lactate production by the lungs is negligible leading to an arteriovenous difference in lactate levels close to zero across the lungs under physiologic conditions.[19] In critically ill patients, Weil and colleagues[20] observed that venous blood samples from a pulmonary artery catheter yielded lactate concentrations equivalent to those in arterial blood. This finding has been replicated in subsequent works in patients with severe sepsis and acute lung injury/acute respiratory distress syndrome,[21–23] as well as in patients without significant hypoxemia.[24]

Similarly, lactate is released in supraphysiologic amounts from the sites of infection and inflammation and is thought to be related to the augmented glycolysis in the recruited and activated leukocytes at the sites of infection. White blood cells have a limited capacity for aerobic (mitochondrial) ATP generation. When activated, these cells rely primarily on augmented anaerobic glycolysis to meet energy requirements, which leads to the production of large amounts of lactate unrelated to oxygen deprivation. In experimental models, following exposure to endotoxin, significant increases were noted in blood lactate levels[25] and were thought to be a result of augmented leukocyte lactate production.

Lactate is metabolized primarily in the liver (60%), kidneys (30%), and heart (10%). In the liver, the periportal hepatocytes directly use lactate to produce glycogen and glucose via the Cori cycle. In patients with chronic liver disease, lactate clearance may be diminished and this can lead to its elevated blood levels.[26,27] Levraut and colleagues[28] challenged hemodynamically stable septic patients with an external lactate load and found that in patients with normal lactate clearance, normal lactate levels were noted. However, mildly elevated levels (2–4 mEq/L) were observed in patients with reduced lactate clearance. In otherwise healthy ambulatory patients with severely impaired liver function, a normal lactate level is the norm. The limited contribution of reduced clearance to elevating lactate levels in critically ill patients was convincingly demonstrated by Revelly and colleagues.[29] They compared 7 patients with septic shock and 7 patients with cardiogenic shock to 7 healthy controls. The subjects were given ^{13}C-radiolabeled lactate and ^{2}H-labeled glucose infusions, and it was noted that the increase in lactate levels resulted from overproduction of lactate and that lactate clearance was similar in all 3 groups.

The renal cortex also uses lactate via the gluconeogenetic pathway to produce glucose.[30] The renal cortex is very sensitive to reduction in renal blood flow, and renal lactate clearance can be impaired in critically ill patients with compromised renal blood flow, leading to elevated lactate levels. Lactate can be excreted by the kidney if the renal threshold is exceeded (approximately 5–6 mmol/L). The serum concentration of lactate is generally less than 2 mmol/L; hence, lactate is not excreted in the urine in physiologic states.

From the ongoing, it is clear that elevated serum lactate levels are a product of some combination of excess production and reduced clearance. Most of the conditions resulting in excess production and reduced clearance of lactate are predominantly pathologic and reflect tissue hypoxia or nonhypoxic tissue injury. This finding is the basis of the use of serum lactate as a biomarker in critically ill patients.

LACTATE AS A BIOMARKER

A biomarker has been defined as "a characteristic that is objectively measured and evaluated as an indicator of normal biologic processes, pathogenic processes, or pharmacologic responses to a therapeutic intervention."[31] The International Sepsis Forum Colloquium on Biomarkers of Sepsis described the roles that may be served by any given biomarker (**Box 2**).[32] In this review of the role of lactate as a biomarker in critically ill patients, the authors describe the performance of serum lactate levels in each of the roles described in **Box 2**.

Lactate as a Diagnostic Biomarker in Critically Ill Patients

For a biomarker to be used in the diagnosis of a clinical condition or pathophysiologic state, the entity to be diagnosed needs to be defined with gold standard criteria or criterion and there has to be a control group in which the condition or pathophysiologic

---

Box 2
Uses of biomarkers

Screening: to identify patients at increased risk of adverse outcome to inform a prophylactic intervention or further diagnostic test

Diagnosis: to establish a diagnosis to inform a treatment decision, and to do so more reliably, more rapidly, or more inexpensively than available methods

Risk stratification: to identify subgroups of patients within a particular diagnostic group, who may experience greater benefit or harm with therapeutic intervention

Monitoring: to measure response to intervention to permit the titration of dose or duration of treatment

Surrogate end point: to provide a more sensitive measure of the consequences of treatment that can substitute for a direct measure of a patient-centered outcome

Data from the Expert Colloquium on Biomarkers of Sepsis. The International Sepsis Forum; Biomarkers Definitions Working Group. Biomarkers and surrogate endpoints: preferred definitions and conceptual framework. Clin Pharmacol Ther 2001;69:89–95; and Marshall JC, Reinhart K. International Sepsis Forum. Biomarkers of sepsis. Crit Care Med 2009;37(7):2290–8.

state is absent. These conditions were infrequently met in the literature reviewed to ascertain the role of lactate as a diagnostic biomarker in critically ill patients. First, the authors have established that elevated serum lactate levels may be because of increased anaerobic or aerobic production, as well as decreased clearance. Further complicating this finding is the fact that increased production may be driven by any of the several organs, and this possibility applies to reductions in clearance as well. Although this review acknowledges the confounding potential aerobic excessive production of lactate and the contribution of reduced lactate clearance in hyperlactinemic patients, it focuses on the use of lactate levels as a diagnostic biomarker for systemic oxygen imbalance.

Hyperlactatemia is typically present in shock states when oxygen consumption becomes critically dependent on oxygen delivery. In this state, accumulated pyruvate from anaerobic metabolism is shunted predominantly toward lactate formation. This shunt leads to cytoplasmic accumulation of lactate and subsequent excretion down its concentration gradient into the circulation. In this state, elevated serum lactate levels are reflective of tissue hypoxia.

Lactate levels as a measure of inadequate perfusion and tissue hypoxia has been supported by observations in both experimental and clinical settings. In experiments in dogs, systemic oxygen delivery was reduced by inducing hypoxia and/or anemia until tissue oxygen demands could no longer be met. Serial lactate levels were obtained, and it was noted that at the point the oxygen consumption in the animals was limited by systemic oxygen delivery, there was a sharp increase in lactate levels.[33,34] Similar results were noted in another experiment with dogs, in which hemodynamic conditions in early septic shock were replicated by inducing a low–cardiac output state and injecting endotoxin.[35] Similar findings have been demonstrated in humans. As far back as 1927, in experiments investigating the responses to exercise in healthy subjects as well as patients with circulatory failure, Meakins and Long[36] reported that once oxygen delivery could not be increased to meet metabolic demands, lactate levels increased in proportion to the severity of the circulatory failure. More recently, Ronco and colleagues[37] were able to replicate in humans the correlation between low systemic oxygen delivery and elevated lactate levels seen in animals. Critically ill patients were examined after life support was discontinued. Oxygen consumption (determined by indirect calorimetry), oxygen delivery (calculated from the Fick equation), and concentrations of arterial plasma lactate were simultaneously determined at 5- to 20-minute intervals while life support was discontinued. It was noted that at the point oxygen consumption became dependent on oxygen delivery, further decrease in systemic oxygen delivery coincided with an increase in lactate levels. Other observations supporting this correlation include the following: (1) Levy and colleagues[38] demonstrated that hemodynamically unstable patients with septic or cardiogenic shock had increased lactate to pyruvate ratio (40:1) compared with controls (10:1) and (2) in the study on early goal-directed therapy in the management of patients with septic shock, elevated lactate levels in severe sepsis or septic shock before resuscitation coincided with a low central venous oxygen saturation ($ScvO_2$), and increases in oxygen delivery were associated with reductions in lactate levels.[39]

Serum Lactate Levels as a Tool for Screening, Risk Stratification, and Prognosis

Clinical evaluation of critically ill patients is limited by the fact that established clinical findings associated with widespread tissue hypoperfusion may not be evident in the early reversible stages of shock.[40,41] Lactate levels may be elevated in hemodynamically stable patients, helping identify a state of occult shock,[42] a condition associated with increased mortality.

Elevated lactate levels may serve as a screening tool by identifying patients with underlying tissue hypoperfusion before the development of clinical findings. It may also be used to distinguish severely ill patients from less severely ill patients. In fulfilling these roles, lactate may serve not only as a screening and risk-stratifying biomarker but also as a prognostic biomarker in critically ill patients. Multiple studies have been conducted on the use of serum lactate levels for screening, risk stratification, and prognostication. The use of lactate measurements or any other biomarker as a screening tool must take into consideration the fact that the posttest probability of an elevated value representing tissue hypoperfusion in a given patient depends on the index patient's pretest probability and likelihood ratio. Given that the patients being tested have been determined by their treating clinicians to be at higher risk for tissue hypoperfusion, elevated lactate levels in these patients are generally accepted to indicate tissue hypoperfusion, and most studies assess the predictive value of lactate levels for outcomes such as mortality. Studies on the use of lactate measurements for prognostic purposes can be divided into 3 distinct time phases:

1. Prehospital setting
2. ED
3. Intensive care unit (ICU).

Prognostic value of lactate levels checked in the prehospital setting

It is acknowledged that early identification of tissue hypoperfusion or shock followed by aggressive early resuscitation is key in improving survival in critically ill patients. The pathophysiologic cascades that result in tissue injury do not necessarily start when patients arrive at the ED. Most prehospital triage systems for trauma and nontrauma patients are based mainly on clinical parameters, which, as discussed previously, leave a lot to be desired. Incorporating lactate measurements in risk stratifying these patients may allow the prompt initiation of life saving therapy. The first study to assess the feasibility of lactate measurements in the prehospital setting was performed by Coats and colleagues,[43] involving the prehospital capillary lactate levels in trauma patients. They observed a moderate correlation ($R^2 = 0.44$) between lactate levels and injury severity in patients who might otherwise be difficult to triage. This study was followed more recently in the study by Jansen and colleagues,[44] in which the venous or capillary blood lactate concentration in 124 patients before hospital arrival was measured by ambulance staff using a handheld battery-powered device. It was reported that the prehospital blood lactate level was associated with in-hospital mortality and provided prognostic information superior to that provided by the patient's vital signs. In study, although higher lactate levels were noted in the patients who died, in multivariate analysis, it was the change in serum lactate levels, between the first measurement in the ambulance and the second on hospital arrival, that was independently associated with death. Based on this work, it can be concluded that lactate levels of 3.5 mmol/L or higher were associated with increased mortality at both time points compared with lactate levels less than 3.5 mmol/L (T1: 41% vs 12% and T2: 47% vs 15%), and in addition, failure to clear lactate may be more significant than an isolated elevated lactate value. The prognostic significance of lactate clearance over time has also been demonstrated in other studies.[45,46] It is the authors' opinion that in the prehospital setting, the ability of a single lactate value to trigger the early initiation of specific treatment algorithm makes it more clinically useful in the prehospital setting than the possible prognostic information derived from lactate clearance measurements. Other works done in the prehospital setting confirm the role of prehospital lactate measurements as a prognostic biomarker.[47,48]

Prognostic value of lactate levels checked in the ED

In a work done by 1 of the authors of this article (P. R. D.),[49] initial serum lactate levels in more than 1100 patients, seen in the ED, the ICU, and general hospital wards of a large teaching hospital were reviewed.

Lactate levels were divided into low (0–2 mmol/L), intermediate (2.1–3.9 mmol/L), and high (≥4.0 mmol/L). A lactate level of 4 mmol/L or more was found to be highly specific (89%–99%) for predicting the acute phase of death and in-hospital death in all 3 groups (**Fig. 2**).

Similar findings were noted in an ED-only population studied by Shapiro and colleagues.[50] They studied 1278 adult patients in an urban academic medical center admitted to the hospital with a suspected infection-related diagnosis, having undergone serum lactate measurements at initial presentation in the ED. Patients were stratified according to lactate levels as low (L), less than 2.5 mmol/L; medium (M), 2.5 to 3.99 mmol/L; and high (H), 4 mmol/L or more. They showed an increasing likelihood of mortality (4%, 9%, and 28.4%, respectively) for each group and calculated 92% specificity for death. Two years later, the same group enrolled normotensive and hypotensive patients presenting to an ED with suspected infection.[51] They showed an odds ratio of death of 2.2 for those patients with intermediate lactate levels and an odds ratio of 7.1 for high lactate levels. These values were independent of hypotension (**Fig. 3**). Although only patients who were subsequently admitted to the hospital were included in the study (allowing for selection bias), it is the authors' contention that those are precisely the patients of interest. More recently, Mikkelson and colleagues[52] studied the prognostic value of an initial lactate measurement obtained in the ED and replicated the findings in the study by Shapiro and colleagues. Based on these studies, and similar studies performed in the ED (**Table 1**), it can be concluded that an elevated lactate level (>4.0 mmol/L) in the ED is predictive of increased mortality in a critically ill patient.

The ED setting presents challenges to designing and performing studies evaluating the prognostic significance of lactate clearance. The time spent by patients in the ED

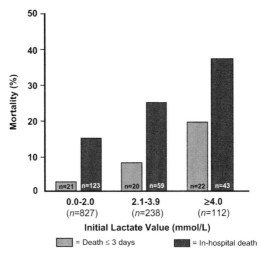

Fig. 2. Acute-phase deaths and in-hospital deaths in infected patients stratified by initial lactate value. The number of acute-phase deaths and in-hospital deaths increased significantly and linearly with increasing lactate concentrations. (*From* Trzeciak S, Dellinger RP, Chansky ME, et al. Serum lactate as a predictor of mortality in patients with infection. Intensive Care Med 2007;33(6):972; with permission.)

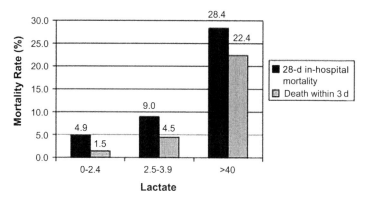

Fig. 3. Lactate as a predictor of mortality. For 28-day in-hospital mortality, 105 (8.2%) of 1278 of patients died; death within 3 days occurred in 55 (4.3%) of 1278 patients. (*From* Shapiro NI, Howell MD, Talmor D, et al. Serum lactate as a predictor of mortality in emergency department patients with infection. Ann Emerg Med 2005;45(5):524–8; with permission.)

may be affected by issues such as bed availability in the ICU, and if fewer ICUs are available, less severely ill patients are likely to be left in the ED for longer periods, leading to a selection bias. Hence, efforts have been made to evaluate the prognostic value of a 2-hour lactate clearance in acute cardiopulmonary insufficiency. In a recent study by Scott and colleagues,[59] 2-hour lactate clearance was evaluated as a prognostic marker in patients presenting to the ED with acute respiratory insufficiency or hemodynamic instability. Patients admitted through the ED into a high-dependency monitoring unit and ICU were included in the study. Arterial lactate levels were measured on ED arrival and at 1, 2, 6, and 24 hours later. The predictive value of 2-hour lactate clearance was evaluated for negative outcomes defined as hospital mortality or need for endotracheal intubation versus positive outcomes defined as discharge or transfer to a general medical ward. From logistic regression and receiver operating characteristic curves, it was found that a 2-hour lactate clearance of more than 15% was a strong predictor of negative outcome ($P<.001$), with a sensitivity of 86% (95% confidence interval [CI], 67%–95%), specificity of 91% (95% CI, 82%–96%), positive predictive value of 80% (95% CI, 61%–92%), and negative predictive value of 92% (95% CI, 84%–98%). In this study, the 2-hour lactate clearance proved more accurate than baseline lactate levels, the shock index, mean arterial pressure (MAP), and the base excess (**Fig. 4**). Notably, the 2-hour clearance was reliable even when the baseline lactate level was only mildly elevated at 3 mmol/L. The results may not be generalizable to all severely ill patients presenting in the ED because the study population was relatively older with multiple comorbidities and reduced physiologic reserves, but they demonstrate the feasibility of obtaining 2-hour lactate clearance in the ED setting, a finding that has been replicated in other studies.[60]

Prognostic value of lactate levels checked in the ICU setting
Multiple studies have evaluated the prognostic value of hyperlactatemia in diverse critically ill populations in the ICU (**Table 2**).

In the ICU setting, area under the receiver operating characteristic curve varied from as low as 0.53[81] to as high as 0.86,[74] which indicates poor to moderately good prognostic performance. Given the time dependency of outcomes in critically ill patients, the limited prognostic values of lactate levels in some patient populations may have been influenced by the pre-ICU management of these patients. Another possibility

Table 1
Prognostic value of blood lactate levels in the ED

Study	N (Mortality, %)	Population	Timing	Cutoff Value	Cutoff a Priori	Sensitivity (%) (95% CI)	Specificity (%) (95% CI)	LR+	LR−	PPV (%) (95% CI)	NPV (%) (95% CI)	AUROC (95% CI)
Sepsis												
Shapiro et al[50]	1278 (8)	Patients with suspected infection	ED admission	2.5	Yes	59 (50–68)	71 (69–74)	2.0	0.5	15 (12–19)	95 (94–96)	0.67
				4.0		36 (27–46)	92 (90–93)	4.5	0.7	28 (21–37)	94 (93–95)	
Shapiro et al[51]	1287 (6)	Patients with suspected infection	ED admission	2.5	Yes	37 (26–49)	73 (71–76)	1.4	0.9	8 (5–11)	95 (94–96)	0.72
				4.0		38 (27–50)	94 (92–95)	6.3	0.7	27 (19–37)	96 (95–97)	
Trzeciak et al[49]	1177 (19)	Patients with infection (60% ED, 22% ICU, 18% non-ICU ward)	In 60% of patients during ED stay (exact timing not available)	2.0	Yes	45 (39–52)	74 (71–77)	1.7	0.7	29 (24–34)	85 (83–88)	—
				4.0		19 (15–23)	93 (91–94)	2.6	0.9	38 (29–48)	83 (81–85)	0.56 (0.53–0.59)
Nguyen et al[53]	111 (42)	Patients with severe sepsis or septic shock	First 6 h of ED stay	10% decrease in 6 h	Yes	45 (30–60)	84 (73–92)	2.8	0.7	68 (49–83)	68 (56–78)	—
Trauma												
Pal et al [54]	5995 (3)	Trauma patients	Trauma service admission	2.0	Yes	85 (79–90)	38 (37–39)	1.4	0.4	4 (3–5)	99 (98–99)	0.72

Study	N (%)	Population	Timing	Cutoff	Gold standard	Sens	Spec	LR+	LR−	PPV	NPV	AUROC (CI)
Dunne et al[55]	15,179 (5)	Trauma patients	Trauma center admission	6.0	Not clear	—	—	—	—	23	98	—
Kaplan and Kellum[56]	282 (23)	Patients with major vascular injury	ED admission	5.0	Not clear	98 (92–100)	—	—	—	—	—	0.98 (0.96–0.99)
Cardiac arrest												
Kliegel et al[57]	394 (51)	Patients post-cardiac arrest (surviving >48 h)	ED admission	2.0	Yes	—	—	—	—	—	—	—
			24 h later			40 (33–47)	68 (61–75)	1.3	0.9	56 (47–64)	52 (46–59)	—
			48 h later			31 (25–38)	86 (80–91)	2.2	0.8	70 (59–79)	55 (49–60)	—
Heterogeneous												
Sankoff et al[58]	176 (11)	Heterogeneous patients with SIRS	ED admission	—	—	—	—	—	—	—	—	0.78 (0.66–0.90)

Abbreviations: AUROC, area under the receiver operating characteristic curve; CI, confidence interval; LR+, positive likelihood ratio; LR−, negative LR; NPV, negative predictive value; PPV, positive predictive value; SIRS, systemic inflammatory response syndrome.

Data from Jansen TC, van Bommel J, Bakker J. Blood lactate monitoring in critically ill patients: a systematic health technology assessment. Crit Care Med 2009;37:2827–39.

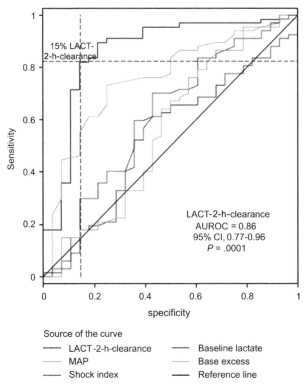

Fig. 4. Receiver operating characteristic curve for LACT-2-h-clearance. AUROC, area under the receiver operating characteristic curve; MAP, mean arterial pressure. (*From* Scott S, Antonaglia V, Guiotto G, et al. Two-hour lactate clearance predicts negative outcome in patients with cardiorespiratory insufficiency. Crit Care Res Pract 2010;2010, Article ID 917053; with permission.)

in a heterogeneous critically ill population is that the prognostic performance of an elevated lactate level may depend on the admitting diagnosis.

A well-designed study by Jansen and colleagues[98] investigated the prognostic value of elevated lactate levels by exploring the association between the degree and duration of elevated lactate levels and Sequential Organ Failure Assessment (SOFA) scores in patients in the ICU. To better reflect the patient population in the ICU, lactate levels were not measured within the first 24 hours, which would exclude measurements in the ED or other non-ICUs. The investigators calculated the area under the lactate curve above 2 mmol/L (lactate$_{AUC>2}$) as well as the daily SOFA scores for days 1 through 28 of ICU stay and obtained initial (day 1), maximal, total, and mean scores. Daily lactate$_{AUC>2}$ was related to both daily SOFA scores and organ subscores. Dividing the ICU stay into an early period (<2.75 days) and a late period (>2.75 days), the relationship between lactate levels and SOFA scores in both the periods was explored. This study found a clear association between lactate levels elevation and SOFA scores, and this association was stronger in the early phase of ICU admission than the late phase. The study also demonstrated an increased risk of multiorgan failure and mortality, with elevated lactate levels of increased duration (**Fig. 5**). When the association between the elevated lactate levels and specific organ SOFA subscores was evaluated, respiratory and coagulation subscores were found to be the most strongly associated (**Tables 3** and **4**). There was no strong correlation between elevated lactate levels and the cardiovascular subscore. These findings raise several interesting thoughts. First, the absence of a strong correlation between elevated lactate levels and cardiovascular SOFA subscores may be related to the fact that cardiovascular SOFA subscores are a measure of macrovascular circulatory adequacy and in some conditions, notably sepsis, microcirculatory dysfunction and exist in spite of acceptable macrocirculatory indices. Second, in critically ill patients, there may be increased production of lactate by nonusual lactate-producing organs, such as the lungs, and the strong association between the elevated lactate level and an increased respiratory SOFA score may reflect the presence of lactate production not related to tissue hypoxia or even acute lung injury, which may significantly alter outcome. Similarly, severe critical illness, especially sepsis, may be associated with dysfunction of the coagulation pathways (which may lead to microcirculatory dysfunction), and in these patients, the SOFA coagulation subscore may reflect the severity of the critical illness, which may explain the strong correlation between lactate levels and coagulation SOFA subscores. From the ongoing, it may be expected that in a diverse ICU population, elevated lactate levels may be more prognostic in disease conditions associated with microcirculatory dysfunction and increased lactate production not related to tissue hypoxia such as severe sepsis. This is consistent with findings reported by Jansen and colleagues[99] in a separate study in which they evaluated the prognostic value of elevated lactate levels in patients in a multidisciplinary ICU and in sepsis as compared with hemorrhage and other low–oxygen-transport states. In 394 patients, the investigators measured blood lactate levels at admission to the ICU (lactate at T0) and the reduction of lactate levels 12 hours later (ΔLacT0–12) and between 12 and 24 hours (ΔLacT12–24) and related these values to in-hospital mortality. They found that regardless of hemodynamic status, lactate levels reduction during the first 24 hours of ICU stay was associated with improved outcome in septic patients; however, it was not the same in patients with other conditions associated with low–oxygen-transport states (including hemorrhagic shock). These findings serve as a rational basis for efforts aimed at guiding therapy in selected populations based on blood lactate levels and are discussed in the following section.

Lactate as a Tool for Monitoring Interventions in the Critically Ill Patient/Lactate-Guided Therapy in the Critically Ill Patient

Efforts are aimed at developing novel biomarkers and surrogates for disease severity to enable clinicians diagnose conditions associated with organ dysfunction early and by early intervention, lead to improved outcomes. The most discriminating biomarker, unless coupled to a rational therapeutic response, is worthless at the bedside. Thus, efforts at studying the role of various biomarkers in critically ill patients need to include a therapeutic response coupled to a predefined elevation in the level of that biomarker. In addition, these studies have to be performed in disease conditions in which lactate levels elevation is more prognostic and preferably early in the course of disease in which outcomes may be changes by the right intervention. Several observational cohort studies have been published describing the implementation of a lactate-guided oxygen delivery therapy algorithm (**Table 5**). In all these studies, guiding therapy based on lactate levels was associated with better outcomes (decreased mortality, decreased infection rates, improved tissue oxygenation indices) in the normolactatemic group. However, these studies are subject to the limitations of observational studies. Also, one of the studies[100] compared the cohort to a historical control group and reported benefits may arguably reflect changes in standards of care over time. It was thus necessary

Table 2
Prognostic value of blood lactate levels in the ICU

Study	N (Mortality, %)	Population	Timing	Cutoff Value	Cutoff a Priori	Sensitivity (95% CI)	Specificity (95% CI)	LR+	LR−	PPV (95% CI)	NPV (95% CI)	AUROC (95% CI)
Infection/sepsis												
Friedman et al[61]	35 (46)	ICU patients with severe sepsis	Timing of start study not clear 24 h after start study	2.0	Yes	81 (54–96) 69 (41–89)	47 (24–71) 84 (60–97)	1.5 4.3	0.4 0.4	57 (34–77) 79 (49–95)	75 (43–99) 76 (53–92)	—
Tamion et al[62]	44 (30)	ICU patients with septic shock	ICU admission	4.5	No	62 (32–86)	68 (49–83)	1.9	0.6	44 (22–69)	81 (61–93)	—
Dondorp et al[63]	268 (17)	ICU patients with severe malaria	ICU admission	—	—	—	—	—	—	—	—	0.66 (0.56–0.76)
Trauma/surgery												
Meregalli et al[42]	44 (16)	Hemodynamically stable surgical ICU patients	ICU admission (T0) and 24 and 48 h later	—	—	—	—	—	—	—	—	T0: 0.58
Singhal et al[64]	30 (50)	Patients with ruptured abdominal aortic aneurysm	Postoperative ICU admission	4.0	No	87 (60–98)	80 (52–96)	4.3	0.2	81 (54–96)	86 (57–98)	—
Maillet et al[65]	325 (5)	Patients post-cardiac surgery	ICU admission During ICU stay	3.0	Yes	69 (38–88) 62	81 (77–86) 75	3.6 2.5	0.4 0.5	15 (7–28) —	98 (96–100) —	0.84 (0.73–0.95) 0.72 (0.57–0.88)
Abramson et al[66]	76 (33)	Multiple trauma patients	24 h after ICU admission 48 h after ICU admission	2.0	Yes	100 (86–100) 76 (55–91)	53 (38–67) 94 (84–99)	2.1 12.7	0 0.3	51 (36–66) 86 (65–97)	100 (87–100) 89 (77–96)	—
Martin et al[67]	1298 (18)	Trauma and emergency surgery patients	ICU admission	2.2	Yes	84 (78–88)	34 (32–37)	1.3	0.5	22 (19–25)	91 (87–93)	0.70 (0.67–0.74)

Study	N	Population	Timing	Lactate	Adjusted	Sensitivity	Specificity					AUC
Blow et al[68]	79 (10%)	Major trauma patients, hemodynamically stable	ICU admission 24 h later	2.5	Yes	100 (63–100) 100 (63–100)	30 (19–42) 92 (83–97)	1.4 12.5	0 0	14 (6–25) 57 (29–82)	100 (84–100) 100 (94–100)	—
Claridge et al[69]	364 (3)	Major trauma patients	ICU admission 24 h later	2.5	Yes	92 (64–100) 54 (25–81)	33 (28–39) 86 (82–89)	1.4 3.9	0.2 0.5	5 (3–8) 12 (5–24)	99 (95–100) 98 (96–99)	—
Wahl et al[70]	169 (11)	Postoperative ICU patients	ICU admission	—	—	—	—	—	—	—	—	0.79
Murillo-Cabezas et al[71]	210 (14)	Hemodynamically stable patients with moderate or severe head injury	During first 48 h ICU stay	2.2	Yes	53 (34–72)	56 (49–63)	1.2	0.8	17 (10–26)	88 (80–93)	—
Liver disease												
Bernal et al[72]	93 (39), 85 at T12	Paracetamol-induced acute liver failure (initial sample)	± ICU admission ±12 h later	3.5 3.0	No	86 (71–95) 82 (65–93)	91 (81–97) 96 (87–100)	9.8 20.5	0.2 0.2	86 (71–95) 93 (77–99)	91 (81–97) 89 (78–96)	— —
	99 (21), 85 at T12	Paracetamol-induced acute liver failure (validation sample)	± ICU admission ±12 h later	3.5 3.0	Yes	67 (43–85) 76 (53–92)	95 (87–99) 97 (89–100)	13.4 25.3	0.3 0.2	78 (52–94) 89 (65–99)	91 (83–96) 93 (83–98)	— —
Watanabe et al[73]	151 (7)	Patients post-liver resection	ICU admission	—	—	—	—	—	—	—	—	0.86
Funk et al[74]	181 (50)	ICU patients with liver cirrhosis	ICU admission	8.9	No	36 (26–46)	99 (94–100)	36.0	0.6	97 (84–100)	61 (53–69)	0.81 (0.75–0.87)
Kruse et al[75]	38 (68)	ICU patients with liver disease	Maximum value during ICU stay	2.2 7.0	No	80 (59–93) 52 (31–72)	62 (32–86) 100 (75–100)	2.1 ∞	0.3 0.5	80 (59–93) 100 (75–100)	62 (32–86) 52 (31–72)	—
Heterogeneous												
Smith et al[76]	T0: 148 (35) T24: 131 (31)	Heterogeneous ICU patients		T0: 1.5 T24: 1.0	No	69 (54–81) 68 (52–82)	77 (68–85) 83 (74–90)	3.0 4.0	0.4 0.4	61 (48–74) 65 (49–79)	82 (73–90) 85 (76–92)	0.78 —

(continued on next page)

Table 2
(continued)

Study	N (Mortality, %)	Population	Timing	Cutoff Value	Cutoff a Priori	Sensitivity (95% CI)	Specificity (95% CI)	LR+	LR−	PPV (95% CI)	NPV (95% CI)	AUROC (95% CI)
Suistomaa et al[77]	98 (13)	Heterogeneous emergency ICU patients	ICU admission (T0) and 24 h later / ICU admission during first 24 h (12 measurements)	2.0	Yes	69 (39–91)	73 (63–83)	2.7	0.4	29 (14–48)	94 (85–98)	—
						77 (46–95)	55 (44–66)	1.7	0.4	21 (10–35)	94 (83–99)	—
Freire et al[78]	319 (25)	Medical ICU patients	During first 24 h of ICU stay	2.0	Yes	77 (66–86)	53 (46–59)	1.6	0.4	35 (28–52)	88 (81–92)	—
				8.0		30 (21–42)	97 (94–99)	10.0	0.7	77 (59–90)	81 (76–85)	—
Cusack et al[79]	100 (31)	Heterogeneous ICU patients	ICU admission	—	—	—	—	—	—	—	—	0.65 (0.52–0.78)
Rocktaeschel et al[80]	300 (28)	Heterogeneous ICU patients	ICU admission	—	—	—	—	—	—	—	—	0.66 (0.59–0.73)
Marik and Bankov[81]	45 (50)	ICU patients requiring PAC	PAC insertion	—	—	—	—	—	—	—	—	0.53
Maynard et al[82]	60 (33)	Heterogeneous ICU patients	Any of 3 time points (ICU admission, 12 or 24 h later)	2.0	Yes	75 (51–91)	55 (38–71)	1.7	0.5	45 (28–64)	81 (62–94)	—
Dubin et al[83]	935 (11)	Heterogeneous ICU patients	ICU admission	2.4	Yes	—	—	—	—	—	—	0.67 (0.61–0.73)
Aduen et al[84]	46 (41)	Hypotensive ICU/ED patients (76% ICU)	During ICU/ED stay	4.0	No	62 (39–84)	88 (71–98)	5.2	0.4	80 (52–96)	77 (59–90)	—
	353 (16)	Nonhypotensive ICU/ED patients (51% ICU)				29 (17–42)	96 (93–98)	7.3	0.7	57 (37–76)	88 (84–91)	—
Levy et al[85]	95 (44%)	Heterogeneous ICU patients	ICU admission 24 h later	2.5	No	72 (55–84)	73 (60–85)	2.7	0.4	68 (52–81)	77 (63–87)	—
Others												
Sasaki et al[86]	41 (44)	ICU patients with RRT	At-onset RRT	3.5	No	83 (59–96)	91 (72–99)	9.2	0.2	88 (64–99)	86 (68–97)	0.74

Children

Source	No. (%)	Population	Timing	Cutoff		Sensitivity	Specificity	LR+	LR−	PPV	NPV	AUROC
Hatherill et al[87]	705 (10)	PICU children	PICU admission	2.0	Yes	46 (34–58)	97 (96–98)	15.3	0.6	64 (49–77)	94 (92–96)	—
	50 (64) from cohort of 705	Hyperlactatemic (>2.0) PICU children	PICU admission			78 (60–90)	89 (65–99)	7.1	0.2	93 (76–99)	70 (47–87)	0.59 (0.43–0.76)
			24 h later									0.86 (0.73–0.99)
Hatherill et al[88]	99 (9)	Children post–cardiac surgery	PICU admission	6.0	No	78 (40–97)	83 (74–90)	4.6	0.3	32 (14–55)	97 (91–100)	—
Hatherill et al[89]	46 (35)	PICU patients with hypotension	PICU admission	5.0	No	75 (49–93)	63 (44–80)	2.0	0.4	52 (31–73)	83 (61–95)	0.83 (0.71–0.95)
	38 (21)		24 h later			25 (3–65)	83 (65–94)	1.5	0.9	29 (4–71)	81 (63–93)	—
Garcia Sanz et al[90]	500 (7)	Heterogeneous PICU patients	PICU admission	2.0	Yes	65 (46–79)	71 (66–75)	2.2	0.5	16 (9–21)	97 (94–98)	0.76 (0.67–0.85)
				3.7	No	56 (38–72)	91 (88–94)	6.2	0.5	33 (21–46)	96 (94–98)	
				5.0	Not clear	47 (30–65)	94 (92–96)	7.8	0.6	41 (24–55)	96 (94–97)	
				7.0	Not clear	32 (19–51)	98 (96–99)	16.0	0.7	52 (31–73)	95 (93–97)	
Balasubramanyan et al[91]	66 (29)	Heterogeneous PICU patients	Not clear	5.0	Not clear	37 (16–62)	87 (74–95)	2.8	0.7	54 (25–81)	77 (64–68)	0.63
Shime et al[92]	141 (8)	Children post–cardiac surgery	PICU admission	3.0	Not clear	64 (31–89)	87 (80–92)	4.9	0.4	29 (13–51)	97 (91–99)	—
				4.0		36 (11–69)	93 (87–96)	5.1	0.7	31 (9–61)	94 (89–98)	
Koliski et al[93]	75 (24)	Heterogeneous PICU patients	PICU admission	2.0	Yes	83 (59–96)	39 (26–52)	1.4	0.4	30 (18–44)	88 (69–98)	—
				2.6	No	71 (47–90)	63 (49–76)	1.9	0.5	38 (22–56)	88 (74–96)	0.68
			12 h later	1.3	No	64	61	1.6	0.6	—	—	0.62
			24 h later	3.0	No	56	97	18.7	0.5	—	—	0.81
Gotay-Cruz et al[94]	10 (20)	Heterogeneous PICU patients	Peak during PICU stay	2.5	Yes	100 (16–100)	63 (24–92)	2.7	0.0	40 (5–85)	100 (46–100)	—
Cheung et al[95]	85 (16)	Infants post–congenital heart surgery	PICU admission	7.0	No	92 (66–100)	69 (57–79)	3.0	0.1	33 (21–55)	98 (89–100)	—
Cheung et al[96]	74 (20)	Neonates treated with ECMO	NICU admission	25	Yes	40 (16–68)	97 (88–100)	13.3	0.6	75 (35–97)	86 (76–94)	—
			12 h later	15		53 (27–79)	100 (94–100)	∞	0.5	100 (63–100)	89 (79–96)	
Durward et al[97]	85 (6)	Children post–cardiac surgery	PICU admission	2.0	Yes	60 (15–95)	83 (72–90)	3.5	0.5	18 (4–43)	97 (90–100)	—
				3.0	No	60	94	9.6		60	94	0.71 (0.44–0.98)
			24 h later	2.0	Yes	60 (15–95)	83 (72–90)	3.5	0.5	18 (4–43)	97 (90–100)	0.80 (0.56–1.00)

Abbreviations: AUROC, area under the receiver operating characteristic curve; LR+, positive likelihood ratio; LR−, negative LR; NICU, neonatal intensive care unit; NPV, negative predictive value; PAC, pulmonary artery catheter; PICU, pediatric intensive care unit; PPV, positive predictive value; RRT, renal replacement therapy.

Data from Jansen TC, van Bommel J, Bakker J. Blood lactate monitoring in critically ill patients: A systematic health technology assessment. Crit Care Med 2009;37(10);2827–39.

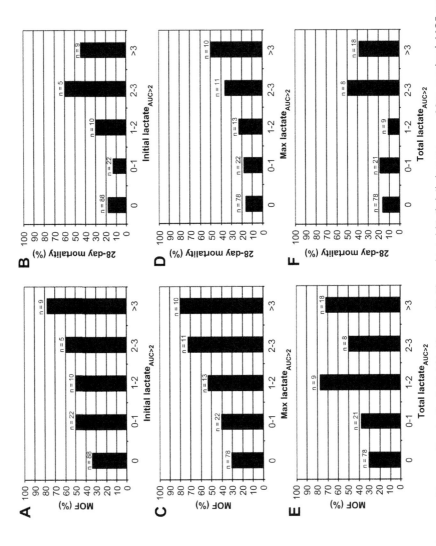

Fig. 5. MOF and 28-day mortality according to the initial (*A, B*), max (*C, D*), and total (*E, F*) daily lactate$_{AUC>2}$. Max, maximal; MOF, multiple organ failure. (*Data from* Jansen TC, van Bommel J, Woodward R, et al. Association between blood lactate levels, Sequential Organ Failure Assessment subscores and 28-day mortality during early and late ICU stay: a retrospective observational study. Crit Care Med 2009;37(8):2369–74.)

Table 3
SOFA organ subscores in normolactatemic and hyperlactatemic patients

SOFA Subscores	Lactate$_{AUC>2}$ = 0	Lactate$_{AUC>2}$>0
Initial		
Respiratory	2 (0–3)	2 (1–4)*
Coagulation	0 (0–1)	1 (0–2)*
Cardiovascular	1 (0–2)	1 (1–4)*
CNS	0 (0–2)	1 (0–4)
Renal	0 (0–0)	0 (0–2)*
Liver	0 (0–0)	0 (0–0)
Maximal		
Respiratory	2 (0–3)	3 (2–4)*
Coagulation	0 (0–1)	1 (0–2)*
Cardiovascular	1 (0–3)	2 (1–4)*
CNS	1 (0–3)	3 (0–4)*
Renal	0 (0–0)	0 (0–2)*
Liver	0 (0–0)	0 (0–1)*
Total		
Respiratory	3.5 (0–17)	9.5 (3–23)*
Coagulation	0 (0–1)	2 (0–5)*
Cardiovascular	1.5 (0–6)	4 (1–13)*
CNS	1 (0–8)	7.5 (0–28)*
Renal	0 (0–0)	0 (0–8)*
Liver	0 (0–0)	0 (0–2)*
Mean		
Respiratory	1.9 (0–2.3)	2.0 (1.3–2.6)*
Coagulation	0 (0–0.5)	0.5 (0–1.1)*
Cardiovascular	0.8 (0–1.1)	1.0 (0.5–2)*
CNS	0.5 (0–2)	1.1 (0–2.8)
Renal	0 (0–0)	0 (0–2)*
Liver	0 (0–0)	0 (0–0.3)*

Initial, maximal, total, and mean values of the individual SOFA organ subscores for patients with hyperlactatemia (lactate$_{AUC>2}$>0, n = 56) compared with the patients without hyperlactatemia (lactate$_{AUC>2}$>0, n = 78).
Abbreviation: CNS, central nervous system.
*P<.05.
Data from Jansen TC, van Bommel J, Woodward R, et al. Association between blood lactate levels, Sequential Organ Failure Assessment subscores and 28-day mortality during early and late ICU stay: a retrospective observational study. Crit Care Med 2009;37:2369–74.

to study the effects of lactate-guided therapy in better-designed studies, in which lactate-guided therapy is compared with currently accepted standards of care. In a study coauthored by one of the authors of this article (P. R. D.),[101] lactate clearance was evaluated against currently recommended targets in the early resuscitation of severely septic patients. Consistent with other studies, the results demonstrated increased mortality with reduced lactate clearance. More importantly, when survivors were compared with nonsurvivors, as a factor associated with increased mortality, failure to clear lactate defined as a lactate clearance of less

Table 4 Relationship between elevated lactate levels and specific organ SOFA subscores						
	Overall		Early		Late	
SOFA Organ Subscore	Effect	P Value	Effect	P Value	Effect	P Value
Respiratory	0.30	<0.001	0.27	0.001	0.34	<0.001
Coagulation	0.13	<0.001	0.08	0.12	0.12	<0.001
Cardiovascular	0.09	0.053	0.22	0.033	0.03	0.60
CNS	0.07	0.14	0.20	0.065	0.03	0.54
Renal	0.04	0.29	0.20	0.017	−0.03	0.95
Liver	0.02	0.21	0.02	0.61	0.04	0.80

Abbreviation: CNS, central nervous system.
Data from Jansen TC, van Bommel J, Woodward R, et al. Association between blood lactate levels, Sequential Organ Failure Assessment subscores and 28-day mortality during early and late ICU stay: a retrospective observational study. Crit Care Med 2009;37:2369–74.

than 10% was as reliable as failing to achieve a superior vena caval oxygen saturation of 70% in the early phase of resuscitation in these patients (**Table 6**). The study did not show a high degree of concordance between achieving lactate clearance and Scvo$_2$ goals. This study served as the basis for further work investigating early goal-directed resuscitation protocols based on lactate clearance.

In the recently published Lactates (lactate clearance vs central venous oxygen saturation as goals of early sepsis therapy) trial,[102] 300 patients with severe sepsis and evidence of hypoperfusion or septic shock, who were admitted to the ED, were randomly assigned to one of the 2 resuscitation protocols in the first 6 hours. One group was resuscitated to normalize central venous pressure (CVP), MAP, and Scvo$_2$ of at least 70%, and the other group was resuscitated to normalize CVP, MAP, and lactate clearance of at least 10%.

Using a primary outcome measure of in-hospital mortality rates, the investigators concluded that in patients with septic shock, who were treated to normalize CVP and MAP, additional management to normalize lactate clearance compared with management to normalize Scvo$_2$ did not result in significantly different in-hospital mortality. The study had its limitations, which the investigators acknowledged in their publication, including the inability to blind the groups, allowing for possible treatment bias, and after CVP and MAP goals were met, in very few patients, Scvo$_2$ was not normalized or lactate clearance failed. Despite these limitations, the conclusions are supported by a more recent publication by Jansen and colleagues.[59]

In the study by Jansen and colleagues,[59] 348 patients with an elevated lactate level (>3.0) and no apparent aerobic cause of lactate levels elevation were randomized to therapy guided by serial lactate level monitoring, the goal being to reduce these levels by 20% every 2 hours or therapy not guided by serial lactate level monitoring. In the study, the proportion of patients in both groups in whom conventional resuscitation goals were achieved was equal. Also, despite management, in one of the groups being guided by lactate clearance, the goal of achieving a 20% or more decrement every 2 hours was achieved equally in both lactate-guided and non–lactate-guided groups. Apart from similarities in both groups, significant differences were also noted. The lactate-guided group received significantly more fluids as well as more vasodilators than the control group (**Table 7**). Of note, the investigators reported a significantly reduced ICU length of stay and also ICU and hospital mortality when adjusting for predefined and commonly accepted risk factors.

Table 5
Observational studies describing the implementation of a lactate-guided oxygen delivery algorithm

Study	N	Patients	Timing	Goals of Therapy	Provided Therapy	Primary End Point	Lactate Level on Entry	Lactate Level After Therapy	Outcome
Rady et al[40]	36	Heterogeneous critically ill patients in the ED	During ED stay (6 ± 3 h)	Lactate <2.0 and $Scvo_2$ ≥65%	22% MV and paralysis, 6% RBCs, 97% fluids, 75% vasoactive agents	Lactate level and $Scvo_2$	4.6 ± 3.8	2.6 ± 2.5, (P<.05 vs entry)	↓ lactate and ↑ $Scvo_2$ (52% ± 18% to 65% ± 13%, P<.05) after Do_2 therapy
Blow et al[98]	79	Hemodynamically stable major trauma patients	First 24 h of ICU stay	Lactate <2.5	Fluids, RBCs, dopamine, dobutamine (amounts not recorded)	In-hospital mortality	58/79 (73%), lactate >2.4	14/79 (18%), lactate >2.4 after 24 h (P<.05 vs entry)	↓ mortality in normolactatemia vs hyperlactatemia after 24 h: 0/65 (0%) vs 6/14 (43%), P<.05
Claridge et al[69]	364	Major trauma patients	First 24 h of ICU stay	Lactate <2.5	Fluids, RBCs, dopamine, dobutamine (amount not recorded)	Infectious complications	246/364 (68%), lactate >2.4	57/364 (16%), lactate >2.4 after 24 h (P<.05 vs entry)	↑ infection rate late (>12 h) vs early (<12 h) lactate normalization: OR, 5.3 (95% CI, 3.1–9.3)
Rossi et al[100]	710 (+1656 historical controls)	Children post–congenital heart surgery	Early hours of ICU stay	Lactate <2.2 or decrease >0.5/h vs no lactate in control group	Any method to ↑ Do_2 or ↓Vo_2 (type/amount not recorded)	In-hospital mortality	Not available	Not available	↓ mortality on comparison with historical control group: 13/710 (2%) vs 61/1656 (4)%, P = .02

Abbreviations: MV, mechanical ventilation; OR, odds ratio; RBCs, red blood cells; ↑, increased; ↓, decreased.

Data from Jansen TC, van Bommel J, Bakker J. Blood lactate monitoring in critically ill patients: a systematic health technology assessment. Crit Care Med 2009;37:2827–39.

Table 6
Multivariate logistic regression analysis of factors associated with in-hospital mortality

Variable	Coefficient	Odds Ratio	95% CI for Odds Ratio
Lactate Nonclearance	1.59	4.9	1.5–15.9
Maximum Scvo$_2$ <70%	1.05	2.7	1.1–7.6
Hypotension despite fluid challenge	0.10	1.1	0.5–2.5

Factors associated with increased mortality on bivariate analysis were evaluated with in-hospital mortality as the dependent variable (n = 148). Logistic regression model was limited to subjects for whom Scvo$_2$ was measured continuously (148/166). Lactate nonclearance, less than 10% decrease in repeat lactate value; hypotension, systolic blood pressure 690 mm Hg after intravenous administration of 20 mL/Kg fluid bolus.

Data from Arnold RC, Shapiro NI, Jones AE, et al. Multicenter study of early lactate clearance as a determinant of survival in patients with presumed sepsis. Shock 2009;32:35–9.

This study is not without its limitations. First, a goal of 20% reduction may be considered somewhat aggressive and could be responsible for the extra fluid resuscitation and vasodilator therapy received by the lactate-guided group, especially in an unblinded study. While acknowledging this concern, it must be noted that the treatment

Table 7
Fluid, inotrope, vasodilator, and red blood cells transfusion therapy in lactate-guided group versus control group

Treatment	Control Group	Lactate-Guided Group	P Value
Fluids (mL)[a]			
0–3 h[b]	2194 ± 1669	2697 ± 1965	0.011
9–72 h[c]	10,043 ± 6141	8515 ± 4987	0.055
Red blood cells transfusion (mL)			
0–8 h[b]	196 ± 495	322 ± 1037	0.15
9–72 h[c]	345 ± 667	423 ± 1300	0.59
Any inotropic agent (%)[d]			
0–8 h[b]	32.9	40.1	0.17
9–72 h[e]	44.2	35.2	0.12
Any vasodilator (%)[f]			
0–8 h[b]	20.2	42.5	<0.001
9–72 h[e]	27.1	43.2	0.005
Any vasopressor (%)[g]			
0–8 h[b]	63.6	69.5	0.25
9–72 h[e]	63.7	71.4	0.16

P values as calculated by 2-sample Student *t* test or the chi-square test, as appropriate.
[a] Sum of crystalloid and colloid fluids.
[b] Values are shown for all patients.
[c] Cumulative values (±SD) are shown for patients who were still admitted to the ICU after 72 h.
[d] Dobutamine, enoximone, or epinephrine.
[e] Proportions are shown for patients who stayed for more than 8 h in the ICU.
[f] Nitroglycerine or ketanserin.
[g] Norepinephrine, dopamine, or phenylephrine.

Data from Jansen TC, van Bommel J, Schoonderbeek FJ, et al. Early lactate-guided therapy in ICU patients: a multicenter, open-label, randomized controlled trial. Am J Respir Crit Care Med 2010; 182:752–61.

algorithm of the lactate-guided group did not result in faster lactate clearance when compared with control group, despite the use of more fluids and vasodilators in the lactate-guided group. Second, although the use of vasodilators for microcirculatory recruitment may be viewed as a departure from standard care and a limitation with regard to the applicability of these results in other settings, in the center where the study was conducted vasodilators represented the local standard of care and were used more in the lactate-guided group simply because of persistent lactate levels elevation.

It is the authors' opinion that the results of these studies provide a rational basis for the use of lactate-guided therapy in critically ill patients, especially those with sepsis-induced tissue hypoperfusion. This argument may be made more strong in settings with limited capability to rapidly place central venous access for Scvo$_2$ measurement. In these cases, rather than blindly administering fluids and vasopressors, lactate-guided therapy may be of clinical relevance.

SUMMARY

Lactate levels are frequently elevated in critically ill patients and correlate well with disease severity. Elevated lactate levels are prognostic in prehospital, ED, and ICU settings and in selected critically ill patients, lactate levels may be used to guide early resuscitation therapy.

REFERENCES

1. Anderson B, Kelly A, Kerr D, et al. Impact of patient and environmental factors on capillary refill time in adults. Am J Emerg Med 2008;26:62–5.
2. Lewin J, Maconochie I. Capillary refill time in adults. Emerg Med J 2008;25: 325–6.
3. Tibby SM, Hatherill M, Murdoch IA. Capillary refill and core–peripheral temperature gap as indicators of haemodynamic status in paediatric intensive care patients. Arch Dis Child 1999;80:163–6.
4. Scheele KW. Opuscula chemica et physica. Leipzig (Germany): Kessinger Publishing Company; 1789. p. 316.
5. Philosophical Magazine Series 4. Taylor & Francis; 1851.
6. Araki T. Ueber die Bildung von Milchsäure und Glycose im Organismus bei Sauerstoffmangel. Z Physiol Chem 1891;15:335–70 [in German].
7. Araki T. Ueber die Bildung von Milchsäure und Glycose im Organismus bei Sauerstoffmangel. Zweite Mittheilung: Ueber die Wirkung von Morphium, Amylnitrit, Cocain. Z Physiol Chem 1891,15.540–01 [in German].
8. Araki T. Ueber die Bildung von Milchsäure und Glycose im Organismus bei Sauerstoffmangel. Dritte Mittheilung. Z Physiol Chem 1892;16:453–9 [in German].
9. Araki T. Ueber Bildung von Glycose und Milchsäure bei Sauerstoff mangel. Entgegnung. Z Physiol Chem 1892;16:201–4 [in German].
10. Zillessen H. Ueber die Bildung von Milchsäure und Glykose in den Organen bei gestörter Circulation und bei der Blausäurevergiftung. Z Physiol Chem 1891;15: 387–404 [in German].
11. Scherer JJ. Chemische und Mikroskopische Untersuchungen zur Pathologie angestellt an den Kliniken des Julius-Hospitales zu Würzburg. Heidelberg (Germany): C.F. Winter; 1843.
12. Scherer JJ. Eine Untersuchung des Blutes bei Leukämie. Verhandlungen der Physikalisch-Medicinischen Gesellschaft im Würzburg 1851;2:321–5 [in German].

13. Folwarczny Carl. Handbuch Der Physiologischen Chemie, Mit Rücksicht Auf Pathologische Chemie Und Analytische Methoden. Wien (Switzerland): Verlag von Sallmayer & Comp; 1863.
14. Mizock BA, Falk JL. Lactic acidosis in critical illness. Crit Care Med 1992;20(1): 80–93.
15. Woods HF, Cohen R. Clinical and biochemical aspects of lactic acidosis. Oxford (UK): Blackwell Scientific; 1976.
16. Gladden LB. Lactate metabolism – a new paradigm for the third millennium. J Physiol 2004;558:5–30.
17. Handy J. Lactate—the bad boy of metabolism, or simply misunderstood? Curr Anaesth Crit Care 2006;17(1–2):71–6.
18. Levy B. Lactate and shock state: the metabolic view. Curr Opin Crit Care 2006; 12(4):315–21.
19. Harris P, Bailey T, Bateman M, et al. Lactate, pyruvate, glucose, and free fatty acid in mixed venous and arterial blood. J Appl Physiol 1963;18:933–6.
20. Weil MH, Michaels S, Rackow EC. Comparison of blood lactate concentrations in central venous, pulmonary artery, and arterial blood. Crit Care Med 1987;15: 489–90.
21. Nimmo GR, Armstrong IR, Grant IS. Sampling site for blood lactate estimation: arterial or mixed venous? Clin Intensive Care 1993;4:8–9.
22. Brown SD, Clark C, Gutierrez G. Pulmonary lactate release in patients with sepsis and the adult respiratory distress syndrome. J Crit Care 1996;11:2–8.
23. Douzinas EE, Tsidemiadou PD, Pitaridis MT, et al. The regional production of cytokines and lactate in sepsis-related multiple organ failure. Am J Respir Crit Care Med 1997;155:53–9.
24. De Backer D, Creteur J, Zhang H, et al. Lactate production by the lungs in acute lung injury. Am J Respir Crit Care Med 1997;156(4 Pt 1):1099–104.
25. Haji-Michael PG, Ladriere L, Senerb A, et al. Leukocyte glycolysis and lactate output in animal sepsis and ex vive human blood. Metabolism 1999;48(6):779–85.
26. Mizock BA. Hyperlactatemia in acute liver failure: decreased clearance versus increased production. Crit Care Med 2001;29(11):2225–6.
27. Bihari D, Gimson AE, Lindridge J, et al. Lactic acidosis in fulminant hepatic failure. Some aspects of pathogenesis and prognosis. J Hepatol 1985;1(4):405–16.
28. Levraut J, Ciebiera JP, Chave S, et al. Mild hyperlactatemia in stable septic patients is due to impaired lactate clearance rather than overproduction. Am J Respir Crit Care Med 1998;157:1021–6.
29. Revelly JP, Tappy L, Martinez A, et al. Lactate and glucose metabolism in severe sepsis and cardiogenic shock. Crit Care Med 2005;33(10):2235–40.
30. Bellomo R. Bench-to-bedside review: lactate and the kidney. Crit Care 2002; 6(4):322–6.
31. Biomarkers Definitions Working Group. Biomarkers and surrogate endpoints: preferred definitions and conceptual framework. Clin Pharmacol Ther 2001;69: 89–95.
32. Marshall JC, Reinhart K, International Sepsis Forum. Biomarkers of sepsis. Crit Care Med 2009;37(7):2290–8.
33. Cain SM. Appearance of excess lactate in anesthetized dogs during anemic and hypoxic hypoxia. Am J Physiol 1965;209:604–8.
34. Cain SM. Oxygen delivery and uptake in dogs during anemic and hypoxic hypoxia. J Appl Physiol 1977;42:228–34.
35. Zhang H, Vincent JL. Oxygen extraction is altered by endotoxin during tamponade-induced stagnant hypoxia in the dog. Circ Shock 1993;40(3):168–76.

36. Meakins J, Long CN. Oxygen consumption, oxygen debt and lactic acid in circulatory failure. J Clin Invest 1927;4(2):273–93.
37. Ronco JJ, Fenwick JC, Tweeddale MG, et al. Identification of the critical oxygen delivery for anaerobic metabolism in critically ill septic and nonseptic humans. JAMA 1993;270(14):1724–30.
38. Levy B, Sadoune LO, Gelot AM, et al. Evolution of lactate/pyruvate and arterial ketone body ratios in the early course of catecholamine-treated septic shock. Crit Care Med 2000;28(1):114–9.
39. Rivers E, Nguyen B, Havstad S, et al. Early goal-directed therapy in the treatment of severe sepsis and septic shock. N Engl J Med 2001;345(19):1368–77.
40. Rady MY, Rivers EP, Nowak RM. Resuscitation of the critically ill in the ED: responses of blood pressure, heart rate, shock index, central venous oxygen saturation, and lactate. Am J Emerg Med 1996;14:218–25.
41. Rixen D, Siegel JH. Bench-to-bedside review: oxygen debt and its metabolic correlates as quantifiers of the severity of hemorrhagic and post-traumatic shock. Crit Care 2005;9:441–53.
42. Meregalli A, Oliveira RP, Friedman G. Occult hypoperfusion is associated with increased mortality in hemodynamically stable, high-risk, surgical patients. Crit Care 2004;8:R60–5.
43. Coats TJ, Smith JE, Lockey D, et al. Early increases in blood lactate following injury. J R Army Med Corps 2002;148:140–3.
44. Jansen TC, van Bommel J, Mulder PG, et al. The prognostic value of blood lactate levels relative to that of vital signs in the pre-hospital setting: a pilot study. Crit Care 2008;12:R160.
45. Bakker J, Coffernils M, Leon M, et al. Blood lactate levels are superior to oxygen-derived variables in predicting outcome in human septic shock. Chest 1991;99(4):956–62.
46. Bakker J, Gris P, Coffernils M, et al. Serial blood lactate levels can predict the development of multiple organ failure following septic shock. Am J Surg 1996; 171(2):221–6.
47. Van Beest PA, Mulder PJ, Oetomo SB. Measurement of lactate in a prehospital setting is related to outcome. Eur J Emerg Med 2009;16(6):318–22.
48. Gunnerson KJ, Brant S, Greenfield N. Pre-hospital lactate levels are better predictors of mortality and hospital admission than traditional vital signs [abstract P84]. Circulation 2009;120:51459.
49. Trzeciak S, Dellinger RP, Chansky ME, et al. Serum lactate as a predictor of mortality in patients with infection. Intensive Care Med 2007;33(6):970–7.
50. Shapiro NI, Howell MD, Talmor D, et al. Serum lactate as a predictor of mortality in emergency department patients with infection. Ann Emerg Med 2005;45(5): 524–8.
51. Shapiro NI, Howell MD, Donnino M, et al. Occult hypoperfusion and mortality in patients with suspected infection. Intensive Care Med 2007;33(11):1892–9.
52. Mikkelsen ME, Miltiades AN, Gaieski DF, et al. Serum lactate is associated with mortality in severe sepsis independent of organ failure and shock. Crit Care Med 2009;37(5):1670–7.
53. Nguyen HB, Rivers EP, Knoblich BP, et al. Early lactate clearance is associated with improved outcome in severe sepsis and septic shock. Crit Care Med 2004; 32:1637–42.
54. Pal JD, Victorino GP, Twomey P, et al. Admission serum lactate levels do not predict mortality in the acutely injured patient. J Trauma 2006;60:583–7 [discussion: 587–9].

55. Dunne JR, Tracy JK, Scalea TM, et al. Lactate and base deficit in trauma: does alcohol or drug use impair their predictive accuracy? J Trauma 2005;58:959–66.

56. Kaplan LJ, Kellum JA. Initial pH, base deficit, lactate, anion gap, strong ion difference, and strong ion gap predict outcome from major vascular injury. Crit Care Med 2004;32:1120–4.

57. Kliegel A, Losert H, Sterz F, et al. Serial lactate determinations for prediction of outcome after cardiac arrest. Medicine 2004;83:274–9.

58. Sankoff JD, Goyal M, Gaieski DF, et al. Validation of the Mortality in Emergency Department Sepsis (MEDS) score in patients with the systemic inflammatory response syndrome (SIRS). Crit Care Med 2008;36:421–6.

59. Jansen TC, van Bommel J, Schoonderbeek FJ, et al. Early lactate-guided therapy in ICU patients: a multicenter, open-label, randomized controlled trial. Am J Respir Crit Care Med 2010;182(6):752–61.

60. Scott S, Antonaglia V, Guiotto G, et al. Two-hour lactate clearance predicts negative outcome in patients with cardiorespiratory insufficiency. Crit Care Res Pract 2010;2010. Article ID 917053.

61. Friedman G, Berlot G, Kahn RJ, et al. Combined measurements of blood lactate concentrations and gastric intramucosal pH in patients with severe sepsis. Crit Care Med 1995;23:1184–93.

62. Tamion F, Le Cam-Duchez V, Menard JF, et al. Erythropoietin and renin as biological markers in critically ill patients. Crit Care 2004;8(5):R328–35.

63. Dondorp AM, Chau TT, Phu NH, et al. Unidentified acids of strong prognostic significance in severe malaria. Crit Care Med 2004;32:1683–8.

64. Singhal R, Coghill JE, Guy A, et al. Serum lactate and base deficit as predictors of mortality after ruptured abdominal aortic aneurysm repair. Eur J Vasc Endovasc Surg 2005;30:263–6.

65. Maillet JM, Le Besnerais P, Cantoni M, et al. Frequency, risk factors, and outcome of hyperlactatemia after cardiac surgery. Chest 2003;123:1361–6.

66. Abramson D, Scalea TM, Hitchcock R, et al. Lactate clearance and survival following injury. J Trauma 1993;35:584–8.

67. Martin MJ, FitzSullivan E, Salim A, et al. Discordance between lactate and base deficit in the surgical intensive care unit: which one do you trust? Am J Surg 2006;191:625–30.

68. Blow O, Magliore L, Claridge JA, et al. The golden hour and the silver day: detection and correction of occult hypoperfusion within 24 hours improves outcome from major trauma. J Trauma 1999;47:964–9.

69. Claridge JA, Crabtree TD, Pelletier SJ, et al. Persistent occult hypoperfusion is associated with a significant increase in infection rate and mortality in major trauma patients. J Trauma 2000;48:8–14 [discussion: 14–5].

70. Wahl W, Pelletier K, Schmidtmann S, et al. [Experiences with various scores in evaluating the prognosis of postoperative intensive care patients]. Chirurg 1996;67:710–7 [discussion: 718] [in German].

71. Murillo-Cabezas F, Amaya-Villar R, Rincon-Ferrari MD, et al. [Evidence of occult systemic hypoperfusion in head injured patients]. Preliminary study. Neurocirugia (Astur) 2005;16:323–32 [in Spanish].

72. Bernal W, Donaldson N, Wyncoll D, et al. Blood lactate as an early predictor of outcome in paracetamol-induced acute liver failure: a cohort study. Lancet 2002;359:558–63.

73. Watanabe I, Mayumi T, Arishima T, et al. Hyperlactemia can predict the prognosis of liver resection. Shock 2007;28:35–8.

74. Funk GC, Doberer D, Kneidinger N, et al. Acid-base disturbances in critically ill patients with cirrhosis. Liver Int 2007;27:901–9.
75. Kruse JA, Zaidi SA, Carlson RW. Significance of blood lactate levels in critically ill patients with liver disease. Am J Med 1987;83:77–82.
76. Smith I, Kumar P, Molloy S, et al. Base excess and lactate as prognostic indicators for patients admitted to intensive care. Intensive Care Med 2001;27:74–83.
77. Suistomaa M, Ruokonen E, Kari A, et al. Time-pattern of lactate and lactate to pyruvate ratio in the first 24 hours of intensive care emergency admissions. Shock 2000;14:8–12.
78. Freire AX, Bridges L, Umpierrez GE, et al. Admission hyperglycemia and other risk factors as predictors of hospital mortality in a medical ICU population. Chest 2005;128:3109–16.
79. Cusack RJ, Rhodes A, Lochhead P, et al. The strong ion gap does not have prognostic value in critically ill patients in a mixed medical/surgical adult ICU. Intensive Care Med 2002;28:864–9.
80. Rocktaeschel J, Morimatsu H, Uchino S, et al. Unmeasured anions in critically ill patients: can they predict mortality? Crit Care Med 2003;31:2131–6.
81. Marik PE, Bankov A. Sublingual capnometry versus traditional markers of tissue oxygenation in critically ill patients. Crit Care Med 2003;31:818–22.
82. Maynard N, Bihari D, Beale R, et al. Assessment of splanchnic oxygenation by gastric tonometry in patients with acute circulatory failure. JAMA 1993;270:1203–10.
83. Dubin A, Menises MM, Masevicius FD, et al. Comparison of three different methods of evaluation of metabolic acid-base disorders. Crit Care Med 2007;35:1264–70.
84. Aduen J, Bernstein WK, Khastgir T, et al. The use and clinical importance of a substrate-specific electrode for rapid determination of blood lactate concentrations. JAMA 1994;272:1678–85.
85. Levy B, Gawalkiewicz P, Vallet B, et al. Gastric capnometry with air-automated tonometry predicts outcome in critically ill patients. Crit Care Med 2003;31:474–80.
86. Sasaki S, Gando S, Kobayashi S, et al. Predictors of mortality in patients treated with continuous hemodiafiltration for acute renal failure in an intensive care setting. ASAIO J 2001;47:86–91.
87. Hatherill M, McIntyre AG, Wattie M, et al. Early hyperlactataemia in critically ill children. Intensive Care Med 2000;26:314–8.
88. Hatherill M, Sajjanhar T, Tibby SM, et al. Serum lactate as a predictor of mortality after paediatric cardiac surgery. Arch Dis Child 1997;77:235–8.
89. Hatherill M, Waggie Z, Purves L, et al. Mortality and the nature of metabolic acidosis in children with shock. Intensive Care Med 2003;29:286–91.
90. Garcia Sanz C, Ruperez Lucas M, Lopez-Herce Cid J, et al. [Prognostic value of the pediatric index of mortality (PIM) score and lactate values in critically-ill children]. An Esp Pediatr 2002;57:394–400 [in Spanish].
91. Balasubramanyan N, Havens PL, Hoffman GM. Unmeasured anions identified by the Fencl-Stewart method predict mortality better than base excess, anion gap, and lactate in patients in the pediatric intensive care unit. Crit Care Med 1999;27:1577–81.
92. Shime N, Ashida H, Hiramatsu N, et al. Arterial ketone body ratio for the assessment of the severity of illness in pediatric patients following cardiac surgery. J Crit Care 2001;16:102–7.

93. Koliski A, Cat I, Giraldi DJ, et al. Blood lactate concentration as prognostic marker in critically ill children. J Pediatr (Rio J) 2005;81:287–92.

94. Gotay-Cruz F, Avilés-Rivera DH, Fernández-Sein A. Lactic acid levels as a prognostic measure in acutely ill patients. P R Health Sci J 1991;10:9–13.

95. Cheung PY, Chui N, Joffe AR, et al. Postoperative lactate concentrations predict the outcome of infants aged 6 weeks or less after intracardiac surgery: a cohort follow-up to 18 months. J Thorac Cardiovasc Surg 2005;130:837–43.

96. Cheung PY, Etches PC, Weardon M, et al. Use of plasma lactate to predict early mortality and adverse outcome after neonatal extracorporeal membrane oxygenation: a prospective cohort in early childhood. Crit Care Med 2002;30: 2135–9.

97. Durward A, Tibby SM, Skellett S, et al. The strong ion gap predicts mortality in children following cardiopulmonary bypass surgery. Pediatr Crit Care Med 2005;6:281–5.

98. Jansen TC, van Bommel J, Woodward R, et al. Association between blood lactate levels, Sequential Organ Failure Assessment subscores and 28-day mortality during early and late ICU stay: a retrospective observational study. Crit Care Med 2009;37(8):2369–74.

99. Jansen TC, van Bommel J, Mulder PG, et al. Prognostic value of blood lactate levels: does the clinical diagnosis at admission matter? J Trauma 2009;66(2): 377–85.

100. Rossi AF, Khan DM, Hannan R, et al. Goal directed medical therapy and point-of-care testing improve outcomes after congenital heart surgery. Intensive Care Med 2005;31:98–104.

101. Arnold RC, Shapiro NI, Jones AE, et al. Multicenter study of early lactate clearance as a determinant of survival in patients with presumed sepsis. Shock 2009; 32(1):35–9.

102. Jones AE, Shapiro NI, Trzeciak S, et al. Lactate clearance vs central venous oxygen saturation as goals of early sepsis therapy. JAMA 2010;303(8): 739–46.

Cardiac Biomarkers in the Critically Ill

Corey E. Ventetuolo, MD[a], Mitchell M. Levy, MD[b],*

KEYWORDS

• Cardiac • Biomarkers • Critical illness

Cardiac biomarkers have well-established roles in acute coronary syndrome and congestive heart failure. In the intensive care unit (ICU), myocardial injury is often unrecognized and leads to increased morbidity and mortality.[1] The diagnosis of myocardial ischemia or left ventricular dysfunction complicating critical illness can be difficult, because patients are often unable to report ischemic symptoms. In the medical ICU (MICU), cardiovascular disease and left ventricular dysfunction commonly predate critical illness and can lead to a complicated clinical course.[2]

Beyond ischemia and heart failure, myocardial damage and the release of biomarkers may be caused by various illnesses frequently encountered in the ICU,[3] including trauma, arrhythmias, pulmonary embolus, renal failure, sepsis, and acute respiratory distress syndrome. In many instances, the detection of cardiac biomarkers may aid in the diagnosis and risk assessment of critically ill patients. In acute respiratory distress syndrome, for example, evidence of myocardial injury from hypoxic vasoconstriction and resultant right ventricular dysfunction may portend a worse outcome.[4,5] Despite increasing interest in the use of cardiac biomarkers in noncardiac critical illness, no clear consensus exists on how and in which settings markers should be measured.[6] This article briefly describes what constitutes an ideal biomarker and focuses on those that have been most well studied in critical illness, specifically troponin, the natriuretic peptides (atrial natriuretic peptide [ANP], brain natriuretic peptide [BNP], and N-terminal proBNP [NT-proBNP]), and heart-type fatty acid–binding protein (H-FABP). The use of these markers in cardiac illness (eg, acute coronary syndrome and congestive heart failure) is beyond the scope of this article, and these are discussed only when relevant to noncardiac critical illness.

[a] Division of Pulmonary, Allergy, and Critical Care Medicine, Department of Medicine, College of Physicians and Surgeons, Columbia University, 622 West 168th Street, PH 8 East, Room 101, New York, NY 10032, USA

[b] Division of Pulmonary and Critical Care Medicine, Department of Medicine, Rhode Island Hospital, The Warren Alpert Medical School of Brown University, 593 Eddy Street, MICU Main 7, Providence, RI 02903, USA

* Corresponding author.

E-mail address: mitchell_levy@brown.edu

Crit Care Clin 27 (2011) 327–343

doi:10.1016/j.ccc.2010.12.004

criticalcare.theclinics.com

0749-0704/11/$ – see front matter © 2011 Elsevier Inc. All rights reserved.

DEFINITIONS AND CRITERIA

The use of biomarkers for diagnostic and prognostic purposes in any illness is appealing given that they are noninvasive, ideally rapidly available, and may be followed over a patient's course of illness. At best, they may serve as potential targets for therapy and surrogates in clinical trials. Assay reliability, the establishment of cut-offs, and timely, affordable processing must be considered and addressed before widespread adoption of a given marker.

A biomarker is defined as "a characteristic that is objectively measured and evaluated as an indicator of normal biological processes, pathogenic processes, or pharmacologic responses to a therapeutic intervention."[7] Before the widespread use of a marker of interest, it must endure validation (ie, have known characteristics, be well standardized, and be accurate) and qualification (ie, be integral to the disease process and have clinically relevant end points).[8] Depending on the intended use, the validation and qualification process may be more or less rigorous (known as the *fit-for-purpose* paradigm in drug development) (**Table 1**).[9]

Some efforts have been made to develop guidelines for the use of cardiac biomarkers in critical illness, and previous reviews have discussed establishing consensus.[6,10] Although cardiac markers (particularly troponin and the BNPs) have been studied in the ICU, sample sizes in these studies have generally been small, and marker assays and cut-offs have varied widely, as have the study populations. Even in the more established areas of acute coronary syndrome and congestive heart failure, these issues have been debated and revised with the evolution of improved, highly sensitive assays.[3,11]

Multiple issues that often arise in critical illness may impact the study (and ultimately bedside application) of cardiac markers. Timing of blood draws, dynamic physiologic changes, such as shifts in intravascular volume and renal failure, and patient

Table 1
The "fit-for-purpose" paradigm of biomarker development

Biomarker	Description	Drug Development Use
Exploration	Biomarker in research and development In vitro and/or preclinical evidence available No or limited data linking biomarker to outcomes in humans	Hypothesis generating
Demonstration	Biomarker with acceptable preclinical sensitivity and specificity Some data supporting association with clinical outcomes	Decision-making
Characterization	Biomarker correlated to clinical outcomes Validity demonstrated by more than one prospective study	Decision-making, dose finding, secondary/tertiary claims
Surrogacy	Biomarker as surrogate for clinical end point	Registration

Data from Wagner JA, Williams SA, Webster CJ. Biomarkers and surrogate end points for fit-for-purpose development and regulatory evaluation of new drugs. Clin Pharmacol Ther 2007;81:104–7.

characteristics (eg, age, gender, body habitus) are just a few of the factors that may impact the validity of a given marker and its measurement. This overview offers clinicians a summary of the current cardiac biomarker literature, and identifies the markers most likely to prove relevant in shaping clinical practice.

SELECTED BIOMARKERS
Troponin

The troponin protein complex (with troponin I, C, and T subunits) modulates calcium-mediated actin and myosin coupling in striated muscle. Each subunit is encoded by different genes with differential specificity for muscle type.[12] Therefore, troponin I and T are highly specific for myocardial contraction and, when detected in the blood, cardiac injury.[3,13] Well established as a useful biomarker in acute myocardial infarction, troponin elevation can be seen in various other circumstances in the ICU, most notably demand ischemia from a host of critical illnesses. According to the most recent consensus statement on the diagnosis of acute myocardial infarction, a positive troponin (I or T) is defined as a value exceeding the 99th percentile of a normal reference population, or the upper reference limit.[3] Assay-specific cut-off values must be determined, and individual assays must show excellent precision (coefficient of variation ≤10%) at the 99th percentile level.[11] Although asymptomatic troponin elevation is seen frequently in patients with renal disease, its detection predicts long-term mortality in the outpatient dialysis setting and in acute illness.[14,15]

Troponin elevation in critical illness (regardless of the clear presence of myocardial infarction) not only is common but also has been associated with worse outcomes in various settings, including the emergency room, MICU, and surgical ICU.[16–23] Even when patients with a history of cardiac disease or evidence of acute coronary syndrome on presentation are excluded from study, troponin elevation is frequent (32%–55%) and may independently predict death.[24,25] In a large (N = 1657) retrospective study of admission troponin levels in patients admitted to a single MICU, troponin elevation was significantly associated with short- and long-term mortality, even after adjustment for severity of illness.[23] In a single-center, prospective study of patients admitted to the MICU, troponin elevation was associated with a longer duration of mechanical ventilation but did not add prognostic value to Acute Physiology and Chronic Health Evaluation (APACHE) II scores.[17] Whether isolated troponin elevation offers additional prognostic information to that gained from current indices of critical illness is unclear. When ICU course is complicated by clinical evidence of cardiac dysfunction (ie, acute myocardial infarction or congestive heart failure), outcomes seem to be worse than with troponin elevation alone.[18,26]

Several small studies have documented an increased risk of death in septic patients who have elevated troponins.[27–31] Degree of hypotension, older age, and severity of illness have been identified as risk factors for myocardial damage in septic patients.[4,29,30,32] Recently, a retrospective analysis of a subset of participants from the Protein C Worldwide Evaluation in Severe Sepsis (PROWESS) trial (N = 598) found that troponin positivity was independently associated with 28-day mortality (odds ratio [OR], 2.02; 95% CI, 1.15–3.54).[32] Whether the detection of troponin in severe sepsis and septic shock indicates true myocardial necrosis or reversible myocardial depression is unknown, although the absence of acute myocardial infarction on autopsy of septic patients argues for the latter.[25,30,33–35]

In acute pulmonary embolism, the presence of right ventricular dysfunction increases the risk of in-hospital complications and death.[36] Troponin positivity has been correlated with echocardiographic right ventricular dysfunction.[37,38] Therefore, troponin may aid in risk stratification of acute pulmonary embolism. A positive troponin has been shown in several prospective studies to be an independent predictor of poor outcomes, but these studies included both hemodynamically stable and unstable patients.[37,39] Perhaps more importantly, several studies have focused on the use of troponin in hemodynamically stable patients, with conflicting results.[40–43] Becattini and colleagues[44] meta-analyzed 20 studies (N = 1985), 16 of which were prospective and 7 of which included normotensive patients only, and found troponin positivity was significantly associated with adverse outcomes and mortality; this association remained significant in the subgroup of patients without shock.

A second meta-analysis pooling nine studies involving only hemodynamically stable patients (N = 1366), however, concluded that an elevated troponin alone does not adequately predict poor outcome in hemodynamically stable pulmonary embolism.[45] Most recently, a highly sensitive troponin assay was shown to accurately prognosticate course in patients with pulmonary embolism who are normotensive (sensitivity and negative predictive value are both 100%) and was superior to older troponin assays and BNP.[46] Taken together, the use of troponin in risk stratification of pulmonary embolism seems to be most valuable when (1) applied to patients without shock and (2) measured with a highly sensitive assay.

The use of troponin for risk assessment in patients with pulmonary arterial hypertension has limited support in the literature and has been studied primarily outside of the ICU.[47] In one small study (N = 55), troponin positivity measured using a highly sensitive assay was highly correlated with echocardiographic right ventricular dysfunction and, more importantly, was more accurate (ie, 100% sensitive and specific) in predicting poor functional class and death than standard troponin assay, NT-proBNP, and H-FABP.[48]

ANP

ANP is released from the atria in response to cardiac stretch from volume loading. Downstream, ANP stimulates peripheral vasodilatation as well as diuresis and natriuresis via renal salt and water handling.[49,50] The N-terminal (pro-ANP) and the midregional portion of ANP's prohormone (MR-proANP) are more stable analytes due to longer half-lives.[51] In critical illness, endogenous ANP may protect against ischemia-reperfusion injury in end-organs as well as maintain endothelial function during acute lung injury.[52,53]

Higher levels of ANP have been associated with the development of myocardial depression in sepsis.[54–57] Increasing levels of ANP also appear to track with worsening hemodynamics and right ventricular dysfunction in critically ill patients, although this has not been clearly documented across all studies.[58–60] In a prospective study of patients admitted to a MICU, elevated pro-ANP levels distinguished survivors from nonsurvivors with similar accuracy as APACHE II scores.[61] Similarly, pro-ANP levels have been shown to predict severity of acute lung injury and survival in patients in the ICU requiring mechanical ventilation.[54,62,63] Pro-ANP and MR-proANP may also be useful in risk stratification of patients with lower respiratory tract infections, particularly community-acquired pneumonia.[64,65] Despite some encouraging preliminary data, the focus of recent research in natriuretic peptides has shifted to BNP and NT-proBNP.

Brain-Type Natriuretic Peptides

Similar to ANP, BNPs play an important role in cardiovascular homeostasis and volume regulation. Secreted in response to myocardial stretch from ventricular pressure and volume loading, the prohormone proBNP is cleaved to BNP and the biologically inactive NT-proBNP. Both biomarkers have been extensively studied in heart failure and emergency room triage, but their role in critical illness is less well defined.[66–68] In heart failure, elevations in NT-proBNP tend to be more pronounced than BNP because of a longer half-life and better stability. NT-proBNP may therefore better discern early cardiac dysfunction without being subject to blood sampling conditions.[69,70] Various patient characteristics can affect BNP and NT-proBNP levels, and appropriate assay cut-offs vary widely. Women and patients with renal dysfunction tend to have higher levels of BNP and NT-proBNP, whereas obese individuals tend to have lower levels.[71–73] In the ICU setting, increasing age, female gender, and renal dysfunction have been correlated with higher concentrations of both peptides.[74–77]

In animals, natriuretic peptides are synthesized in response to inflammatory cytokines important in sepsis pathogenesis.[78] Elevations in BNP (and NT-proBNP) may be seen across all shock states and may track with traditional inflammatory biomarkers, such as C-reactive protein and white blood cell count.[79,80] Although increases in BNP and NT-proBNP have been reported in severe sepsis and septic shock, high levels do not necessarily correlate with sepsis-induced cardiac dysfunction or outcome.[60,79,81–85] Experts have proposed that the catabolic pathway for natriuretic peptides is altered in sepsis, leading to impaired clearance and detectable elevations in septic patients.[86]

In undifferentiated shock, BNP levels do not clearly correlate with left heart filling pressures, but low levels do seem to be useful for ruling out cardiac dysfunction (reported negative predictive value, 93%–95%).[87–89] In several small studies of patients without preexisting cardiac dysfunction admitted with shock, high levels of BNP predicted death.[81,88] Marked elevations in NT-proBNP (>1000 pg/mL) have been shown to independently predict mortality in unselected critically ill patients and patients with septic shock, although this finding has not been replicated across all studies.[63,70,89–93] Compared with BNP, NT-proBNP seems to more accurately detect the presence of cardiac dysfunction (measured hemodynamically) and poor outcomes in the critically ill.[89,92] In two studies with unselected and predominantly critically ill cardiac patients, NT-proBNP predicted survival and illness severity scores (APACHE II and Simplified Acute Physiology II scores, respectively).[93,94]

Without measurement of left heart filling pressures, acute lung injury can be difficult to distinguish from pulmonary edema, especially when a critically ill patient has a history of cardiac dysfunction. Low levels of BNP support the diagnosis of acute lung injury but do not completely exclude cardiogenic edema.[76] Absolute or serial measurements do not clearly track with volume status or pulmonary artery occlusion pressure, however, and current evidence does not support the routine use of natriuretic peptides to differentiate acute lung injury/acute respiratory distress syndrome from heart failure.[76,77,89,95]

The prognostic value of BNP and NT-proBNP has also been studied in acute pulmonary embolus. Both peptides are elevated in hemodynamically stable patients with evidence of echocardiographic right ventricular dysfunction.[96–100] In one of the larger, multicenter studies of normotensive patients with pulmonary embolism, NT-proBNP (>300 pg/mL) independently predicted adverse outcomes with reasonable accuracy, and outperformed troponin and H-FABP (negative predictive value, 100%; 95% CI, 91%–100%).[101] These findings have not been duplicated across all studies, however, and previous data suggest that higher NT-proBNP cut-off values (>1000 pg/mL) are more appropriate.[43,99,102,103] Although elevated BNP has been shown to predict the presence of echocardiographic right ventricular dysfunction, a reliable cut-off has not been established.[100,104–107] Several meta-analyses have shown that both peptides are useful in diagnosing right ventricular dysfunction and independently predict hospital complications and at least short-term mortality.[97,98,108] Overall, BNP and NT-proBNP are probably most useful for their ability to predict a benign course in pulmonary embolism (ie, rule-out complications) when normal or low.

Although both natriuretic peptides have been correlated to disease progression and survival in patients with pulmonary artery hypertension,[109–112] the use of natriuretic peptides has not been well studied in these critically ill patients. In a single study of patients with pulmonary artery hypertension admitted to an ICU with acute right ventricular failure, elevated BNP at baseline predicted ICU mortality.[113]

H-FABP

H-FABP is a low–molecular weight cytoplasmic protein involved in the buffering and metabolism of fatty acids released from damaged myocardium.[114] Present in high concentrations in the heart only, H-FABP appears in the blood within 90 minutes of myocardial ischemia and returns to baseline within 24 hours.[115] Several rapid sandwich enzyme-linked immunosorbent assays (ELISAs) have been shown to have excellent reliability.[116–118] Point-of-care assays have also been developed and validated against sandwich ELISA, although these assays may have less precision and have not been widely studied.[119–122] H-FABP increases with age and declining renal function, and may be higher in men than in women.[116,123]

H-FABP has not yet been widely studied in critical illness. Given that it is a fairly novel marker, the literature supporting its use in acute coronary syndrome warrants reviewing. Despite the advent of more sensitive troponin assays, H-FABP seems to be more sensitive (but less specific) than troponin in early detection of acute myocardial infarction.[124–128] In patients with confirmed acute coronary syndrome, H-FABP independently predicts adverse cardiovascular outcomes and death, and seems to identify high-risk patients who are troponin I–negative.[117,129] Most recently, Viswanathan and colleagues[130] duplicated these findings in a large cohort of low- to intermediate-risk patients with suspected acute coronary syndrome, suggesting that H-FABP may complement traditional biomarkers in the diagnosis and risk stratification of myocardial ischemia. These studies have used different ELISA kits with variable cut-offs for H-FABP (between 5.3 and 8 ng/mL) based on 99th percentile values for the normal population and assay characteristics.[116,129]

H-FABP may also be useful in risk stratification for patients with acute pulmonary embolism. Several small prospective studies have show that baseline H-FABP elevation (>6 ng/mL) independently predicts adverse outcomes in both hemodynamically stable and unstable patients, and may be more informative than troponin or NT-proBNP.[102,131]

More recently, Dellas and colleagues[132] prospectively studied the use of H-FABP in normotensive patients (N = 126). Elevated H-FABP (>6 ng/mL) successfully predicted major complications, including death, at 30 days (OR, 25.9; 95% CI, 2.9–229.3; P = .003); outperformed troponin T, NT-proBNP, and echocardiographically documented right ventricular dysfunction; and was independently associated with long-term mortality, although the overall event rate was low in this study.[132] Similar associations have been shown in patients with pulmonary embolism and documented echocardiographic right ventricular dysfunction.[133] A single study examined the use of H-FABP in patients with chronic thromboembolic pulmonary hypertension (CTEPH).[134] Persistent elevations in H-FABP independently predicted an adverse outcome (CTEPH-related death, need for lung transplantation, or pulmonary hypertension after pulmonary endarterectomy) and, in the patients who underwent pulmonary endarterectomy, baseline HFABP elevation (>2.7 ng/mL) was associated with a lower probability of event-free survival.[134]

A small study examined the use of H-FABP levels from cerebrospinal fluid in subarachnoid hemorrhage and found associations with hemorrhage severity and poor outcome.[135] Elevated H-FABP levels have also been correlated to aortic aneurysm size but not the presence of hemodynamic instability or end-organ dysfunction.[122] Finally, patients with pulmonary infections resulting in multiorgan dysfunction may have increased levels of circulating H-FABP.[136] Although H-FABP has been increasingly recognized as a useful biomarker in acute coronary syndrome and pulmonary embolism, whether it will ultimately be used in critical care settings remains to be seen.

Other Potential Markers of Interest

Although other cardiac biomarkers have not been extensively studied in an ICU setting, several novel markers may have potential for future study and use in critical illness. Myocardial ischemia decreases the ability of albumin's N-terminal to bind cobalt and other transition metals; this ischemia-modified albumin (IMA) can be detected in the blood through quantifying albumin cobalt binding, and may be an early marker of myocardial damage before the development of frank necrosis.[137] Although preliminary studies of the role of IMA in diagnosing acute coronary syndrome suggest that it may be a fairly sensitive biomarker, thus far it seems to be poorly specific and, in the largest prospective study to date, it did not add diagnostic value to standard measures.[137–141] Although several small studies suggest that IMA may be a useful marker for identifying ischemia in other organs, such as the cerebrovasculature, mesentery, and limbs, and for detecting venous thromboembolism, current literature does not support the routine use of IMA in critical illness.[142–147]

Although not a cardiac biomarker per se, adrenomedullin and its prohormone proadrenomedullin are ubiquitous peptides that have been isolated from the heart and are synthesized and released from the endothelium.[148] These peptides cause potent vasodilatation and natriuresis, and enhanced cardiac contractility and nitric oxide synthesis.[149,150] The midregion fragment of the prohormone, MR-proadrenomedullin, may be a more ideal biomarker than its parent peptides.[151] These markers may have prognostic value in acute myocardial infarction and heart failure.[152–154] Both adrenomedullin and MR-proadrenomedullin are elevated in patients with systemic inflammatory response syndrome and in sepsis, and levels may track with severity of illness.[151,155–159] Experts have proposed that adrenomedullin plays an important role in the cardiovascular response and endothelial regulation during sepsis.[160] In a prospective study of septic patients, MR-proadrenomedullin elevation predicted survival with similar accuracy to illness severity scores.[157] Elevated levels of MR-proadrenomedullin may also be useful in risk stratification in community-acquired pneumonia, particularly in high-risk patients (as defined by the pneumonia severity index).[64,161,162]

SUMMARY

Critical illness is frequently complicated by preexisting cardiovascular disease and heart failure. Similarly, the development of ischemia and myocardial suppression from common ICU conditions complicates a patient's course. Therefore, well-established cardiac biomarkers might be useful in the ICU setting for the diagnosis and risk assessment of cardiac disease complicating critical illness. Although elevated troponin and natriuretic peptides likely signal a poor prognosis in shock (including septic shock), whether they should be routinely incorporated into clinical practice is currently unclear. Although the natriuretic peptides may be useful in differentiating acute lung injury from heart failure, these markers do not clearly track with filling pressures or volume status.

In acute pulmonary embolism, identifying patients at high-risk for a complicated course and early death remains challenging. Current guidelines recommend replacing terminology such as *massive* and *submassive* pulmonary embolism to avoid assigning risk based on anatomic characteristics and clot burden.[163] However, the patients who will benefit the most from a biomarker-guided strategy are those who present without shock but may have evidence of early right ventricular ischemia (potentially detected by troponin or H-FABP) or right ventricular pressure loading (with release of natriuretic peptides).[164] Although how biomarkers should be incorporated into clinical decision making in pulmonary embolism is unclear, currently they are probably most useful for predicting a benign course in patients without shock. Highly sensitive troponin assays and H-FABP may prove to be the most valuable biomarkers in this setting.

Cardiac biomarkers may ultimately play an important role in critical care, with several caveats. First, specific assays have limitations, assay cut-offs have not been clearly established, and measurements during dynamic critical illness may be problematic. Second, biomarker interpretation may vary depending on individual patient characteristics and ICU diagnosis. Last, any marker measured in isolation is unlikely to surpass careful bedside assessment.

REFERENCES

1. Guest TM, Ramanathan AV, Tuteur PG, et al. Myocardial injury in critically ill patients: a frequently unrecognized complication. JAMA 1995;273(24): 1945–9.
2. Marcelino PA, Marum SM, Fernandes AP, et al. Routine transthoracic echocardiography in a general intensive care unit: an 18 month survey in 704 patients. Eur J Intern Med 2009;20(3):e37–42.
3. Thygesen K, Alpert JS, White HD, et al. Universal definition of myocardial infarction. Eur Heart J 2007;28(20):2525–38.
4. Bajwa EK, Boyce PD, Januzzi JL, et al. Biomarker evidence of myocardial cell injury is associated with mortality in acute respiratory distress syndrome. Crit Care Med 2007;35(11):2484–90.
5. Bull TM, Clark B, McFann K, et al, NIH NHLBI ARDS Network. Pulmonary vascular dysfunction is associated with poor outcomes in patients with acute lung injury. Am J Respir Crit Care Med 2010;182(9):1123–8.
6. NACB Writing Group Members, Wu AH, Jaffe AS, et al. National academy of clinical biochemistry laboratory medicine practice guidelines: use of cardiac troponin and B-type natriuretic peptide or N-terminal proB-type natriuretic peptide for etiologies other than acute coronary syndromes and heart failure. Clin Chem 2007;53(12):2086–96.
7. The Biomarker Definitions Working Group. Biomarkers and surrogate endpoints: preferred definitions and conceptual framework. Clin Pharmacol Ther 2001;69: 89–95.
8. Wagner JA, Williams SA, Webster CJ. Biomarkers and surrogate end points for fit-for-purpose development and regulatory evaluation of new drugs. Clin Pharmacol Ther 2007;81:104–7.

9. Lee JW, Devanarayan V, Barrett YC, et al. Fit-for-purpose method development and validation for successful biomarker measurement. Pharm Res 2006;23: 312–28.

10. Noveanu M, Mebazaa A, Mueller C. Cardiovascular biomarkers in the ICU. Curr Opin Crit Care 2009;15(5):377–83.

11. NACB Writing Group Members, Apple FS, Jesse RL, et al. National Academy of Clinical Biochemistry and IFCC Committee for Standardization of Markers of Cardiac Damage Laboratory Medicine practice guidelines: analytical issues for biochemical markers of acute coronary syndromes. Circulation 2007; 115(13):e352–5.

12. Parmacek MS, Solaro RJ. Biology of the troponin complex in cardiac myocytes. Prog Cardiovasc Dis 2004;47(3):159–76.

13. Adams JE III, Bodor G, Davila-Roman V, et al. Cardiac troponin I. A marker with high specificity for cardiac injury. Circulation 1993;88(1):101–6.

14. Apple FS, Murakami MM, Pearce LA, et al. Predictive value of cardiac troponin I and T for subsequent death in end-stage renal disease. Circulation 2002; 106(23):2941–5.

15. Kang EW, Na HJ, Hong SM, et al. Prognostic value of elevated cardiac troponin I in ESRD patients with sepsis. Nephrol Dial Transplant 2009;24(5): 1568–73.

16. Baillard C, Boussarsar M, Fosse J, et al. Cardiac troponin I in patients with severe exacerbation of chronic obstructive pulmonary disease. Intensive Care Med 2003;29:584–9.

17. King DA, Codish S, Novack V, et al. The role of cardiac troponin I as a prognosticator in critically ill medical patients: a prospective observational cohort study. Crit Care 2005;9(4):31.

18. Kollef MH, Ladenson JH, Eisenberg PR. Clinically recognized cardiac dysfunction: An independent determinant of mortality among critically ill patients. Chest 1997;111(5):1340–7.

19. Noble J, Reid A, Jordan L, et al. Troponin I and myocardial injury in the ICU. Br J Anaesth 1999;82:41–6.

20. Relos RP, Hasinoff IK, Beilman GJ. Moderately elevated serum troponin concentrations are associated with increased morbidity and mortality rates in surgical intensive care unit patients. Crit Care Med 2003;31(11):2598–603.

21. Turley AJ, Gedney JA. Role of cardiac troponin as a prognosticator in critically ill patients. Crit Care 2005;9(6):E30.

22. Wright RS, Williams BA, Cramner H, et al. Elevations of cardiac troponin I are associated with increased short term mortality in noncardiac critically ill emergency department patients. Am J Cardiol 2002;90(6):634–6.

23. Babuin L, Vasile VC, Rio Perez JA, et al. Elevated cardiac troponin is an independent risk factor for short- and long-term mortality in medical intensive care unit patients. Crit Care Med 2008;36(3):759–65.

24. Quenot JP, Le Teuff G, Quantin C, et al. Myocardial injury in critically ill patients. Chest 2005;128(4):2758–64.

25. Ammann P, Maggiorini M, Bertel O, et al. Troponin as a risk factor for mortality in critically ill patients without acute coronary syndromes. J Am Coll Cardiol 2003; 41:2004–9.

26. Lim W, Qushmaq I, Cook D, et al. Elevated troponin and myocardial infarction in the intensive care unit: a prospective study. Crit Care 2005;9(6):R636–44.

27. Spies C, Haude V, Overbeck M, et al. Serum cardiac troponin T as a prognostic marker in early sepsis. Chest 1998;113(4):1055–63.

28. Turner A, Tsamitros M, Bellomo R. Myocardial cell injury in septic shock. Crit Care Med 1999;27(9):1775–80.
29. Arlati S, Brenna S, Prencipe L, et al. Myocardial necrosis in ICU patients with acute non-cardiac disease: a prospective study. Intensive Care Med 2000; 26(1):31–7.
30. ver Elst KM, Spapen HD, Nguyen DN, et al. Cardiac troponins I and T are biological markers of left ventricular dysfunction in septic shock. Clin Chem 2000;46(5):650–7.
31. Mehta NJ, Khan IA, Gupta V, et al. Cardiac troponin I predicts myocardial dysfunction and adverse outcome in septic shock. Int J Cardiol 2004;95(1):13–7.
32. John J, Woodward DB, Wang Y, et al. Troponin-I as a prognosticator of mortality in severe sepsis patients. J Crit Care 2010;25(2):270–5.
33. Ammann P, Fehr T, Minder EI, et al. Elevation of troponin I in sepsis and septic shock. Intensive Care Med 2001;27(6):965–9.
34. Wu AH. Increased troponin in patients with sepsis and septic shock: myocardial necrosis or reversible myocardial depression? Intensive Care Med 2001;27(6): 959–61.
35. Fernandes CJ, Akamine N, Knobel E. Cardiac troponin: a new serum marker of myocardial injury in sepsis. Intensive Care Med 1999;25(10):1165–8.
36. Goldhaber SZ, Visani L, De Rosa M. Acute pulmonary embolism: Clinical outcomes in the international cooperative pulmonary embolism registry (ICOPER). Lancet 1999;353(9162):1386–9.
37. Konstantinides S, Geibel A, Olschewski M, et al. Importance of cardiac troponins I and T in risk stratification of patients with acute pulmonary embolism. Circulation 2002;106(10):1263–8.
38. Meyer T, Binder L, Hruska N, et al. Cardiac troponin I elevation in acute pulmonary embolism is associated with right ventricular dysfunction. J Am Coll Cardiol 2000;36(5):1632–6.
39. Giannitsis E, Muller-Bardorff M, Kurowski V, et al. Independent prognostic value of cardiac troponin T in patients with confirmed pulmonary embolism. Circulation 2000;102(2):211–7.
40. Douketis JD, Leeuwenkamp O, Grobara P, et al. The incidence and prognostic significance of elevated cardiac troponins in patients with submassive pulmonary embolism. J Thromb Haemost 2005;3(3):508–13.
41. Pruszczyk P, Bochowicz A, Torbicki A, et al. Cardiac troponin T monitoring identifies high-risk group of normotensive patients with acute pulmonary embolism. Chest 2003;123(6):1947–52.
42. Jimenez D, Diaz G, Molina J, et al. Troponin I and risk stratification of patients with acute nonmassive pulmonary embolism. Eur Respir J 2008; 31(4):847–53.
43. Kostrubiec M, Pruszczyk P, Bochowicz A, et al. Biomarker-based risk assessment model in acute pulmonary embolism. Eur Heart J 2005;26(20): 2166–72.
44. Becattini C, Vedovati MC, Agnelli G. Prognostic value of troponins in acute pulmonary embolism: a meta-analysis. Circulation 2007;116(4):427–33.
45. Jimenez D, Uresandi F, Otero R, et al. Troponin-based risk stratification of patients with acute nonmassive pulmonary embolism: systematic review and meta-analysis. Chest 2009;136(4):974–82.
46. Lankeit M, Friesen D, Aschoff J, et al. Highly sensitive troponin T assay in normotensive patients with acute pulmonary embolism. Eur Heart J 2010;31(15): 1836–44.

47. Torbicki A, Kurzyna M, Kuca P, et al. Detectable serum cardiac troponin T as a marker of poor prognosis among patients with chronic precapillary pulmonary hypertension. Circulation 2003;108:844–8.

48. Filusch A, Giannitsis E, Katus HA, et al. High-sensitive troponin T: a novel biomarker for prognosis and disease severity in patients with pulmonary arterial hypertension. Clin Sci (Lond) 2010;119(5):207–13.

49. Weidmann P, Hasler L, Gnadinger MP, et al. Blood levels and renal effects of atrial natriuretic peptide in normal man. J Clin Invest 1986;77(3):734–42.

50. de Zeeuw D, Janssen WM, de Jong PE. Atrial natriuretic factor: its pathophysiological significance in humans. Kidney Int 1992;41(5):1115–33.

51. Morgenthaler NG, Struck J, Thomas B, et al. Immunoluminometric assay for the midregion of pro-atrial natriuretic peptide in human plasma. Clin Chem 2004; 50(1):234–6.

52. Birukova AA, Xing J, Fu P, et al. Atrial natriuretic peptide attenuates LPS-induced lung vascular leak: Role of PAK1. Am J Physiol Lung Cell Mol Physiol 2010;299(5):L652–63.

53. Nakamoto M, Shapiro JI, Shanley PF, et al. In vitro and in vivo protective effect of atriopeptin III on ischemic acute renal failure. J Clin Invest 1987;80(3):698–705.

54. Mazul-Sunko B, Zarkovic N, Vrkic N, et al. Pro-atrial natriuretic peptide hormone from right atria is correlated with cardiac depression in septic patients. J Endocrinol Invest 2001;24(7):22–4.

55. Hartemink KJ, Groeneveld AB, de Groot MC, et al. Alpha-atrial natriuretic peptide, cyclic guanosine monophosphate, and endothelin in plasma as markers of myocardial depression in human septic shock. Crit Care Med 2001;29(1):80–7.

56. Witthaut R, Busch C, Fraunberger P, et al. Plasma atrial natriuretic peptide and brain natriuretic peptide are increased in septic shock: impact of interleukin-6 and sepsis-associated left ventricular dysfunction. Intensive Care Med 2003; 29(10):1696–702.

57. Mitaka C, Hirata Y, Makita K, et al. Endothelin-1 and atrial natriuretic peptide in septic shock. Am Heart J 1993;126(2):466–8.

58. Boldt J, Menges T, Kuhn D, et al. Alterations in circulating vasoactive substances in the critically ill–a comparison between survivors and non-survivors. Intensive Care Med 1995;21(3):218–25.

59. Bein T, Pfeifer M, Keyl C, et al. Right ventricular function and plasma atrial natriuretic peptide levels during fiberbronchoscopic alveolar lavage in critically ill, mechanically ventilated patients. Chest 1995;108(4):1030–5.

60. Ueda S, Nishio K, Akai Y, et al. Prognostic value of increased plasma levels of brain natriuretic peptide in patients with septic shock. Shock 2006;26(2):134–9.

61. Morgenthaler N, Struck J, Christ-Crain M, et al. Pro-atrial natriuretic peptide is a prognostic marker in sepsis, similar to the APACHE II score: an observational study. Crit Care 2005;9(1):R37–45.

62. Tanabe M, Ueda M, Endo M, et al. Effect of acute lung injury and coexisting disorders on plasma concentrations of atrial natriuretic peptide. Crit Care Med 1994;22(11):1762–8.

63. Berdal JE, Stavem K, Omland T, et al. Prognostic merit of N-terminal-proBNP and N-terminal-proANP in mechanically ventilated critically ill patients. Acta Anaesthesiol Scand 2008;52(9):1265–72.

64. Schuetz P, Wolbers M, Christ-Crain M, et al. Prohormones for prediction of adverse medical outcome in community-acquired pneumonia and lower respiratory tract infections. Crit Care 2010;14(3):R106–14.

65. Muller B, Suess E, Schuetz P, et al. Circulating levels of pro-atrial natriuretic peptide in lower respiratory tract infections. J Intern Med 2006;260(6):568–76.

66. Lainchbury JG, Troughton RW, Strangman KM, et al. N-terminal pro-B-type natriuretic peptide-guided treatment for chronic heart failure: results from the BATTLESCARRED (NT-proBNP-assisted Treatment To Lessen Serial Cardiac Readmissions And Death) trial. J Am Coll Cardiol 2009;55(1):53–60.

67. Januzzi JJ, Camargo CA, Anwaruddin S, et al. The N-terminal pro-BNP investigation of dyspnea in the emergency department (PRIDE) study. Am J Cardiol 2005;95(8):948–54.

68. Maisel AS, McCord J, Nowak RM, et al. Bedside B-type natriuretic peptide in the emergency diagnosis of heart failure with reduced or preserved ejection fraction: results from the breathing not properly multi-national study. J Am Coll Cardiol 2003;41(11):2010–7.

69. Hunt PJ, Richards AM, Nicholls MG, et al. Immunoreactive amino-terminal pro-brain natriuretic peptide (NT-proBNP): a new marker of cardiac impairment. Clin Endocrinol 1997;47(3):287–96.

70. Brueckmann M, Huhle G, Lang S, et al. Prognostic value of plasma N-terminal pro-brain natriuretic peptide in patients with severe sepsis. Circulation 2005; 112(4):527–34.

71. Redfield MM, Rodeheffer RJ, Jacobsen SJ, et al. Plasma brain natriuretic peptide concentration: impact of age and gender. J Am Coll Cardiol 2002; 40(5):976–82.

72. Anwaruddin S, Lloyd-Jones DM, Baggish A, et al. Renal function, congestive heart failure, and amino-terminal pro-brain natriuretic peptide measurement: results from the Pro-BNP Investigation of Dyspnea in the Emergency Department (PRIDE) Study. J Am Coll Cardiol 2006;47(1):91–7.

73. Das SR, Drazner MH, Dries DL, et al. Impact of body mass and body composition on circulating levels of natriuretic peptides: results from the Dallas Heart Study. Circulation 2005;112(14):2163–8.

74. Bal L, Thierry S, Brocas E, et al. B-type natriuretic peptide (BNP) and N-terminal-proBNP for heart failure diagnosis in shock or acute respiratory distress. Acta Anaesthesiol Scand 2006;50(3):340–7.

75. McLean AS, Huang SJ, Nalos M, et al. The confounding effects of age, gender, serum creatinine, and electrolyte concentrations on plasma B-type natriuretic peptide concentrations in critically ill patients. Crit Care Med 2003;31(11):2611–8.

76. Rana R, Vlahakis N, Daniels C, et al. B-type natriuretic peptide in the assessment of acute lung injury and cardiogenic pulmonary edema. Crit Care Med 2006;34:1941–6.

77. Forfia PR, Watkins SP, Rame JE, et al. Relationship between B-type natriuretic peptides and pulmonary capillary wedge pressure in the intensive care unit. J Am Coll Cardiol 2005;45(10):1667–71.

78. Tanaka T, Kanda T, Takahashi T, et al. Interleukin-6-induced reciprocal expression of SERCA and natriuretic peptides MRNA in cultured rat ventricular myocytes. J Int Med Res 2004;32(1):57–61.

79. Rudiger A, Gasser S, Fischler M, et al. Comparable increase of B-type natriuretic peptide and amino-terminal pro-B-type natriuretic peptide levels in patients with severe sepsis, septic shock, and acute heart failure. Crit Care Med 2006;34(8):2140–4.

80. Rudiger A, Fischler M, Harpes P, et al. In critically ill patients, B-type natriuretic peptide (BNP) and N-terminal pro-BNP levels correlate with C-reactive protein values and leukocyte counts. Int J Cardiol 2008;126(1):28–31.

81. Charpentier J, Luyt CE, Fulla Y, et al. Brain natriuretic peptide: a marker of myocardial dysfunction and prognosis during severe sepsis. Crit Care Med 2004;32(3):660–5.
82. Roch A, Allardet-Servent J, Michelet P, et al. NH2 terminal pro-brain natriuretic peptide plasma level as an early marker of prognosis and cardiac dysfunction in septic shock patients. Crit Care Med 2005;33(5):1001–7.
83. Hoffmann U, Brueckmann M, Bertsch T, et al. Increased plasma levels of nt-proANP and NT-proBNP as markers of cardiac dysfunction in septic patients. Clin Lab 2005;51(7/8):373–9.
84. Maeder M, Fehr T, Rickli H, et al. Sepsis-associated myocardial dysfunction: Diagnostic and prognostic impact of cardiac troponins and natriuretic peptides. Chest 2006;129(5):1349–66.
85. McLean AS, Huang SJ, Hyams S, et al. Prognostic values of B-type natriuretic peptide in severe sepsis and septic shock. Crit Care Med 2007; 35(4):1019–26.
86. Pirracchio R, Deye N, Lukaszewicz AC, et al. Impaired plasma B-type natriuretic peptide clearance in human septic shock. Crit Care Med 2008;36(9):2542–6.
87. McLean AS, Tang B, Nalos M, et al. Increased B-type natriuretic peptide (BNP) level is a strong predictor for cardiac dysfunction in intensive care unit patients. Anaesth Intensive Care 2003;31(1):21–7.
88. Tung RH, Garcia C, Morss AM, et al. Utility of B-type natriuretic peptide for the evaluation of intensive care unit shock. Crit Care Med 2004;32(8):1643–7.
89. Jefic D, Lee JW, Jefic D, et al. Utility of B-type natriuretic peptide and N-terminal pro B-type natriuretic peptide in evaluation of respiratory failure in critically ill patients. Chest 2005;128(1):288–95.
90. Almog Y, Novack V, Megralishvili R, et al. Plasma level of N terminal pro-brain natriuretic peptide as a prognostic marker in critically ill patients. Anesth Analg 2006;102(6):1809–15.
91. Coquet I, Darmon M, Doise JM, et al. Performance of N-terminal-pro-B-type natriuretic peptide in critically ill patients: a prospective observational cohort study. Crit Care 2008;12(6):6.
92. Januzzi JL, Morss A, Tung R, et al. Natriuretic peptide testing for the evaluation of critically ill patients with shock in the intensive care unit: a prospective cohort study. Crit Care 2006;10(1):R37.
93. Kotanidou A, Karsaliakos P, Tzanela M, et al. Prognostic importance of increased plasma amino-terminal pro-brain natriuretic peptide levels in a large noncardiac, general intensive care unit population. Shock 2009;31(4):342–7.
94. Meyer B, Huelsmann M, Wexberg P, et al. N-terminal pro-B-type natriuretic peptide is an independent predictor of outcome in an unselected cohort of critically ill patients. Crit Care Med 2007;35(10):2268–73.
95. Levitt J, Vinayak A, Gehlbach B, et al. Diagnostic utility of B-type natriuretic peptide in critically ill patients with pulmonary edema: a prospective cohort study. Crit Care 2008;12(1):R3.
96. Vuilleumier N, Righini M, Perrier A, et al. Correlation between cardiac biomarkers and right ventricular enlargement on chest CT in non massive pulmonary embolism. Thromb Res 2008;121(5):617–24.
97. Cavallazzi R, Nair A, Vasu T, et al. Natriuretic peptides in acute pulmonary embolism: a systematic review. Intensive Care Med 2008;34(12):2147–56.
98. Klok FA, Mos IC, Huisman MV. Brain-type natriuretic peptide levels in the prediction of adverse outcome in patients with pulmonary embolism: a systematic review and meta-analysis. Am J Respir Crit Care Med 2008;178(4):425–30.

99. Pruszczyk P, Kostrubiec M, Bochowicz A, et al. N-terminal pro-brain natriuretic peptide in patients with acute pulmonary embolism. Eur Respir J 2003;22(4): 649–53.

100. Pieralli F, Olivotto I, Vanni S, et al. Usefulness of bedside testing for brain natriuretic peptide to identify right ventricular dysfunction and outcome in normotensive patients with acute pulmonary embolism. Am J Cardiol 2006;97(9): 1386–90.

101. Vuilleumier N, Le Gal G, Verschuren F, et al. Cardiac biomarkers for risk stratification in non-massive pulmonary embolism: a multicenter prospective study. J Thromb Haemost 2009;7(3):391–8.

102. Puls M, Dellas C, Lankeit M, et al. Heart-type fatty acid-binding protein permits early risk stratification of pulmonary embolism. Eur Heart J 2007;28(2):224–9.

103. Binder L, Pieske B, Olschewski M, et al. N-terminal pro-brain natriuretic peptide or troponin testing followed by echocardiography for risk stratification of acute pulmonary embolism. Circulation 2005;112(11):1573–9.

104. ten Wolde M, Tulevski II, Mulder JW, et al. Brain natriuretic peptide as a predictor of adverse outcome in patients with pulmonary embolism. Circulation 2003; 107(16):2082–4.

105. Kruger S, Graf J, Merx MW, et al. Brain natriuretic peptide predicts right heart failure in patients with acute pulmonary embolism. Am Heart J 2004;147(1): 60–5.

106. Ray P, Maziere F, Medimagh S, et al. Evaluation of B-type natriuretic peptide to predict complicated pulmonary embolism in patients aged 65 years and older: brief report. Am J Emerg Med 2006;24(5):603–7.

107. Kucher N, Printzen G, Goldhaber SZ. Prognostic role of brain natriuretic peptide in acute pulmonary embolism. Circulation 2003;107(20):2545–7.

108. Lega JC, Lacasse Y, Lakhal L, et al. Natriuretic peptides and troponins in pulmonary embolism: a meta-analysis. Thorax 2009;64(10):869–75.

109. Fijalkowska A, Kurzyna M, Torbicki A, et al. Serum N-terminal brain natriuretic peptide as a prognostic parameter in patients with pulmonary hypertension. Chest 2006;129(5):1313–21.

110. Leuchte HH, Holzapfel M, Baumgartner RA, et al. Clinical significance of brain natriuretic peptide in primary pulmonary hypertension. J Am Coll Cardiol 2004; 43(5):764–70.

111. Souza R, Jardim C, Julio Cesar Fernandes C, et al. NT-proBNP as a tool to stratify disease severity in pulmonary arterial hypertension. Respir Med 2007; 101(1):69–75.

112. Nagaya N, Nishikimi T, Okano Y, et al. Plasma brain natriuretic peptide levels increase in proportion to the extent of right ventricular dysfunction in pulmonary hypertension. J Am Coll Cardiol 1998;31(1):202–8.

113. Sztrymf B, Souza R, Bertoletti L, et al. Prognostic factors of acute heart failure in patients with pulmonary arterial hypertension. Eur Respir J 2010; 35(6):1286–93.

114. Alhadi HA, Fox KA. Do we need additional markers of myocyte necrosis: the potential value of heart fatty-acid-binding protein. QJM 2004;97(4):187–98.

115. Glatz JF, van Bilsen M, Paulussen RJ, et al. Release of fatty acid-binding protein from isolated rat heart subjected to ischemia and reperfusion or to the calcium paradox. Biochim Biophys Acta 1988;961(1):148–52.

116. Bathia DP, Carless DR, Viswanathan K, et al. Serum 99th centile values for two heart-type fatty acid binding protein assays. Ann Clin Biochem 2009;46(6): 464–7.

117. Kilcullen N, Viswanathan K, Das R, et al. Heart-type fatty acid-binding protein predicts long-term mortality after acute coronary syndrome and identifies high-risk patients across the range of troponin values. J Am Coll Cardiol 2007;50(21):2061–7.
118. Ohkaru Y, Asayama K, Ishii H, et al. Development of a sandwich enzyme-linked immunosorbent assay for the determination of human heart type fatty acid-binding protein in plasma and urine by using two different monoclonal antibodies specific for human heart fatty acid-binding protein. J Immunol Methods 1995;178(1):99–111.
119. Chan CP, Sum KW, Cheung KY, et al. Development of a quantitative lateral-flow assay for rapid detection of fatty acid-binding protein. J Immunol Methods 2003; 279(1/2):91–100.
120. Liao J, Chan CP, Cheung Y, et al. Human heart-type fatty acid-binding protein for on-site diagnosis of early acute myocardial infarction. Int J Cardiol 2009; 133(3):420–3.
121. Watanabe T, Ohkubo Y, Matsuoka H, et al. Development of a simple whole blood panel test for detection of human heart-type fatty acid-binding protein. Clin Biochem 2001;34(4):257–63.
122. Hazui H, Negoro N, Nishimoto M, et al. Serum heart-type fatty acid-binding protein concentration positively correlates with the length of aortic dissection. Circ J 2005;69(8):958–61.
123. Niizeki T, Takeishi Y, Takabatake N, et al. Circulating levels of heart-type fatty acid-binding protein in a general Japanese population: effects of age, gender, and physiologic characteristics. Circ J 2007;71(9):1452–7.
124. Seino Y, Ogata K, Takano T, et al. Use of a whole blood rapid panel test for heart-type fatty acid-binding protein in patients with acute chest pain: comparison with rapid troponin T and myoglobin tests. Am J Med 2003;115(3):185–90.
125. Reichlin T, Hochholzer W, Bassetti S, et al. Early diagnosis of myocardial infarction with sensitive cardiac troponin assays. N Engl J Med 2009;361(9):858–67.
126. Valle HA, Riesgo LG, Bel MS, et al. Clinical assessment of heart-type fatty acid binding protein in early diagnosis of acute coronary syndrome. Eur J Emerg Med 2008;15(3):140–4.
127. Haltern G, Peiniger S, Bufe A, et al. Comparison of usefulness of heart-type fatty acid binding protein versus cardiac troponin T for diagnosis of acute myocardial infarction. Am J Cardiol 2010;105(1):1–9.
128. McCann CJ, Glover BM, Menown IB, et al. Novel biomarkers in early diagnosis of acute myocardial infarction compared with cardiac troponin T. Eur Heart J 2008;20(23):2843 50.
129. O'Donoghue M, de Lemos JA, Morrow DA, et al. Prognostic utility of heart-type fatty acid binding protein in patients with acute coronary syndromes. Circulation 2006;114(6):550–7.
130. Viswanathan K, Kilcullen N, Morrell C, et al. Heart-type fatty acid-binding protein predicts long-term mortality and re-infarction in consecutive patients with suspected acute coronary syndrome who are troponin-negative. J Am Coll Cardiol 2010;55(23):2590–8.
131. Kaczynska A, Pelsers MM, Bochowicz A, et al. Plasma heart-type fatty acid binding protein is superior to troponin and myoglobin for rapid risk stratification in acute pulmonary embolism. Clin Chim Acta 2006;371(1/2):117–23.
132. Dellas C, Puls M, Lankeit M, et al. Elevated heart-type fatty acid-binding protein levels on admission predict an adverse outcome in normotensive patients with acute pulmonary embolism. J Am Coll Cardiol 2010;55(19):2150–7.

133. Boscheri A, Wunderlich C, Langer M, et al. Correlation of heart-type fatty acid-binding protein with mortality and echocardiographic data in patients with pulmonary embolism at intermediate risk. Am Heart J 2010;160(2):294–300.

134. Lankeit M, Dellas C, Panzenbock A, et al. Heart-type fatty acid-binding protein for risk assessment of chronic thromboembolic pulmonary hypertension. Eur Respir J 2008;31(5):1024–9.

135. Zanier ER, Longhi L, Fiorini M, et al. Increased levels of CSF heart-type fatty acid-binding protein and tau protein after aneurysmal subarachnoid hemorrhage. Acta Neurochir Suppl 2008;102:339–43.

136. Yan GT, Lin J, Hao XH, et al. Heart-type fatty acid-binding protein is a useful marker for organ dysfunction and leptin alleviates sepsis-induced organ injuries by restraining its tissue levels. Eur J Pharmacol 2009;616(1–3):244–50.

137. Christenson RH, Duh SH, Sanhai WR, et al. Characteristics of an albumin cobalt binding test for assessment of acute coronary syndrome patients: a multicenter study. Clin Chem 2001;47(3):464–70.

138. Sinha MK, Roy D, Gaze DC, et al. Role of ischemia modified albumin, a new biochemical marker of myocardial ischaemia, in the early diagnosis of acute coronary syndromes. Emerg Med J 2004;21(1):29–34.

139. Anwaruddin S, Januzzi JL Jr, Baggish AL, et al. Ischemia-modified albumin improves the usefulness of standard cardiac biomarkers for the diagnosis of myocardial ischemia in the emergency department setting. Am J Clin Pathol 2005;123(1):140–5.

140. Keating L, Benger JR, Beetham R, et al. The PRIMA Study: presentation ischaemia-modified albumin in the emergency department. Emerg Med J 2006;23(10):764–8.

141. Lin RM, Fatovich DM, Grasko JM, et al. Ischaemia modified albumin cannot be used for rapid exclusion of acute coronary syndrome. Emerg Med J 2010;27(9):668–71.

142. Gunduz A, Turedi S, Mentese A, et al. Ischemia-modified albumin levels in cerebrovascular accidents. Am J Emerg Med 2008;26(8):874–8.

143. Gunduz A, Mentese A, Turedi S, et al. Serum ischaemia-modified albumin increases in critical lower limb ischaemia. Emerg Med J 2008;25(6):351–3.

144. Mentese A, Mentese U, Turedi S, et al. Effect of deep vein thrombosis on ischaemia-modified albumin levels. Emerg Med J 2008;25(12):811–4.

145. Turedi S, Gunduz A, Mentese A, et al. Value of ischemia-modified albumin in the diagnosis of pulmonary embolism. Am J Emerg Med 2007;25(7):770–3.

146. Gunduz A, Turedi S, Mentese A, et al. Ischemia-modified albumin in the diagnosis of acute mesenteric ischemia: a preliminary study. Am J Emerg Med 2008;26(2):202–5.

147. Turedi S, Gunduz A, Mentese A, et al. The value of ischemia-modified albumin compared with d-dimer in the diagnosis of pulmonary embolism. Respir Res 2008;9:49.

148. Sugo S, Minamino N, Kangawa K, et al. Endothelial cells actively synthesize and secrete adrenomedullin. Biochem Biophys Res Commun 1994;201(3):1160–6.

149. Shimosawa T, Fujita T. Hypotensive effect of a newly identified peptide, proadrenomedullin N-terminal 20 peptide. Hypertension 1996;28(3):325–9.

150. Szokodi I, Kinnunen P, Tavi P, et al. Evidence for cAMP-independent mechanisms mediating the effects of adrenomedullin, a new inotropic peptide. Circulation 1998;97(11):1062–70.

151. Struck J, Tao C, Morgenthaler NG, et al. Identification of an adrenomedullin precursor fragment in plasma of sepsis patients. Peptides 2004;25(8):1369–72.

152. Khan SQ, O'Brien RJ, Struck J, et al. Prognostic value of midregional pro-adrenomedullin in patients with acute myocardial infarction. The LAMP (Leicester Acute Myocardial Infarction Peptide) Study. J Am Coll Cardiol 2007;49(14):1525–32.
153. Maisel A, Mueller C, Nowak R, et al. Mid-region pro-hormone markers for diagnosis and prognosis in acute dyspnea. Results from the BACH (Biomarkers In Acute Heart Failure) Trial. J Am Coll Cardiol 2010;55(19):2062–76.
154. Richards AM, Doughty R, Nicholls MG, et al. Plasma N-terminal pro-brain natriuretic peptide and adrenomedullin: prognostic utility and prediction of benefit from carvedilol in chronic ischemic left ventricular dysfunction. Australia-New Zealand Heart Failure Group. J Am Coll Cardiol 2001;37(7):1781–7.
155. Ueda S, Nishio K, Minamino N, et al. Increased plasma levels of adrenomedullin in patients with systemic inflammatory response syndrome. Am J Respir Crit Care Med 1999;160(1):132–6.
156. Nishio K, Akai Y, Murao Y, et al. Increased plasma concentrations of adrenomedullin correlate with relaxation of vascular tone in patients with septic shock. Crit Care Med 1997;25(6):953–7.
157. Christ-Crain M, Morgenthaler NG, Struck J, et al. Mid-regional pro-adrenomedullin as a prognostic marker in sepsis: an observational study. Crit Care 2005;9(6):15.
158. Wang RL, Kang FX. Prediction about severity and outcome of sepsis by pro-atrial natriuretic peptide and pro-adrenomedullin. Chin J Traumatol 2010; 13(3):152–7.
159. Guignant C, Voirin N, Venet F, et al. Assessment of pro-vasopressin and pro-adrenomedullin as predictors of 28-day mortality in septic shock patients. Intensive Care Med 2009;35(11):1859–67.
160. Wang P. Adrenomedullin and cardiovascular responses in sepsis. Peptides 2001;22(11):1835–40.
161. Christ-Crain M, Morgenthaler NG, Stolz D, et al. Pro-adrenomedullin to predict severity and outcome in community-acquired pneumonia. Crit Care 2006; 10(3):28.
162. Huang DT, Angus DC, Kellum JA, et al. Midregional proadrenomedullin as a prognostic tool in community-acquired pneumonia. Chest 2009;136(3):823–31.
163. Members AT, Torbicki A, Perrier A, et al. Guidelines on the diagnosis and management of acute pulmonary embolism. Eur Heart J 2008;29(18):2276–315.
164. Goldhaber SZ. Fine-tuning risk stratification for acute pulmonary embolism with cardiac biomarkers. J Am Coll Cardiol 2010;55(19):2158–9.

Sepsis Biomarkers in Polytrauma Patients

Charles A. Adams Jr, MD[a,b,c],*

KEYWORDS

• Trauma • Biomarker • Sepsis

Trauma is the leading cause of death during the first 4 decades of life and kills more Americans than diseases such as cancer, heart disease, and lung disease combined over this time span.[1] Each year, more than 2 million people encounter traumatic injuries, and of these people, more than 150,000 die as a result of their injuries. Although this toll is shocking, when one considers the lost economic productivity of trauma patients coupled with the expense of caring for them, the numbers become truly staggering and exceed more than $130 billion annually.[1] Classically, death caused by trauma follows a trimodal distribution: immediate, early, and late.[2,3] The immediate deaths occur in the field and are caused by lethal injuries, such as massive head trauma, or exsanguination from devastating injuries, such as torn aortas or hepatic avulsions. Early trauma deaths occur in the first few hours following injury and are caused by traumatic brain injury and herniation or ongoing hemorrhage. The last group of deaths, the late group, typically occurs in the intensive care unit several days after trauma because of septic complications and multiorgan failure. In this last group of patients, the early detection of infectious complications through the application of suitable biomarkers can have, perhaps, its greatest effect on improved outcomes following severe trauma.

A biomarker can be defined as a clinical indicator that can be directly measured and evaluated as a sign of a physiologic, pathogenic, or pharmacologic response.[4] For the biomarker to have real clinical relevance, it needs to be sensitive and specific, or else it will only serve to add yet another piece of conflicting clinical information to an already complex and confusing medical picture. In simpler terms, a biomarker can be considered as a laboratory test that is readily available and can accurately point to a clinical condition of interest, such as an infection or sepsis.[5] Unlike ordinary sepsis, which annually affects roughly 750,000 Americans who are more likely to be elderly

The author has nothing to disclose.

[a] Warren Alpert School of Medicine of Brown University, Providence, RI, USA

[b] Division of Trauma and Surgical Critical Care, Rhode Island Hospital, 593 Eddy Street, APC 453, Providence, RI 02903, USA

[c] Surgical and Trauma Intensive Care Units, Rhode Island Hospital, Providence, RI 02903, USA

* Corresponding author. Division of Trauma and Surgical Critical Care, Rhode Island Hospital, 593 Eddy Street, APC 453, Providence, RI 02903.

E-mail address: Cadams1@lifespan.org

Crit Care Clin 27 (2011) 345–354

doi:10.1016/j.ccc.2010.12.002

0749-0704/11/$ – see front matter © 2011 Elsevier Inc. All rights reserved.

criticalcare.theclinics.com

or have predisposing medical comorbidities, sepsis following trauma occurs in a younger cohort who typically have far fewer comorbidities. Outwardly, this observation would suggest that diagnosing sepsis in trauma patients ought to be easier and that a trauma biomarker would be readily available; however, the physiologic responses to injury are often indistinguishable from sepsis and therefore render this assumption invalid.

Traumatic injury spans a continuum from minor localized injuries to overwhelming severe polytrauma affecting nearly every organ and tissue in the body. Hemorrhagic shock and subsequent resuscitation expose the individual to whole-body ischemia-reperfusion injury, can incite the activation of multiple cell lines and generation of numerous proinflammatory and antiinflammatory cytokines, and prime the patient for additional physiologic insults or hits that can produce an exaggerated physiologic response.[6,7] Even a relatively moderate injury such as a closed femur fracture typically results in the systemic inflammatory response syndrome (SIRS).[8] Thus, tachycardia, tachypnea, leukocytosis, and low-grade fever following such an injury are part of the normal physiologic response to injury rather than signs of infection. Therefore, the classically accepted biomarkers such as temperature, white blood cell count, heart rate, or respiratory rate following trauma are greatly diminished in their ability to indicate infection. In this confusing setting of both normal and abnormal signs and conflicting clinical data, a trauma biomarker should stand out as a sensitive yet specific marker of infection.

Because inflammation following trauma is the norm, some investigators have attempted to quantify the degree of inflammation, the time it takes to return to baseline, or late spikes in inflammatory markers as predictors of organ failure or death. Much of this work has focused on the early inflammatory (T-helper cell [T_H] 1) cytokines such as IL (interleukin) 1, IL-6, IL-8, and tumor necrosis factor (TNF),[9–14] but the preponderance of the literature supports IL-6 as the biomarker of choice in trauma.[15] IL-6 is a ubiquitous, multifunctional, regulatory cytokine that is important to initiating the acute phase response in an organism. IL-6 plasma levels have been shown to correlate with the severity of injury[16–20] and can predict complications such as pneumonia[21] and even death[20] as a result of major trauma. Despite some of the promising results with IL-6 as a biomarker, it fails to fulfill many of the tenets required of an ideal biomarker because it is relatively insensitive, lacks specificity, and is not readily available to most bedside clinicians. The same limitations are true for the other inflammatory cytokines that are part of the T_H1 inflammatory response and hinder their use as biomarkers.[22]

Initially, most investigators focused on the early proinflammatory response to trauma and attempted to use these markers to predict outcome with little tangible success.[10–22] Over time, it has become apparent that following traumatic injury, the immune system progresses from an initial hyperinflammatory state to a compensatory antiinflammatory state, resulting in profound immune suppression.[23] It is not by coincidence that most late trauma deaths occur during this period of posttraumatic immune dysfunction, thus further demonstrating the need for an accurate biomarker in this state. Some of the more common mediators of the posttraumatic immune-suppressed state are IL-4, IL-10, prostaglandin E_2 (PGE_2), and transforming growth factor β (TGF-β).[24] Among these mediators, IL-10 is perhaps the most important regulatory cytokine and has a major effect on T lymphocytes, causing their suppression.[24] PGE_2 is another important regulatory mediator and is responsible for macrophage downregulation and for suppressing the production of TNF and the inflammatory cytokine IL-12.[25] Although all these mediators are important components of the immune-suppressed state, none of them are capable of functioning as an effective biomarker, nor are they sensitive enough to discern infection against the background of generalized immune dysfunction.

Despite the tremendous advancements made in the understanding of the complex interactions between the innate and humoral immune systems, particularly as they relate to the responses to acute illness and injury, the definitive biomarker of infection in the confusing milieu of varying posttraumatic inflammation has not yet been found. With each new discovery of a putative mediator of trauma-induced hyperinflammation or hypoinflammation, it is hoped that the so-called Holy Grail or ultimate biomarker would be found. The search for the ultimate biomarker has taken an interesting turn as of late, with the growing concept of the "danger signal" model in immunology.[26] According to this model, immune system activation is dependent on signals derived from damaged or dying cells, both foreign and endogenous, and trauma (and other similar stimuli) can result in SIRS in addition to the expected immunologic responses to infection. As noted previously, SIRS is the expected response to trauma and makes the distinction between infection and sterile sepsis exceedingly difficult.[27,28] No clear-cut biomarker has emerged as a result of this paradigm shift in immunology, but there are several promising candidates that have been appropriately named the alarmins.[29,30] The alarmins and other danger signals hold great promise as potential biomarkers, but the experimental and clinical data to support this optimism are limited.

There are many so-called endogenous danger molecules that are liberated as a result of tissue injury, including the intracellular chaperones or heat shock proteins, defensins, annexins, S-100 protein, cathelicidin, eosinophil-derived neurotoxin, and high mobility group box nuclear protein 1 (HMGB1).[29–31] Among these molecules, HMGB1 is emerging as a leading biomarker of tissue injury and by default, an ostensible trauma biomarker. HMGB1 is an intracellular protein than can translocate to the nucleus where it binds to DNA and regulates gene expression; however, under certain pathologic conditions, such as those that cause cellular necrosis, it can be released into the bloodstream where it has different immunomodulating properties.[32] HMGB1 is a true danger signal in that its most powerful effects on the immune system occur when it is released in response to cellular necrosis and not apoptosis.[32] Thus, unregulated cell death is a far more potent trigger for the role of HMGB1 in the immune system than programmed or apoptotic cell death. Plasma HMGB1 levels have been shown to correlate with mortality in both sepsis[33] and trauma.[34] Although data are limited, HMGB1 levels seem to correlate with the severity of injury, tissue hypoperfusion as measured by base deficit, and levels of other inflammatory cytokines such as IL-6, as well as with the likelihood of developing multiple-organ dysfunction syndrome and death following trauma.[34] In this regard, HMGB1 shows great potential as an overall prognostic indicator after trauma, but its ability to predict infectious complications of trauma remains undetermined at present.

The role of HMGB1 in stratifying mortality in septic patients is not clear, with some conflicting studies from humans and animals showing that it may or may not correlate well with the likelihood of dying of sepsis.[35,36] HMGB1 may be a much better candidate as a trauma biomarker than as a biomarker for critical illness or sepsis because its expression seems to be at the highest following hemorrhagic shock.[37] Indeed, experimental animal data further indicate the importance of HMGB1 in hemorrhagic shock, because blocking HMGB1 in vivo results in decreased organ failure and mortality caused by hemorrhage.[38,39] Whether HMGB1 plays a role in susceptibility to bacterial infection and sepsis following hemorrhagic shock remains to be demonstrated in humans, but animal data suggest that it is intricately associated with inflammation, following a "2-hit" model of hemorrhage followed by bacterial challenge.[40]

Out of the myriad of potential biomarkers of posttraumatic sepsis and death, the current leading candidate would have to be procalcitonin (PCT). PCT is the peptide precursor of the hormone calcitonin, which is normally produced by parafollicular C cells of the thyroid and is important to calcium homeostasis.[41] However, in response to bacterial infection, PCT is released from various cell types outside the thyroid and has been shown to be a reliable indicator of bacterial infection and sepsis.[42,43] PCT levels have been shown to be elevated in septic patients who have undergone total thyroidectomy, and elevated PCT levels do not subsequently result in the elevation of serum calcium levels.[44] PCT seems to be an intermediary marker of infectious inflammation because its levels peak 3 to 4 hours after an infectious insult, whereas the cytokine IL-6 and TNF are produced in the first hour or so.[45] Thus, PCT secretion is dependent on IL-6 and TNF, but the cytokines do not seem to be appreciably affected by PCT release.[45]

PCT's importance to the septic response is borne out by evidence showing that it is a reliable early indicator of severe postoperative complications[46–48] and that its levels correlate with the incidence and severity of multiorgan failure.[49,50] It is not uncommon for PCT levels to increase by a factor of more than 1000 times in response to endotoxin or inflammatory cytokine exposure. Because the half-life of PCT is roughly 22 hours, a decrease in its level can also be viewed as a biomarker of resolving infection, which is another characteristic that adds to its overall utility as a biomarker. Serial sampling of PCT after trauma has revealed that PCT levels are typically elevated shortly after traumatic injury, but this elevation typically subsides unless a subsequent bacterial infection occurs.[51] Elevations in PCT levels immediately after traumatic injury seem to predict that the patient is at increased risk for sepsis during hospitalization and should prompt an anticipatory approach to infection in that patient.[51]

Because PCT levels are intimately related to the presence (or absence) of bacterial endotoxin in the circulation, it is a far more sensitive biomarker of infection than nonspecific markers, such as C-reactive protein (CRP).[52,53] CRP belongs to the family of acute phase reactants, is synthesized primarily in the liver and lung, and is important to the function of complement and for the opsonization and phagocytosis of bacteria.[54] IL-6, which is predominantly released by macrophages, promotes the release of CRP in response to virtually all sources of systemic inflammation, including infections or trauma.[55] Before the advent of more sophisticated biomarkers such as PCT, CRP was the most extensively investigated biomarker in critically ill patients. CRP was used in establishing a diagnosis of sepsis, because of its prognostic ability in septic patients, and as an indicator of the severity of sepsis.[5] CRP levels are easily determined and reliable; commercially available assays can rapidly determine the serum level of CRP. However, when compared with PCT, CRP is far less sensitive, thus limiting its role as a useful biomarker for infection following traumatic injury. Head-to-head comparisons and analyses have borne this out, thus further supporting PCT, rather than CRP, as a leading biomarker for infection following traumatic injury.[56]

PCT has another valuable role in the care of trauma patients besides its ability to indicate bacterial infection that seems incongruent with its correlation to bacterial infection. Several investigators have shown that PCT levels spike shortly after major traumatic injury and that the magnitude of this level correlates with the propensity to develop multiorgan failure.[57–59] Elevated PCT levels following trauma have been shown to coincide more with blunt abdominal trauma than trauma to other body regions.[60,61] One possible explanation for the observed linkage between abdominal trauma and elevation of PCT levels centers on a direct effect on the bowel itself, breaching gut barrier integrity and allowing luminal bacteria to gain access to the bloodstream. Alternatively, traumatic shock, particularly hemorrhagic shock, often results in bacteremia or endotoxemia unexplained by direct injury to the gastrointestinal tract and has been cited as evidence for the controversial concept of gut barrier failure and bacterial translocation.[62–64] Whatever the inciting stimulus is, the association of PCT with abdominal trauma lends further credence to its role as a trauma-specific biomarker and as a predictor of organ failure and bacterial infection following major traumatic injury.

Other gut-derived substances have been identified and have many similarities to PCT both in terms of the predictive ability as a biomarker and in the pattern of release following traumatic injury. Pancreatic stone peptide/regenerating peptide (PSP/reg) was initially discovered in the pancreas but was then subsequently detected in the bloodstream of patients with severe pancreatitis.[65] PSP/reg is a lectin-binding acute phase protein, whose release is promoted by IL-6. The protein has been isolated from several extrapancreatic tissues.[66] PSP/reg is incredibly similar to PCT in that its low-level constitutive expression from its native tissue is vastly upregulated in response to the inflammatory cytokines of the septic response, and this induced expression occurs in tissues outside the site of its constitutive expression. Once in the bloodstream, PSP/reg causes the activation of leukocytes and has been shown to be a sensitive indicator of sepsis.[67] In a study comparing PCT with PSP/reg in moderately to severely injured trauma patients, PSP/reg seemed to be a better sign of infectious complications in the confusing hyperinflammatory postinjury state. In addition, PSP/reg shows some ability to differentiate between localized and systemic infection.[67] The high signal-to-noise ability of PSP/reg for sepsis coupled with its capacity to discern local from systemic infection renders it an encouraging trauma biomarker, but like all biomarkers, more data are required to truly identify its proper role.

Emerging data about cellular biomarkers such as peripheral endothelial progenitor cells (EPCs) also hold great promise for the role of these biomarkers in clarifying the immune state following severe trauma. EPCs have shown some ability to make the straightforward distinction between SIRS, sepsis, and severe sepsis because their levels seem to closely parallel this infectious continuum. EPCs are released from the bone marrow in response to infection and have shown correlation with the severity of sepsis; thus, they should serve a useful role as a trauma biomarker, although the timing of the appearance of EPCs in response to infection remains to be elucidated.[68] Certainly, EPCs warrant further investigation as a sepsis biomarker in trauma patients, but it is unclear what their true utility will be in light of trauma's profound negative effect on the function and cellular components of the bone marrow.[69]

A second cellular biomarker is $CD4^+CD25^+$ regulatory T (T_{reg}) cells, which are responsible for controlling the immune response to infection. Under normal conditions, T_{reg} cells comprise no more than 5% to 10% of the circulating $CD4^+$ T cells, but their levels are greatly elevated in septic patients but not in those with SIRS. Like EPCs, T_{reg} cells may be useful biomarkers in the complex and changing posttraumatic immune state, which should prove particularly useful in caring for survivors of the most severe trauma.[70] However, because T_{reg} cell activity is dependent on direct cellular interactions that seem to be partially mediated by TGF-β, it is much more likely that T_{reg} cells are powerful effectors of the postinjury immunocompromised state rather than true symbols of infection.[71] It seems that T_{reg} cells are partly responsible for the immune paralysis that follows many shock states and probably contribute to T-cell anergy as well, but these activities alone are probably not suitable for their role as a biomarker, other than to confirm the postshock immunocompromised state.[72]

Recently, yet another promising biomarker that shares many of the positive traits of PCT and PSP/reg has been identified. This new biomarker is the N-terminal fragment of the precursor of C-type natriuretic peptide (CNP), or NT-proCNP. The natriuretic group of peptides is a diverse group of proteins that are released by the heart and central nervous system and have various important physiologic properties. Atrial natriuretic peptide (ANP) is produced by atrial myocytes, and brain (or B-type) natriuretic peptide (BNP) is predominantly produced by ventricular myocytes.[73] Both ANP and BNP are released in response to cardiac-wall stretch, foment natriuresis and diuresis, and oppose the action of many inflammatory and sympathetic neuroendocrine mediators.

CNP was initially identified in the central nervous system but has subsequently been localized to the endothelium of the vascular system.[74] CNP release from the endothelium is driven by most of the inflammatory cytokines of the T_H1 response, such as IL-1 and TNF, and CNP functions to preserve the flow through the vasculature by opposing the action of the potent vasoconstrictors endothelin 1 and angiotensin II.[75] Both ANP and BNP serve as potent stimulators of CNP release, but unlike ANP and BNP, CNP has essentially no effect on natriuresis, diuresis, or the renin-angiotensin system. Because the inflammatory septic cytokines promote CNP release from the endothelium, CNP's precursor NT-proCNP should be a potential biomarker of infection. Indeed, continuous sampling of NT-proCNP in severely injured trauma patients showed a dramatic increase in its level nearly 2 days before the development of a septic event.[76] Enthusiasm for use of NT-proCNP as a posttraumatic marker of infection must be tempered by the fact that traumatic brain injury, which commonly occurs after blunt trauma, may dramatically affect CNP and NT-proCNP levels in response to septic insults, thus affecting its sepsis predicting abilities.[76]

The ongoing search for the ideal biomarker in trauma patients is beginning to be successful as more sensitive and specific indicators of the posttrauma immune state emerge. Confounding this search is the fact that the normal physiologic response to major injury is immune activation followed by immune suppression, both of which have attributes mirroring the septic condition. A reliable biomarker is desperately needed for severely injured trauma patients because they are at increased risk for sepsis and sepsis-related mortality. In fact, in some studies, these patients have a mortality rate approaching 40%.[77]

Clinical work relating to sepsis biomarkers remains in the earliest stages, but even at this early juncture, the number of would-be biomarkers is astounding. To date, there have been more than 3300 publications involving nearly 180 different sepsis biomarkers, but the leading trauma biomarker candidates can be narrowed to PCT, PSP/reg, and NT-proCNP.[78] Remarkably, all 3 of these putative biomarkers share similar traits such that all 3 are constitutively expressed by 1 cell type but are radically upregulated and released from different cells in response to a bacterial infection. Of these 3 biomarkers, PSP/reg and NT-proCNP seem especially promising candidates for the Grail because they seem to be more sensitive than PCT for infection following trauma, but it is not known yet whether these biomarkers will stand the test of time as the clinical and scientific data surrounding their use grow.

REFERENCES

1. Available at: www.cdc.gov/Injury/Publications/FactBook. Accessed November 12, 2010.
2. Baker CC, Oppenheimer L, Stephens B, et al. Epidemiology of trauma deaths. Am J Surg 1980;140:144–50.
3. Trunkey DD. Trauma. Accidental and intentional injuries account for more years of life lost in the U.S. than cancer and heart disease. Among the prescribed

remedies are improved preventive efforts, speedier surgery and further research. Sci Am 1983;249:28–35.

4. The Biomarker Definitions Working Group. Biomarkers and surrogate endpoints: preferred definitions and conceptual framework. Clin Pharmacol Ther 2001;69: 89–95.

5. Ventetuolo CE, Levy MM. Biomarkers: diagnosis and risk assessment in sepsis. Clin Chest Med 2008;29:591–603.

6. Lenz A, Franklin GA, Cheadle WA. Systemic inflammation after trauma. Injury 2007;38:1336–45.

7. Keel M, Trentz O. Pathophysiology of polytrauma. Injury 2005;36:691–709.

8. Hauser CJ, Zhou X, Joshi P, et al. The immune microenvironment of human fracture/soft-tissue hematomas and its relationship to systemic immunity. J Trauma 1997;42:895–903.

9. Maier B, Lefering R, Lehnert M, et al. Early versus late onset of multiple organ failure is associated with differing patterns of plasma cytokine biomarker expression and outcome after severe trauma. Shock 2007;28:668–74.

10. Morganti-Kosmann MC, Rancan M, Otto VI, et al. Role of cerebral inflammation after traumatic brain injury: a revised concept. Shock 2001;16:165–77.

11. Strecker W, Gebhard F, Rager J, et al. Early biochemical characterization of soft-tissue trauma and fracture trauma. J Trauma 1999;47:358–64.

12. Roumen RM, Redl H, Schlag G, et al. Inflammatory mediators in relation to the development of multiple organ failure in patients after severe blunt trauma. Crit Care Med 1995;23:474–80.

13. Roumen RM, Hendriks T, van der Ven-Jongekrijg J, et al. Cytokine patterns in patients after major vascular surgery, hemorrhagic shock, and severe blunt trauma. Relationship with subsequent adult respiratory distress syndrome and multiple organ failure. Am Surg 1993;218:769–76.

14. Maier B, Schwerdtfeger K, Mautes A, et al. Differential release of interleukins 6, 8, and 10 in cerebrospinal fluid and plasma after traumatic brain injury. Shock 2001; 15:421–6.

15. Lausevic Z, Lausevic M, Trbojevic-Stankovic J, et al. Predicting multiple organ failure in patients with severe trauma. Can J Surg 2008;51:97–102.

16. Gebhard F, Pfetsch H, Steinbach G, et al. Is interleukin-6 an early marker of injury severity following major trauma in humans? Arch Surg 2000;135:291–5.

17. Stensballe J, Christiansen M, Tonnesen E, et al. The early IL-6 and IL-10 response in trauma is correlated with injury severity and mortality. Acta Anaesthesiol Scand 2009;53:515–21.

18. Giannoudis PV, Hildebrand F, Pape HC. Inflammatory serum markers in patients with multiple trauma. Can they predict outcome? J Bone Joint Surg Br 2004;86: 313–23.

19. Mimasaka S, Hashiyada M, Nata M, et al. Correlation between serum IL-6 levels and death: usefulness in diagnosis of "traumatic shock?" Tohoku J Exp Med 2001;193:319–24.

20. Johannes F, Marcus M, Jochen K, et al. Circulating inflammatory and metabolic parameters to predict organ failure after multiple trauma. Eur J Trauma 2002; V28:333–9.

21. Woiciechowsky C, Schoning B, Cobanov J, et al. Early IL-6 plasma concentrations correlate with severity of brain injury and pneumonia in brain-injured patients. J Trauma 2002;52:339–45.

22. Heizmann O, Koeller M, Muhr G, et al. Th1- and Th2-type cytokines in plasma after major trauma. J Trauma 2008;65:1374–8.

23. Tschoeke SK, Ertel W. Immunoparalysis after multiple trauma. Injury 2007;38: 1346–57.
24. Couper KN, Blount DG, Riley EM. IL-10: the master regulator of immunity to infection. J Immunol 2008;180:5771–7.
25. Ertel W, Morrison MH, Ayala A, et al. Blockade of prostaglandin production increases cachectin synthesis and prevents depression of macrophage functions after hemorrhagic shock. Ann Surg 1991;213:265–71.
26. Matzinger P. Friendly and dangerous signals: is the tissue in control? Nat Immunol 2007;8:11–3.
27. Marshall J. Both the disposition and the means of cure: 'severe SIRS', 'sterile shock', and the ongoing challenge of description. Crit Care Med 1997;25:1765–6.
28. Moore FA, Moore EE. Evolving concepts in the pathogenesis of postinjury multiple organ failure. Surg Clin North Am 1995;75:257–77.
29. Bianchi ME. DAMPs, PAMPs and alarmins: all we need to know about danger. J Leukoc Biol 2007;81:1–5.
30. Oppenheim JJ, Yang D. Alarmins: chemotactic activators of immune response. Curr Opin Immunol 2005;17:359–65.
31. Klune JR, Dhupar R, Cardinal J, et al. HMGB1: endogenous danger signaling. Mol Med 2008;14:476–84.
32. Fink MP. Bench-to-bedside review: high-mobility group box 1 and critical illness. Crit Care 2007;11:229.
33. Gibot S, Massin F, Cravoisy A, et al. High-mobility group box 1 protein plasma concentrations during septic shock. Intensive Care Med 2007;33:1347–53.
34. Cohen MJ, Brohi K, Calfee CS, et al. Early release of high mobility group box nuclear protein 1 after severe trauma in humans: role of injury severity and tissue hypoperfusion. Crit Care 2009;13:R174.
35. Sunden-Cullberg J, Norrby-Teglund A, Rouhiainen A, et al. Persistent elevation of high mobility group box-1 potein (HMGB1) in patients with severe sepsis and septic shock. Crit Care Med 2005;33:564–73.
36. Wang H, Bloom O, Zhang M, et al. HMG-1 as a late mediator of endotoxin lethality in mice. Science 1999;285:248–51.
37. Ombrellino M, Wang H, Ajemian MS, et al. Increased serum concentrations of high-mobility group protein 1 in hemorrhagic shock. Lancet 1999;354:1446–7.
38. Yang R, Harada N, Mollen KP, et al. Anti-HMGB1 neutralizing antibody ameliorates gut barrier dysfunction and improves survival after hemorrhagic shock. Mol Med 2006;12:104–14.
39. Kim JY, Park JS, Strassheim D, et al. HMGB1 contributes to the development of acute lung injury after hemorrhage. Am J Physiol Lung Cell Mol Physiol 2005;288:958–65.
40. Guo F, Shi Y, Xu H, et al. High mobility group box 1 as a mediator of endotoxin administration after hemorrhagic shock-primed lung injury. Braz J Med Biol Res 2009;42:804–11.
41. Mueller B, White JC, Nylen ES, et al. Ubiquitous expression of the calcitonin-1 gene in multiple tissues in response to sepsis. J Clin Endocrinol Metab 2001; 56:396–404.
42. Clec'h C, Ferriere F, Karoubi P, et al. Diagnostic and prognostic value of procalcitonin in patients with septic shock. Crit Care Med 2004;32:1166–9.
43. Uzzan B, Cohen R, Nicolas P, et al. Procalcitonin as a diagnostic test for sepsis in critically ill adults and after surgery or trauma: a systematic review and meta-analysis. Crit Care Med 2006;34:1996–2003.
44. Assicot M, Gendrel D, Carsin H, et al. High serum procalcitonin concentrations in patients with sepsis and infection. Lancet 1993;341:515–8.

45. Dahaba AA, Metzler H. Procalcitonin's role in the sepsis cascade. Is procalcitonin a sepsis marker or mediator? Minerva Anestesiol 2009;75:447–52.
46. Reith HB, Mittelkowtter U, Debus ES, et al. Procalcitonin in early detection of postoperative complications. Dig Surg 1998;15:260–5.
47. Dahaba AA, Hagara B, Fall A, et al. Procalcitonin for early prediction of survival outcome in postoperative critically ill patients with severe sepsis. Br J Anaesth 2006;97:503–8.
48. Mokart D, Merlin M, Sannini A, et al. Procalcitonin, interleukin 6 and systemic inflammatory response syndrome (SIRS): early markers of postoperative sepsis after major surgery. Br J Anaesth 2005;94:767–73.
49. Schroeder J, Staubach KH, Zabel P, et al. Procalcitonin as a marker of severity in septic shock. Langenbecks Arch Surg 1999;384:33–8.
50. Vincent JL, de Mendonca A, Cantraine F, et al. Use of the SOFA score to assess the incidence of organ dysfunction/failure in intensive care units: results of a multicenter, prospective study. Working group on "sepsis-related problems" of the European Society of Intensive Care Medicine. Crit Care Med 1998;26:1793–800.
51. Castelli GP, Pognani C, Cita M, et al. Procalcitonin as a prognostic and diagnostic tool for septic complications after major trauma. Crit Care Med 2009;37:1845–9.
52. Meisner M, Adina H, Schmidt J. Correlation of procalcitonin and C-reactive protein to inflammation, complications, and outcome during the intensive care unit course of multiple-trauma patients. Crit Care 2006;10:R1.
53. Balci C, Sivaci R, Akbulut G, et al. Procalcitonin level as an early marker in patients with multiple trauma under intensive care. J Int Med Res 2009;37: 1709–17.
54. Szalai AJ, Briles DE, Volnakis JE. Role of complement in C-reactive-protein-mediated protection of mice from *Streptococcus pneumoniae*. Infect Immun 1996;64:4850–3.
55. Biffl WL, Moore EE, Moore FA, et al. Interleukin-6 in the injured patient. Marker of injury or mediator of inflammation? Ann Surg 1996;224:647–64.
56. Herzum I, Renz H. Inflammatory markers in SIRS, sepsis and septic shock. Curr Med Chem 2008;15:581–7.
57. Hensler T, Sauerland S, Lefering R, et al. The clinical value of procalcitonin and neopterin in predicting sepsis and organ failure after major trauma. Shock 2003;20:420–6.
58. Wanner GA, Keel M, Steckholzer U, et al. Relationship between procalcitonin plasma levels and severity of injury, sepsis, organ failure, and mortality in injured patients. Crit Care Med 2000;28:950–7.
59. Rodl H, Schlag G, Togel E, et al. Procalcitonin release patterns in a baboon model of trauma and sepsis: relationship to cytokines and neopterin. Crit Care Med 2000;28:3659–63.
60. Maier M, Wutzler S, Lehnert M, et al. Serum procalcitonin levels in patients with multiple injuries including visceral trauma. J Trauma 2009;66:243–9.
61. Sauerland S, Hensler T, Bouillon B, et al. Plasma levels of procalcitonin and neopterin in multiple trauma patients with or without brain injury. J Neurotrauma 2003; 10:953–60.
62. Rush BF Jr, Sori AJ, Murphy TF, et al. Endotoxemia and bacteremia during hemorrhagic shock. The link between trauma and sepsis. J Trauma 1988;207:549–54.
63. Deitch EA. Bacterial translocation of the gut flora. J Trauma 1990;30:S184–9.
64. Deitch EA, Xu D, Franko L, et al. Evidence favoring the role of the gut as a cytokine-generating organ in rats subjected to hemorrhagic shock. Shock 1994;1:141–5.

65. Schmiegel W, Burchert M, Kalthoff H, et al. Immunochemical characterization and quantitative distribution of pancreatic stone protein in sera and pancreatic secretions in pancreatic disorders. Gastroenterology 1990;99:1421–30.
66. Dusetti NJ, Ortiz EM, Mallo GC, et al. Pancreatitis-associated protein I (PAP I), an acute phase protein induced by cytokines. Identification of two functional interleukin-6 response elements in the rat PAP I promoter region. J Biol Chem 1995;330:129–32.
67. Keel M, Harter L, Reding T, et al. Pancreatic stone protein is highly increased during posttraumatic sepsis and activates neutrophil granulocytes. Crit Care Med 2009;37:1642–8.
68. Becchi C, Pillozzi S, Fabbri LP, et al. The increase of endothelial progenitor cells in the peripheral blood: a new parameter for detecting onset and severity of sepsis. Int J Immunopathol Pharmacol 2008;21:697–705.
69. Livingston DH, Anjaria D, Wu J, et al. Bone marrow failure following severe injury in humans. Ann Surg 2003;238:748–53.
70. Saito K, Wagatsuma T, Toyama H, et al. Sepsis is characterized by the increase in percentages of circulating CD4$^+$CD25$^+$ regulatory T cells and plasma levels of soluble CD25. Tohoku J Exp Med 2008;216:61–8.
71. Ni Choileain N, MacConmara M, Zang Y, et al. Enhanced regulatory T cell activity is an element of the host response to injury. J Immunol 2006;176:225–36.
72. Hein F, Massin F, Cravoisy-Popovic A, et al. The relationship between CD4$^+$CD25$^+$CD127$^-$ regulatory T cells and inflammatory response and outcome during shock states. Crit Care 2010;14:R19.
73. Suttner SW, Boldt J. Natriuretic peptide system: physiology and clinical utility. Curr Opin Crit Care 2004;10:336–41.
74. Barr CS, Rhodes P, Struthers AD. C-type natriuretic peptide. Peptides 1996;17:1243–51.
75. Nazario B, Hu RM, Komatsu Y, et al. Cytokine induced C-type natriuretic peptide (CNP) secretion from vascular endothelium cells – evidence for CNP as a novel autocrine/paracrine regulator from endothelial cells. Endocrinology 1993;133:3038–41.
76. Bahrami S, Pelink L, Khadem A, et al. Circulating NT-proCNP predicts sepsis in multiple traumatized patients without brain injury. Crit Care Med 2010;38:161–6.
77. Osborn TM, Tracy JK, Dunne JR, et al. Epidemiology of sepsis in patients with traumatic injury. Crit Care Med 2004;32:2234–40.
78. Pierrakos C, Vincent JL. Sepsis biomarkers: a review. Crit Care 2010;14:R15.

Biomarkers in Acute Lung Injury: Insights into the Pathogenesis of Acute Lung Injury

L.J. Mark Cross, MRCP, PhD[a], Michael A. Matthay, MD[b,c,d],*

KEYWORDS

- Biomarkers • Acute lung injury
- Acute respiratory distress syndrome • Pathophysiology

The ability of the lung to perform gas exchange is made possible in part by the effective relationship between the alveolar epithelium and the endothelium of the pulmonary microvasculature.[1–4] When either barrier is injured, interstitial and alveolar edema may develop. Based on experimental in vitro and in vivo models, dysfunction of the normal endothelial–epithelial barriers plays a fundamental role in the development of acute lung injury (ALI).[2,5–13] ALI is characterized by noncardiogenic pulmonary edema and is associated with high mortality and morbidity associated with several clinical disorders including pneumonia, nonpulmonary sepsis, aspiration syndromes, and major trauma and shock.[2,14–17] Despite several clinical trials, no pharmacologic intervention has been shown to be effective in reducing mortality.[18–20] The selection and design of novel therapeutic interventions target should be achieved by understanding of the pathophysiological mechanisms involved in ALI.[2,19,20] Studies of biomarkers of lung and systemic injury in patients with ALI (and in animal models) can provide more insight into the pathogenesis of ALI and potentially help in the design of novel therapeutic approaches and objectively assessing the response to new

Disclosure: LJMC has received funding from Northern Ireland HSC Research and Development Fellowship.

[a] Centre for Infection and Immunity, Queen's University of Belfast, Room 01/014, Health Sciences Building, 97 Lisburn Road, Belfast, BT9 7BL, Northern Ireland, UK
[b] Cardiovascular Research Institute, University of California, San Francisco, 505 Parnassus Avenue, M-917, San Francisco, CA 94143-0624, USA
[c] Department of Medicine, Division of Pulmonary and Critical Care, University of California, San Francisco, 505 Parnassus Avenue, San Francisco, CA 94143-2202, USA
[d] Department of Anesthesia, University of California, San Francisco, 505 Parnassus Avenue, San Francisco, CA 94143-2202, USA
* Corresponding author. 505 Parnassus Avenue, Moffitt Hospital, M-917, University of California, San Francisco, CA 94143-0624.
E-mail address: michael.matthay@ucsf.edu

Crit Care Clin 27 (2011) 355–377
doi:10.1016/j.ccc.2010.12.005
0749-0704/11/$ – see front matter © 2011 Elsevier Inc. All rights reserved.

therapies as a surrogate marker. The ideal biomarker also should possess both high sensitivity and high specificity for predicting clinical outcomes (**Box 1**).[21]

Over the past 20 years, focus on biomarkers in ALI has yielded important information regarding the pathophysiology of the lung injury and repair and has highlighted which cells and their mediators have been involved.[22–28] Studies of biomarkers also have led indirectly to the generation of new ideas regarding potential novel therapeutic targets.[19,20,29] These biomarkers in ALI can reflect either cellular activation or cell injury, as well as ongoing acute activation of the inflammatory, coagulation, and fibrinolytic systems. Some of the biologic markers may possess pleiotropic effects and may have a role in the repair process. Some of these biomarkers have been investigated as potential surrogate markers for the development of ALI as well as clinical outcomes, such as ventilator-free days, morbidity, and mortality.[22,24] Currently, biomarkers in ALI remain primarily within the domain of a research tool to aid in the delineation of the pathophysiologic mechanisms involved in ALI and its subsequent repair, although they have been shown to have prognostic value also. The validation of readily measurable biomarkers that may have a role in the design of future clinical trials or in selecting subgroups of patients with ALI is an important long-term objective. In addition to clinical criteria for ALI, biomarkers could be of value in evaluating and testing new pharmacologic or cell-based therapies for ALI.[22,24]

This article reviews some of the biomarkers that have been investigated in ALI, with a focus on biomarkers in groups that reflect their primary function (**Table 1**). In ALI, there are at least two different phases.[2] Initially there is an exudative phase occurring early, associated with diffuse alveolar damage, microvascular injury with subsequent pulmonary edema, type 1 pneumocyte necrosis, and the influx of inflammatory cells and mediator release. This phase is followed by a fibro-proliferative phase, during which there is proliferation of fibroblasts and type 2 pneumocyte hyperplasia and lung repair.[2] To date, the mechanisms of epithelial repair at the alveolar level has focused mostly on the role of the alveolar type 2 cell type and how these cells and the progenitor cells spread, migrate, and proliferate and what mechanisms are involved in this process and if any of these mechanisms could lead to therapeutic targets in the future.[30] The mechanisms that are important in lung epithelial repair include interactions with the extracellular matrix components, structural components, cellular signaling pathways leading to spreading and/or migration, and other mediators that might be important in progenitor cell selection, proliferation, or recruitment.[30]

INFLAMMATION

The inflammatory responses in ALI can either be directly related to an ongoing primary infectious stimulus such as pneumonia or there may be systemic inflammation that is being amplified by the lung injury.[2,31] The inflammatory cascade involves inflammatory cells and the release of inflammatory mediators.[31] Comparing the ratio of cytokines in serum with bronchoalveolar lavage fluid (BALF) suggests that most of the

---

Box 1
Biomarkers for acute lung injury: the ideal properties

High sensitivity and specificity in predicting clinical outcome

Sample has to be easily and safely collected from critically ill patients and the biomarker has to be able to be easily measured with reproducible results across multiple sites

Has a defined role in the pathogenesis of acute lung injury and repair

inflammatory mediators have a pulmonary origin and are not just the effect of the exudative phase of ALI with the flooding of the alveolar environment with serum mediators. There are both proinflammatory and anti-inflammatory mediators; therefore it maybe more the balance of these mediators and their biologic inhibitors in the surrounding milieu that regulate much of the development of lung injury and repair, which may have implications for their use as biomarkers in isolation or in combination.[30,31] Most publications have focused on the significance of antigenic levels of inflammatory biomarkers rather than determination of the net inflammatory balance (use of molar ratios), which maybe be of greater physiologic and clinical importance. Inflammatory mediators have been measured both in the plasma or serum, or locally in BALF or undiluted pulmonary edema fluid.[2,24,32,33] These mediators may be actively secreted from cells that have been recruited into the air spaces in response to the inflammatory cascade or may appear due to release from cellular death.[2,24,32–34] These inflammatory mediators include the proinflammatory cytokines such as interleukin (IL)-1β, tumor necrosis factor (TNF)α, IL-6, and IL-8 which possess potent proinflammatory actions, as well as the anti-inflammatory interleukins including IL-1ra, IL-10, and IL-13 (**Fig. 1**).

One of the most biologically active cytokines in the early phases of ALI is IL-1β, which is elevated in plasma and is predictive of clinical outcomes.[35–37] IL-1β is a potent inducer of lung fibrosis[38–40] and causes release of various proinflammatory chemokines (eg, monocyte chemotactic protein [MCP]-1, macrophage inflammatory protein [MIP] -1α, IL-6, and IL-8) with subsequent recruitment of inflammatory cells[41–45] into the air spaces. Additionally, IL-1β can alter endothelial–epithelial barrier permeability and fluid transport, leading to edema (which is mediated in part via the αvβ5/β6 integrin pathway).[46] IL-1β is elevated in plasma and BALF in patients with ALI, but also is elevated in higher tidal volume and lower positive end-expiratory pressure (PEEP) ventilation.[47,48] Due to these important clinical findings in patients with ALI and the understanding of IL-1 biology, including the knowledge of the existence of the presence of the naturally occurring inhibitors of IL-1 signaling, namely IL-1Ra or sIL-1RII,[49,50] it is proposed that these could be putative novel therapeutic targets. The existence of polymorphisms of IL-1Ra gives some clinical insight into the relevance of IL-1 biology in the role of ALI.[51] IL-1Ra has been demonstrated to be elevated in BALF of patients with ALI.[52,53] However, it may be important to investigate the ratio between the levels of proinflammatory IL-1β and anti-inflammatory IL-1Ra, because this ratio determines the net inflammatory effect of IL-1β.[50] The ratio of IL-1β/IL-1Ra influences the production of other mediators that may be important in epithelial repair, such as hepatocyte growth factor (HGF) via a cyclooxygenase 2 (COX-2)/prostaglandin E2 dependent mechanism.[54] However, one study demonstrated that there was a significant relationship between an IL-1β functional bioassay and the antigenic measurement of IL-1β, and the presence of the antagonists IL-1Ra or sIL-1RII did not correlate with IL-1β biologic activity.[50]

Another early proinflammatory cytokine that is in both plasma and BALF in the early phase of ALI is TNFα. It is postulated that resident alveolar macrophages stimulated by pathogen recognition generate much of the production of the early cytokines, IL-1β and TNF-α, which in turn stimulate neighboring cells to produce a battery of chemokines that mediate the recruitment of neutrophils, monocytes, and lymphocytes into the alveolar space.[55–58] The alveolar macrophages may initially be important therefore in the proinflammatory stage, but they also have been postulated to have important anti-inflammatory activity in the resolution/repair phase via phagocytosis of apoptotic neutrophils and cell debris as well as secreting epithelial growth factors in a TNFα-dependent mechanism. TNFα also has been demonstrated to indirectly

Table 1
Summary table of biomarkers that have been investigated in acute lung injury

Biomarker	System Classification	Predictive of Clinical Outcome	Evidence as Role as Biomarker from Multicenter Studies	Biologic Sample Source	Summary of Pathogenesis Role in +	Summary of Cellular Mechanisms as Potential Therapeutic Targets
IL-1β	Proinflammatory	Positive	No	Plasma BALF	↑ permeability of alveolar barrier; Induction of inflammatory cytokines and chemokines; Recruitment of inflammatory cells; Profibrotic; Epithelial repair	αvβ5/β6 integrins pathway; IL-1R/Toll-like receptor activation via RhoA; ↑ COX-2 producing PGE-2 that activates EP-3 receptors; EGF/TGF-a pathway and MAPK
IL-1Ra / sIL-1RII and their ratio with IL-1β	Anti-inflammatory	Negative	No	Plasma BALF	Anti-inflammatory antagonist of IL-1β	↓ in IL-1β bioavailability
TNF-α	Pleiotropic	Positive	No	Plasma BALF	Induction of inflammatory cytokines and chemokines; Recruitment of inflammatory cells; Indirectly promote pulmonary edema; ↑ permeability of alveolar barrier; Repair mechanisms	Activation of TNF-α receptors TNF-R1, TNF-R2 and sTNF-R and subsequent pathways; Production of ROS, which ↓ ENaC and Na+-K+ATPase; RhoA/ROCK; Phagocytosis of apoptotic neutrophils and debris
sTNFr-I and II	Anti-inflammatory	Positive	Yes	Plasma BALF	Modulates TNF-α activity	Binds TNF and reduces its bioavailability to bind to its cellular receptors

IL-8	Pro-inflammatory	Positive	Plasma BALF (not reliable predictor source)	Yes	Recruitment of inflammatory cells Activation and priming of neutrophils Upregulation of adhesion molecules Activation of the endothelium	CXCR1 and CXCR2 receptors via G_i CXCR1 and CXCR2 via Rho and Rac
Anti-IL-8 autoantibody/IL-8 immune complexes	Proinflammatory	Positive	Plasma BALF	No	Complement activation Dysfunction of epithelial and endothelial Modulation of IL-8 bioactivity	FCγRIIa pathway via ERK, Syk, Src, PI3-K
IL-6	Pleiotropic	Positive	Plasma BALF	Yes	Lymphocyte differentiation and activation–both B cell and T cell Monocyte/macrophage activation Epithelial repair and endothelial cytoprotective	ERK pathway via JAK/STAT, Ras/ERK and PI3-K/Akt Cross talk with cytokines and inactivation of proapoptotic proteins via PI3-K/Akt
sIL-6R and ratio with IL-6	Proinflammatory	Positive	Plasma	No	Enhancement of IL-6 effects	IL-6 agonist activity binds with IL-6 to promote gp130 dimerization
IL-18	Proinflammatory	Not determined	Plasma	Preclinical and experimental models	Neutrophil recruitment and activation Cofactor for lymphocyte differentiation and activation	Induction of IFN-γ via activation of the IL-1 receptor (R)/Toll receptor family
IL-10	Anti-inflammatory	Negative	Plasma	Yes	Inhibition of T_H differentiation	Inhibition of NF-κβ

(continued on next page)

Table 1 (*continued*)

Biomarker	System Classification	Predictive of Clinical Outcome	Biologic Sample Source	Evidence as Role as Biomarker from Multicenter Studies	Summary of Pathogenesis Role in +	Summary of Cellular Mechanisms as Potential Therapeutic Targets
					Inhibition of chemokine and cytokine release Neutrophil suppression	
IL-4	Anti-inflammatory	No	Plasma BALF	No	Epithelial repair Inhibits synthesis of proinflammatory cytokines Increases production of IL-1Ra Pulmonary fibrosis	IRS-1 or -2
IL-13	Pleitropic	Negative	Plasma	No	Suppresses pro-inflammatory cytokine production Increases production of IL-1Ra	Inhibition of NF-κβ
TGF-β	Pleitropic	Negative	Plasma	No	Inhibits expression of proinflammatory adhesion molecules	Via Smad proteins
Protein C	Coagulation	Positive	Plasma	Yes	Endogenous anticoagulant Improves endothelial permeability Suppression of proinflammatory cytokines	Activation of the sphigosine-1-phosphate pathway Induced transcription of antiapoptotic proteins
PAI-1	Coagulation	Positive	Plasma BALF	Yes	Regulate fibrinolysis and dissolution of fibrin clots Directly inhibits integrin-mediated cell migration	Inhibits plasminogen activator

Thrombomodulin	Coagulation	Positive	BALF	No	↓ fibrin deposition ↓ leukocyte accumulation ↓ alveolar permeability and pulmonary edema	Cofactor in thrombin-induced activation of protein C
HGF	Growth factor	Positive	BALF	No	Alveolar epithelial cell mitogen Epithelial repair	C-Met receptor and activation of PI-3 K pathway or tyrosine kinase activation
KGF	Growth factor	Not determined	BALF	No	Alveolar epithelial cell mitogen Epithelial repair	FGF receptor and activation of tyrosine kinase
VGEF	Growth factor	Positive	Plasma BALF (decreased levels)	No	↑ vascular permeability ↑ endothelial cell survival and proliferation	Via VEGF tyrosine kinase family of receptors
Ang-2/Ang-1	Growth factor	Positive	Plasma	No	Promotes endothelial and epithelial apoptosis Causes barrier dysfunction	Tie-2 receptor tyrosine kinase
Surfactant D	Epithelial cell type 2 marker	Positive	Plasma BALF	Yes	↓ surface tension Confer innate immunity	Physical properties of the molecule and induce phagocytosis
RAGE	Epithelial cell-type 1 marker	Positive	Plasma BALF	Yes	Production of proinflammatory cytokines, ROS and protease production	Binds EN-RAGE or HMGB-1 and activates NFκB
VWF	Endothelial cell marker	Positive	Plasma BALF	Yes	Hemostasis and role in platelet function	Intrinsic activity

Abbreviations: ↑, increased; ↓, decreased BALF, bronchoalveolar lavage fluid; COX-2, cyclooxygenase 2; EGF, epidermal growth factor; ERK, extracellular signal-regulated kinase; HMGB, high-mobility group box; IFN, interferon; IL, interleukin; JAK/STAT, Janus kinase/signal transducer and activator of transcription; RAGE, receptor for advanced glycation end products TGF, transforming growth factor; TNF, tumor necrosis factor; VEGF, vascular endothelial growth factor.

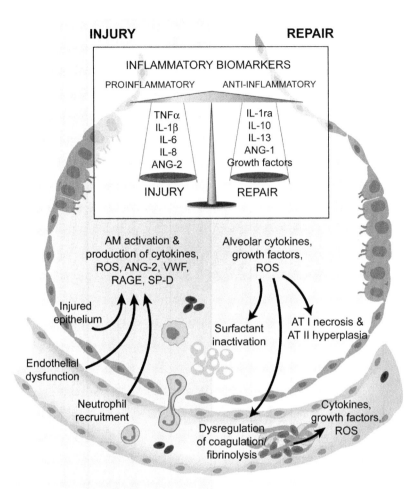

Fig. 1. The injured alveolus in the acute phase (left hand side) and the repair phase in acute lung injury (ALI). In the acute exudative phase, there is activation of resident alveolar macrophages, which results in production of several proinflammatory molecules. These stimulate chemotaxis and activation of neutrophils that release various mediators that further increase the proinflammatory environment of the injured alveolus and are associated with alveolar endothelial and epithelial injury. Some of the mechanisms that play a role repair in ALI are illustrated (right hand side). Alveolar type 2 cells undergo hyperplasia, and there is also recruitment of fibroblasts (not shown). There is release of growth factors and anti-inflammatory cytokines involved in repair. These mediators as well as cell-specific activation/injury can be measured as biomarkers. AM, alveolar macrophage; ANG, angiopoietin; AT, alveolar epithelial cell type; IL, interleukin; IL-1ra, interleukin 1 receptor antagonist, RAGE, receptor for advanced glycation end products, reactive oxygen species, SPD, surfactant D; VWF, von Willebrand factor.

promote pulmonary edema by producing reactive oxygen species that subsequently decrease the expression of ENaC and the Na$^+$-K$^+$-ATPase.[59] The dysregulation of the microcirculation leading to increased permeability occurs in part by a RhoA/ROCK-dependent destabilization of the microtubules.[60] There is some evidence that TNFα is increased in plasma and BALF and is predictive of outcome in single center studies.[36,61] The lack of correlation of TNFα with outcomes in multicenter studies may relate to the timing of measurement and the source of measurement, as well as the effect that the presence of the soluble TNFα receptors (sTNFr) 1 and 2, which can bind TNF and compete with its binding to the cellular receptor, thus reducing its bioavailability of TNFα.[62] sTNFr 1 and 2 are elevated in the plasma and have been demonstrated to be predictive of a poor outcome.[28,62] TNFα has been modulated by the use of pharmacologic agents in experimental models including inhibitors of TNF-α mRNA transcription (eg, pentoxifylline), accelerators of TNF-α mRNA degradation (eg, thalidomide), inhibitors of TNF-α protein translation (eg, tetravalent guanylhydrazones), and the metalloproteinase inhibitors that prevent the cleavage of the membrane-bound protein to the active moiety.[20,63–68] In the last decade there have been substantive investigations of these inhibitors in preclinical models of ALI, with some of these inhibitors being taken into further drug development in the form of early clinical trials but with little evidence of outcome data.[18]

IL-6 and IL-8 are two other proinflammatory cytokines that have been demonstrated to be elevated in both plasma and BALF and are predictive of poor outcomes in ALI patients.[61,69] IL-8 has a role in neutrophil and monocyte chemotaxis and inhibits neutrophil apoptosis and elevated levels correlates well with number of neutrophils and total protein (a surrogate marker for permeability of the alveolar barrier) in BALF and also are elevated in nonsurvivors compared with survivors in single-center and multicenter studies.[61,70] The BALF levels of IL-8 have yielded varying results in different studies, in which there have been significant differences between survivors and nonsurvivors.[53,57,71] Other studies, however, have not demonstrated this difference.[72,73] This result is similar to various other proinflammatory cytokines (eg, IL-6, MCP-1), perhaps reflecting the heterogeneous group of ALI patients utilized in these studies, the timing of the collection of the BALF, and the uncertain relationship to the timing of the onset of ALI. BALF IL-8 levels recently were demonstrated to be negatively correlated with lung compliance and positively correlated with changes in Sequential Organ Failure Assessment score (SOFA).[33] Recently, BALF IL-8 levels were demonstrated to be independently associated with mortality in a multivariate analysis of patients with infection-induced ALI in a single center study.[33] Obviously BALF measurement requires an invasive procedure, and the use of plasma IL-8 may be easier and safer for these critically ill patients. Indeed in children with septic shock, plasma levels less than 220 pg/mL identify patients with a low risk for death with a negative predictive value of 94% to 95% for 28-day mortality.[74] However, in a recent paper investigating the role of plasma IL-8 in the adult population with ALI, the correlation with 28-day mortality and the plasma IL-8 levels above 220 pg/mL was much weaker in the adult group than in the pediatric population.[75] These differences probably can be explained in part by the heterogeneity of ALI patients in the adult population, who were selected prospectively for septic shock and the differences in comorbidities that occur in the adult population that will affect the mediators and clinical outcomes. Finally, the timing of the onset of sepsis was not recorded in the adult population, whereas within the pediatric population the IL-8 was recorded at 24 hours after admission to the intensive care unit (ICU). Another difference is that of adult obesity and elevated body mass index (BMI). One group of investigators reported that within the adult population with ALI the plasma IL-8 levels fall with increasing BMI, but this did not correspond to improvement in clinical outcomes.[76] Several studies have evaluated the role of the anti-IL-8 autoantibody/IL-8 immune complexes in ALI.[77] These complexes are present in patients who have been just admitted to ICU and before the inflammatory cascade with influx of neutrophils or resultant lung injury.[78] A mixture of IL-8 and IL-8 autoantibodies (in excess) has inhibitory actions on neutrophil recruitment and activation; however, IL-8 autoantibody/IL-8 immune complexes from patients with ALI have the ability via the FCγRIIa to possess proinflammatory activities.[79–81] It also has been demonstrated that blocking the FCγRIIa pathway suppresses the in vitro proinflammatory actions of this immune complex.[80] The immune complex evokes complement activation and interaction with human epithelial and endothelial cells, leading to loss of integrity via cellular dysfunction. The IL-8 autoantibody/IL-8–FCγRIIa pathway signaling molecules could act as potential therapeutic targets for future development (eg, Src, spleen tyrosine kinase [Syk], phosphoinositide 3-kinases [PI3-K], and extracellular signal-regulated kinase [ERK]).[80,82] In one study, the levels of these immune complexes were higher in those patients who developed ALI, and there was a correlation with mortality in patients who already had developed ALI.[78]

IL-6 is another cytokine involved in ALI that signals through the ERK pathway[83] and can activate multiple signal transduction pathways including Janus kinase/signal transducer and activator of transcription (JAK/STAT), rat sarcoma/extracellular signal-regulated kinase (Ras/ERK), and the PI3-K/Akt.[83–85] IL-6 is critical for B cell differentiation and maturation with secretion of immunoglobulins, cytotoxic T cell differentiation, macrophage and monocyte function, and production of acute phase proteins. Elevated levels of IL-6 in plasma and BALF have been reported in both single center studies as well as larger multicenter studies to predict mortality in ALI.[61,69] Although IL-6 activates both proinflammatory and anti-inflammatory mechanisms, IL-6 primarily has a proinflammatory profile. The presence of the IL-6 agonist sIL-6R also has been investigated in ALI, and higher molar ratio of IL-6/sIL-6R is associated with a higher risk of death.[50] Additionally, IL-6 has been investigated in ALI as a candidate gene with studies that have focused on IL-6 single-nucleotide polymorphism (SNPs) in the -174 promoter region and other gene polymorphisms of IL-6.[86–88] Currently there has been no uniform finding from these studies, and further research is required, as the IL-6 polymorphisms may be stimulus specific.[88–90] IL-6 is protective in hyperoxia-induced lung injury, in which IL-6 is cytoprotective to endothelial cells via inactivation of types of proapoptotic proteins (eg, B-cell lymphoma 2 [Bcl-2]-associated X protein [Bax]) via phosphorylation via the PI3 K/Akt pathway.[91] IL-6 has also been demonstrated to possess pleiotropic effects in vitro and in vivo and has been suggested to play an important role in the repair of the alveolar epithelium. These pleiotropic effects are reported to be due to the cross talk with other cytokines in the alveolar environment and the particular cell types present that express the receptor for IL-6.[92,93]

There are other cytokines that possess anti-inflammatory actions (eg, IL-10, transforming growth factor-β [TGF-β], IL-13, and IL-4). Novel therapeutic targets could be designed around such mediators, which can in vivo attenuate the injury to the lung. IL-10 has preventative value in lipopolysaccharide (LPS)-induced ALI via its anti-inflammatory actions including its inhibition of T_H1 differentiation, suppression of neutrophil activation, and chemokine down-regulation.[92] This effect may be achieved by the destabilization of mRNA of proinflammatory chemokines and preventing degradation of IκB-α, therefore inhibiting the activation of NF-κB, a proinflammatory intracellular signal moiety.[93–95] The timing of IL-10 administration in relationship to the injury is influential on its ability to possess anti-inflammatory activities. In a multicenter trial, the presence of increased plasma levels of IL-10 was a negative predictor of a poor outcome.[69] IL-13 is another pleiotropic cytokine that possesses potent anti-inflammatory properties. It is mostly produced from T_H2 cells and also from T_H1 cells to a lesser extent and suppresses TNF-α, IL-1β, IL-8, and chemokine production and like IL-10 inhibits the activation of NFκB, but can also enhance the production of the anti-inflammatory moiety IL-1Ra.[95–97] In addition to the anti-inflammatory cytokines, there is also an important effect of endogenous anti-inflammatory soluble receptors and other moieties that may bind with the proinflammatory cytokine, hence reducing its bioavailability and adjusting the net balance between proinflammatory and anti-inflammatory effects. Within the local environment there will be an influence of the cells (that constitute the alveolar microenvironment) by the variable expression of cellular receptors, which therefore bind and influence the bioavailability of the mediators, a process that may have differing effects depending on the timing of the ligand receptor interaction during ALI, especially if the cytokine possesses pleiotropic effects. The inflammatory cascade has an important effect on the inflammatory cells that are recruited into the alveoli and via their mediator release can elicit injury to the epithelial and endothelial barriers, but in certain instances can also be important in the repair and resolution phase as highlighted by IL-6. Additionally, the inflammatory cascade is important in leading to hemorrhage within the alveoli, in part related to the interactions with the coagulation and fibrinolytic cascades and platelets.

Coagulation and Fibrinolysis

Activation of the inflammatory cascade results in the activation of the coagulation system, which in turn can influence inflammatory responses by effecting expression of IL-1, IL-6, and IL-8 and migration of inflammatory cells across the endothelial and epithelial barriers into the alveoli.[98–100] The proinflammatory events also may inhibit fibrinolysis and also induce platelet activation.[99–104] Several coagulation biomarkers have been demonstrated to be abnormal in ALI including protein C, plasminogen activator inhibitor (PAI-1) and thrombomodulin.[26,98,105,106] Thrombomodulin activates protein C, leading to the formation of a thrombus. The alveolar epithelium contains thrombomodulin, which can activate protein C, leading to formation of activated protein C (APC), an important endogenous anticoagulant. APC can improve endothelial permeability via activation of the sphigosine-1-phosphate pathway and suppression of proinflammatory cytokines. In ALI, the plasma and BALF levels of protein C (part of the APC complex) are low, and the plasma levels of PAI-1 are elevated. Both of these findings have been associated with increased mortality.[26,98,105,106] Therefore, there was a rationale for drug trials in patients with ALI with therapeutic interventions focused on administering pharmacologic doses of human recombinant APC.[107–110] Based on in vitro studies, APC can protect the endothelial barrier via protease-activated receptor-1 (PAR-1)-dependent mechanisms. In the PROWESS trial of APC for severe sepsis, APC was anticipated to have anticoagulant and anti-inflammatory effects that may have benefited patients with more severe sepsis.[109,111] A recent phase 2 trial, in which patients with ALI from nonseptic causes were studied, APC was not effective in increasing VFDs but did decrease pulmonary dead space.[110] The mortality rate in this study was only 13 % compared with other ALI studies that included patients with sepsis in whom the mortality is higher, approximately 25%. The results of this trial agree with the results of the ADDRESS and RESOLVE trials in which patients had no benefit from APC, but their severity of illness was less than in the original trial of severe sepsis in PROWESS.[112,113] PROWESS-SHOCK is a large phase 3 clinical trial that is testing the efficacy of APC in patients with persistent septic shock and high risk of death. Recruitment is expected to be finished by summer of 2011.[114,115]

Fibrinolytic activity is decreased in patients with ALI, which may in part be related to high BALF levels of PAI-1 as well as decreased fibrinolysis. There is also the occurrence of increased fibrin production.[99,100,106,116] PAI-1 is secreted by various cells such as endothelial cells, epithelial cells, macrophages, and fibroblasts. The significantly higher plasma levels of PAI-1 in ALI patients who do not survive may reflect a greater impairment in the fibrinolytic system in these patients.

Platelets also play a crucial role in hemostasis and thrombosis as well as the coagulation and fibrinolytic system. However, over the last decade it has been documented that the platelets have a diverse and extended role via their ability to release mediators to recruit inflammatory cells and progenitor cells, release proinflammatory and anti-inflammatory cytokines, as well angiogenic factors, all of which may contribute to the pathobiology of ALI. All of these pathways utilize various active moieties including chemokines, P-selectins, and other adhesion molecules as well as signaling molecules such as Src kinases, all of which may be future therapeutic targets. The selectins have been studied in small single center studies are expressed on the vascular endothelium and platelets and along with adhesion molecules help facilitate the interactions between inflammatory cells, platelets, and vascular endothelium.[117–119] The contribution of these cells in the pathophysiology of ALI are influenced by various mediators already outlined, but they also are regulated by growth factors and components of the extracellular milieu which will be briefly discussed in the next sections.

Growth Factors

Growth factors appear to play a major role in the repair and resolution of ALI.[120] The repair of the damaged alveolar epithelium is an incompletely understood process that involves hyperplasia of type 2 pneumocytes (and perhaps type 1 pneumocytes), migration along the basement membrane by the type 2 cells to form a new epithelial barrier, and complex interactions with extracellular matrix and other cells such as alveolar macrophages.[43,121,122] Various growth factors promote repair of the alveolar epithelium including keratinocyte growth factor (KGF), hepatocyte growth factor (HGF), epidermal growth factor (EGF), acidic fibroblast growth factor (FGF), retinoic acid, transforming growth factor-α (TGF-α), and insulin-like growth factor (IGF-1). Lung endothelial repair is promoted by vascular endothelial growth factor (VEGF). Repair can be accompanied by fibrosis that may be promoted by TGF-β, activin-A, platelet-derived growth factor (PDGF), basic FGF, and IGF-1 but inhibited by HGF and interferon-γ (IFN-γ). There are at least two major pathways that growth factors utilize in ALI, either tyrosine kinase receptor mediation (eg, KGF, HGF, FGF, VEGF, EGF and PDGF), or serine-threonine kinase receptors such as TGFβ1, which tend to have an opposing effect on the upregulation that occurs when the tyrosine kinase receptor pathway is utilized.[44,123] Some of these growth factors have been studied as biomarkers in ALI.

KGF and HGF are potent mitogens for type 2 pneumocytes and are postulated to play an important role in the repair of the epithelium following lung injury.[124,125] KGF and HGF are elevated in BALF from patients with ALI.[124] HGF can be produced by alveolar neutrophils, macrophages, endothelial cells, and fibroblasts and upregulated by various proinflammatory cytokines such as IL-1β and TNFα via a COX_2/PGE_2-dependent mechanism.[125,126] HGF also can be released by the proteolytic activity of proteases that cleave the HGF from the extracellular matrix. In a single center study, elevation of HGF was associated with worse clinical outcomes.[124] HGF mediates its effects via the c-Met receptor, which initiates several downstream effects such as protecting cells from DNA damage (via PI-3 K pathway) and enhancing epithelial cell motility Gab-1 recruitment (Ras/Rac and PI-3 K).[54,127] There is a need to investigate how the combined effects of these growth factors occur such as the synergistic effect of HGF with VGEF on endothelial cell activity and the combined effect of HGF with KGF in the repair of lung injury.

In the lung, VEGF is produced primarily by epithelial cells. VEGF seems to increase microvascular permeability in ALI, but also during the repair phase has an important role in increasing endothelial cell proliferation and survival. The levels of VEGF are increased in plasma from patients with ALI, but are decreased in BALF compared with healthy controls. Subsequently BALF VEGF increases during the resolution of the lung injury.[128–132] The role of VEGF in ALI is not fully delineated but the low levels of VEGF in BALF from ALI patients and patients with hydrostatic edema may indicate that the low levels are due to a dilutional effect from alveolar flooding in the exudative edema fluid.[132] Certain single studies have shown increased plasma VEGF and decreased BALF VEGF levels are associated with worse clinical outcomes.

Among vascular growth factors that have been demonstrated to be linked to outcome in ALI patients are the angiopoietin peptides angiopoietin 1 (Ang-1) and angiopoietin 2 (Ang-2) and in particular the ratio of Ang-2/Ang-1.[133,134] These peptides bind to the Tie-2 receptor tyrosine kinase and act in an agonist/antagonist manner.[135] Ang-1 via the Tie-2 receptor stabilizes the endothelium by dampening inflammation and inhibiting apoptosis of the endothelial cell, whereas Ang-2 promotes endothelial and epithelial apoptosis, phosphorylates myosin light chains, and causes barrier dysfunction.[134,135] Both of these peptides work to modify the integrity of the microvascular endothelium. One recent study reported that a high ratio of Ang-2/Ang-1 was an independent predictor of mortality in patients with ALI, even after adjustment for other variables associated with poor outcomes.[134]

Biomarkers of Alveolar Epithelial/Endothelial Injury

Because alveolar epithelial injury plays an important role in determining the severity of ALI, investigators have studied biochemical markers that may reflect injury to either the type 1 or type 2 alveolar epithelial cell. Surfactant proteins are primarily secreted by type 2 pneumocytes and are amphiphilic lipoproteins that help maintain low alveolar surface tension preventing alveolar collapse and they have a role in the innate immune defense of the lung. Surfactant protein D is primarily a product of type 2 cells, and the receptor for advanced glycation end products (RAGE) is released primarily by type 1 cells.[136–138] RAGE belongs to the immunoglobulin superfamily and binds calgranulin (also called EN-RAGE) or high-mobility group box-1 (HMGB-1), which activates NF$\kappa\beta$ leading to the production of proinflammatory cytokines, reactive oxygen species, and protease production.[28,139–142] Both of these proteins are elevated in the plasma in ALI patients and have been associated with worse clinical outcomes.[136–138] Elevated levels of plasma RAGE early in ALI seem to identify patients with more alveolar epithelial injury, and it is those patients who benefited most from low tidal volume ventilation in the randomized ARDS net trial. Another epithelial protein that has been studied as a potential biomarker is an epithelial mucin protein, called Kerbs von den Lungren-6 (KL-6), which is unregulated during injury on the surface of the type 2 pneumocytes.[143] KL-6 has been demonstrated to be increased in interstitial lung disease in which there is disarray of the alveolar structure, and it is correlated with increased barrier permeability.[144] Early pulmonary edema levels of KL-6 have been demonstrated to be elevated in patients with ALI who did not survive compared with patients with ALI who have better mortality, but increased KL-6 levels are not able to predict those patients who are at risk of developing ALI.[143,145,146] As well as the important role the alveolar epithelium type 1 and 2 play in ALI and repair, there is one other cell type that produces a protein that may have an important role as a biomarker, namely the Clara cell and the protein called Clara cell-specific protein (CC-16).[147] This has been evaluated in a single center study in which elevated CC-16 serum level was associated with increased risk of mortality. This may prove to be a biomarker of interest in the future.

Not only is there epithelial injury, but endothelial dysfunction plays a central role in lung injury and repair (see **Fig. 1**), not only in contributing to the influx of inflammatory cells and mediators during the exudative phase but as an active source of growth factors and mediators that can affect vascular tone, cellular proliferation, and angiogenesis. The endothelium is also the site in which the above systems of inflammation, coagulation and fibrinolysis cross talk can occur and therefore influences directly the outcome of these systems. Endothelial activity is detected again by the use of various potential biomarkers including von Willebrand factor (VWF), angiotensin converting enzyme, or tissue factor pathway inhibitor, and many studies have focused on these in ALI as has been reviewed recently.[148] VWF has been well documented both in multi-center trials and single center trials to be increased in plasma and BALF of patients with ALI as well as be associated with being predictive of outcome of these patients.[107,149,150] VWF is a glycoprotein that is secreted by both the megakaryocytes and the vascular endothelium, and it has a pivotal role in hemostasis by being the carrier protein for clotting factors such as factor 9 as well as acting as a mechanical bridging component between the platelets and the endothelium. There have been two major studies that have indicated that the plasma levels of VWF are not predictive of the onset of ALI.[107,149] However, more recently[150] in a study with patients in the early phase of ALI, the pulmonary edema fluid and the plasma levels of VWF were associated with clinical outcome, demonstrating that the endothelium activation is associated with increased mortality.

The study of proteins in the alveolar compartment may be a useful research tool to help delineate mechanisms that are involved in the lung injury and repair process. Proteomics is useful, as it not only permits the identification and quantification of novel proteins that are present in the process but also can identify structural changes that may occur to some of these proteins that will directly effect the native biologic activity. These are post-translational modification, such as glycation, glycosylation, phosphorylation, or sulphation, which can regulate the activity of the proteins, which can be missed when relying on identification of proteins simply by antigenic recognition.[151–153]

SUMMARY

Studies of biomarkers in ALI have provided valuable insights into the pathogenesis of lung injury and repair. Currently, it is not possible to identify a single biomarker that is specific or sensitive enough to be incorporated into routine clinical practice. However, in the future, measurement of plasma biomarkers may help stratify ALI patients for clinical trials. As illustrated in one recent study,[24] the combination of clinical predictors and elevated levels of two to three plasma biomarkers may prove useful to predict prognosis in patients with ALI, as well as to select patients for clinical trials of new therapeutic modalities.

ACKNOWLEDGMENTS

Thanks to Professor DF McAuley for help in manuscript preparation.

REFERENCES

1. Bernard GR, Brigham KL. Pulmonary edema: pathophysiologic mechanisms and new approaches to therapy. Chest 1986;89:594–600.

2. Ware LB, Matthay MA. The acute respiratory distress syndrome. N Engl J Med 2000;342:1334–49.

3. Orfanos SE, Mavrommati I, Korovesi I, et al. Pulmonary endothelium in acute lung injury: from basic science to the critically ill. Intensive Care Med 2004;30: 1702–14.

4. Diaz JV, Brower R, Calfee CS, et al. Therapeutic strategies for severe acute lung injury. Crit Care Med 2010;38(8):1644–50.

5. Tomashefski JF. Pulmonary pathology of adult respiratory distress syndrome. Clin Chest Med 2000;21(3):435–66.

6. Dudek SM, Birukov KG, Zhan X, et al. Novel interaction of cortactin with endothelial cell myosin light chain kinase. Biochem Biophys Res Commun 2002; 298(4):511–9.

7. Birukov KG, Birukova AA, Dudek SM, et al. Shear stress-mediated cytoskeletal remodeling and cortactin translocation in pulmonary endothelial cells. Am J Respir Cell Mol Biol 2002;26(4):453–64.

8. Pugin J, Verghese G, Widmer MC, et al. The alveolar space is the site of intense inflammatory and profibrotic reactions in the early phase of acute respiratory distress syndrome. Crit Care Med 1999;27:304–12.

9. Wiener-Kronish JP, Albertine KH, Matthay MA. Differential responses of the endothelial and epithelial barriers of the lung in sheep to *Escherichia coli* endotoxin. J Clin Invest 1991;88:864–75.

10. Sznajder JI. Strategies to increase alveolar epithelial fluid removal in the injured lung. Am J Respir Crit Care Med 1999;160:1441–2.

11. Matute-Bello G, Frevert CW, Martin TR. Animal models of acute lung injury. Am J Physiol Lung Cell Mol Physiol 2008;295(3):L379–99.

12. Matthay MA, Zimmerman GA. Acute lung injury and the acute respiratory distress syndrome: four decades of inquiry into pathogenesis and rational management. Am J Respir Cell Mol Biol 2005;33:319–27.

13. Ware LB. Modeling human lung disease in animals. Am J Physiol Lung Cell Mol Physiol 2008;294(2):L149–50.

14. Brattström O, Granath F, Rossi P, et al. Early predictors of morbidity and mortality in trauma patients treated in the intensive care unit. Acta Anaesthesiol Scand 2010;54:1007–17.

15. Brun-Buisson C, Minelli C, Bertolini G, et al. Epidemiology and outcome of acute lung injury in European intensive care units. Results from the ALIVE study. Intensive Care Med 2004;30(1):51–61.

16. Rubenfeld GD, Caldwell E, Peabody E, et al. Incidence and outcomes of acute lung injury. N Engl J Med 2005;353(16):1685–93.

17. Cheung AM, Tansey CM, Tomlinson G, et al. Two-year outcomes, health care use, and costs of survivors of acute respiratory distress syndrome. Am J Respir Crit Care Med 2006;174(5):538–44.

18. Adhikare N, Burns KE, Meade MO. Pharmacologic therapies for adults with acute lung injury and acute respiratory distress syndrome. Cochrane Database Syst Rev 2004;4:CD004477.

19. Bosma KJ, Taneja R, Lewis JF. Pharmacotherapy for prevention and treatment of acute respiratory distress syndrome: current and experimental approaches. Drugs 2010;70(10):1255–82.

20. Frank AJ, Thompson BT. Pharmacological treatments for acute respiratory distress syndrome. Curr Opin Crit Care 2010;16(1):62–8.

21. Moriates C, Maisel A. The utility of biomarkers in sorting out the complex patient. Am J Med 2010;123(5):393–9.

22. Levitt JE, Gould MK, Ware LB, et al. The pathogenetic and prognostic value of biologic markers in acute lung injury. J Intensive Care Med 2009;24(3): 151–67.

23. Fremont RD, Koyama T, Calfee CS, et al. Acute lung injury in patients with traumatic injuries: utility of a panel of biomarkers for diagnosis and pathogenesis. J Trauma 2010;68(5):1121–7.

24. Ware LB, Koyama T, Billheimer DD, et al. Prognostic and pathogenetic value of combining clinical and biochemical indices in patients with acute lung injury. Chest 2010;137(2):288–96.

25. Liu KD, Glidden DV, Eisner MD, et al. Predictive and pathogenetic value of plasma biomarkers for acute kidney injury in patients with acute lung injury. Crit Care Med 2007;35(12):2755–61.

26. Ware LB, Matthay MA, Parsons PE, et al. Pathogenetic and prognostic significance of altered coagulation and fibrinolysis in acute lung injury/acute respiratory distress syndrome. Crit Care Med 2007;35(8):1821–8.

27. Calfee CS, Ware LB. Biomarkers of lung injury in primary graft dysfunction following lung transplantation. Biomark Med 2007;1(2):285–91.

28. Calfee CS, Eisner MD, Ware LB, et al. Trauma-associated lung injury differs clinically and biologically from acute lung injury due to other clinical disorders. Crit Care Med 2007;35:2243–50.

29. Black SM. New insights into acute lung injury. Vascul Pharmacol 2010;52:171–4.

30. Crosby LM, Waters CM. Epithelial repair mechanisms in the lung. Am J Physiol Lung Cell Mol Physiol 2010;298(6):L715–31.

31. Galani V, Tatsaki E, Bai M, et al. The role of apoptosis in the pathophysiology of acute respiratory distress syndrome (ARDS): an up-to-date cell-specific review. Pathol Res Pract 2010;206(3):145–50.

32. Frank JA, Parsons PE, Matthay MA. Pathogenetic significance of biological markers of ventilator-associated lung injury in experimental and clinical studies. Chest 2006;130(6):1906–14.

33. Lin WC, Lin CF, Chen CL, et al. Prediction of outcome in patients with acute respiratory distress syndrome by bronchoalveolar lavage inflammatory mediators. Exp Biol Med (Maywood) 2010;235(1):57–65.

34. Dos Santos CC. Advances in mechanisms of repair and remodeling in acute lung injury. Intensive Care Med 2008;34(4):619–30.

35. Hoshino T, Okamoto M, Sakazaki Y, et al. Role of proinflammatory cytokines IL-18 and IL-1 beta in bleomycin-induced lung injury in humans and mice. Am J Respir Cell Mol Biol 2009;41(6):661–70.

36. Pugin J, Ricou B, Steinberg KP, et al. Proinflammatory activity in bronchoalveolar lavage fluids from patients with ARDS: a prominent role for interleukin-1. Am J Respir Crit Care Med 1996;153:1850–6.

37. Olman MA, White KE, Ware LB, et al. Microarray analysis indicates that pulmonary edema fluid from patients with acute lung injury mediates inflammation, mitogen gene expression, and fibroblast proliferation through bioactive interleukin-1. Chest 2002;121:69S–70S.

38. Zhang Y, Lee TC, Guillemin B, et al. Enhanced IL-1 beta and tumor necrosis factor-alpha release and messenger RNA expression in macrophages from idiopathic pulmonary fibrosis or after asbestos exposure. J Immunol 1993;150(9): 4188–96.

39. Kolb M, Margetts PJ, Anthony DC, et al. Transient expression of IL-1beta induces acute lung injury and chronic repair leading to pulmonary fibrosis. J Clin Invest 2001;107:1529–36.

40. Bonniaud P, Margetts PJ, Ask K, et al. TGF-beta and Smad 3 signaling link inflammation to chronic fibrogenesis. J Immunol 2005;175:5390–5.

41. Ward PA. Role of complement, chemokines, and regulatory cytokines in acute lung injury. Ann N Y Acad Sci 1996;796:104–12.

42. Goodman RB, Pugin J, Lee JS, et al. Cytokine-mediated inflammation in acute lung injury. Cytokine Growth Factor Rev 2003;14:523–35.

43. Geiser T, Jarreau PH, Atabai K, et al. Interleukin-1 beta augments in vitro alveolar epithelial repair. Am J Physiol Lung Cell Mol Physiol 2000;279: L1184–90.

44. Geiser T, Atabai K, Jarreau PH, et al. Pulmonary edema fluid from patients with acute lung injury augments in vitro alveolar epithelial repair by an IL-1 beta-dependent mechanism. Am J Respir Crit Care Med 2001;163:1384–8.

45. Strieter RM, Kunkel SL. Acute lung injury: the role of cytokines in the elicitation of neutrophils. J Med 1994;42(4):640–51.

46. Ganter MT, Roux J, Miyazawa B, et al. Interleukin-1 beta causes acute lung injury via alphavbeta5 and alphavbeta6 integrin-dependent mechanisms. Circ Res 2008;102(7):804–12.

47. Ranieri VM, Suter PM, Tortorella C, et al. Effect of mechanical ventilation on inflammatory mediators in patients with acute respiratory distress syndrome: a randomized controlled trial. JAMA 1999;282(1):54–61.

48. Ranieri VM, Giunta F, Suter PM, et al. Mechanical ventilation as a mediator of multisystem organ failure in acute respiratory distress syndrome. JAMA 2000; 284(1):43–4.

49. Frank JA, Pittet J-F, Wray C, et al. Protection from experimental ventilator-induced acute lung injury by IL-1 receptor blockade. Thorax 2008;63: 147–53.

50. Park WY, Goodman RB, Steinberg KP. Cytokine balance in the lungs of patients with acute respiratory distress syndrome. Am J Respir Crit Care Med 2001;164: 1896–903.

51. Patwari PP, O'Cain P, Goodman DM, et al. Interleukin-1 receptor antagonist intron 2 variable number of tandem repeats polymorphism and respiratory failure in children with community-acquired pneumonia. Pediatr Crit Care Med 2008;9(6):553–9.

52. Donnelly SC, Strieter RM, Reid PT, et al. The association between mortality rates and decreased concentrations of interleukin-10 and interleukin-1 receptor antagonist in the lung fluids of patients with the adult respiratory distress syndrome. Ann Intern Med 1996;125:191–6.

53. Goodman RB, Strieter RM, Martin DP, et al. Inflammatory cytokines in patients with persistence of the acute respiratory distress syndrome. Am J Respir Crit Care Med 1996;154:602–11.

54. Quesnel C, Marchand-Adam S, Fabre A, et al. Regulation of hepatocyte growth factor secretion by fibroblasts in patients with acute lung injury. Am J Physiol Lung Cell Mol Physiol 2008;294(2):L334–40.

55. Leeper-Woodford SK, Carey PD, Byrne K, et al. Tumour necrosis factor. Alpha and beta subtypes appear in circulation during onset of sepsis-induced lung injury. Am Rev Respir Dis 1991;143:1076–82.

56. Sheridan BC, McIntyre RC, Meldrum DR, et al. Pentoxifylline treatment attenuates pulmonary vasomotor dysfunction in acute lung injury. J Surg Res 1997;71:150–4.

57. Meduri GU, Kohler G, Headley S, et al. Inflammatory cytokines in the BAL of patients with ARDS. Persistent elevation over time predicts poor outcome. Chest 1995;108:1303–14.

58. Borelli E, Roux-Lombard P, Gray GE, et al. Plasma concentration of cytokines, their soluble receptors, and antioxidant vitamins can predict the development of multiple organ failure in patients at risk. Crit Care Med 1996;24:392–7.

59. Dada LA, Sznajder JI. Hypoxic inhibition of alveolar fluid reabsorption. Adv Exp Med Biol 2007;618:159–68.

60. Petrache I, Birukova A, Ramirez SI, et al. The role of the microtubules in tumour necrosis factor-alpha-induced endothelial permeability. Am J Respir Cell Mol Biol 2003;28(5):574–81.

61. Meduri GU, Headley S, Kohler G, et al. Peristent elevation of inflammatory cytokines predicts a poor outcome in ARDS. Plasma IL-1 beta and IL-6 levels are consistent and efficient predictors of outcome over time. Chest 1995;107: 1062–73.

62. Parsons PE, Matthay MA, Ware LB, et al. Elevated plasma levels of soluble TNF receptors are associated with morbidity and mortality in patients with acute lung injury. Am J Physiol Lung Cell Mol Physiol 2005;288(3):L426–31.

63. Michetti C, Coimbra R, Hoyt DB, et al. Pentoxifylline reduces acute lung injury in chronic endotoxemia. J Surg Res 2003;115(1):92–9.

64. Oliveira-Junior IS, Oliverira WR, Cavassani SS, et al. Effects of pentoxifylline on inflammation and lung dysfunction in ventilated septic animals. J Trauma 2010; 68(4):822–66.

65. Lima ML, Castro P, Machado AL, et al. Synthesis and anti-inflammatory activity of phthalimide derivatives, designed as new thalidomide analogues. Bioorg Med Chem 2002;10:3067–73.

66. Rocco PRM, Momesso DP, Figueira RC, et al. Thereapeutic potential of a new phosphodiesterase inhibitor in acute lung injury. Eur Respir J 2003;22:20–7.

67. Tracey KJ. Suppression of TNF and other proinflammatory cytokines by the tetravalent guanylhydrazone CNI-1493. Prog Clin Biol Res 1998;397:335–43.

68. Murumkar PR, DasGupta S, Chandani SR, et al. Novel TACE inhibitors in drug discovery: a review of patented compounds. Expert Opin Ther Pat 2010; 20(1):31–57.

69. Parsons PE, Eisner MD, Thompson BT, et al. Lower tidal volume ventilation and plasma cytokine markers of inflammation in patients with acute lung injury. Crit Care Med 2005;33:1–6.

70. McClintock D, Zhuo H, Wickersham N, et al. Biomarkers of inflammation, coagulation, and fibrinolysis predict mortality in acute lung injury. Crit Care 2008; 12:R41.

71. Agouridakis P, Kyriakou D, Alexandrakis MG, et al. The predictive role of serum and bronchoalveolar lavage cytokines and adhesion molecule for acute respiratory distress: development and outcome. Respir Res 2002;3:25–33.

72. Baughman RP, Gunther KL, Rashkin MC, et al. Changes in the inflammatory response of the lung during acute respiratory distress syndrome: prognostic indicators. Am J Respir Crit Care Med 1996;154:76–81.

73. Schutte H, Lohmeyer J, Rosseau S, et al. Bronchoalveolar and systemic cytokine profiles in patients with ARDS, severe pneumonia and cardiogenic pulmonary oedema. Eur Respir J 1996;9:1858–67.

74. Wong HR, Cvijanovich N, Wheeler DS, et al. Interleukin 8 as a stratification tool for interventional trials involving pediatric septic shock. Am J Respir Crit Care Med 2008;178:276–82.

75. Calfee CS, Thompson BT, Parsons PE, et al. Plasma interleukin-8 is not an effective risk stratification tool for adults with vasopressor-dependent septic shock. Crit Care Med 2010;38(6):1436–41.

76. Stapleton RD, Dixon AE, Parsons PE, et al. The association between BMI and plasma cytokine levels in patients with acute lung injury. Chest 2010;138(3):568–77.
77. Kurdowska A, Miller EJ, Baughman RP, et al. Anti-interleukin-8 autoantibodies in alveolar fluid from patients with the adult respiratory distress syndrome. J Immunol 1996;157:2699–706.
78. Kurdowska A, Noble JM, Grant IS, et al. Anti-interleukin-8 autoantibodies in patients at risk for acute respiratory distress syndrome. Crit Care Med 2002; 30(10):2335–7.
79. Fudala R, Krupa A, Stankowska D, et al. Anti-interleukin-8 autoantibody: interleukin-8 immune complexes in acute lung injury/acute respiratory distress syndrome. Clin Sci (Lond) 2008;114:403–12.
80. Fudala R, Krupa A, Stanlowska D, et al. Does activation of the FcγRIIa play a role in the pathogenesis of the acute lung injury/acute respiratory distress syndrome? Clin Sci (Lond) 2010;118:519–26.
81. Krupa A, Kato H, Matthay MA, et al. Proinflammatory activity of anti-IL-8 autoantibody: IL-8 complexes in alveolar edema fluid from patients with acute lung injury. Am J Physiol Lung Cell Mol Physiol 2004;286(6):L1105–13.
82. Fudala R, Krupa A, Matthay MA, et al. Anti-IL-8 autoantibody: IL-8 immune complexes suppress spontaneous apoptosis of neutrophils. Am J Physiol Lung Cell Mol Physiol 2007;293:L364–74.
83. Horvath CM. The Jak-STAT pathway stimulates by interleukin-6. Sci STKE 2004; 260:TR9.
84. Hirano T, Nakajima K, Hibi M. Signaling mechanisms through gp130: a model of the cytokine system. Cytokine Growth Factor Rev 1997;8:241–52.
85. Hirano T, Ishihara K, Hibi M. Roles of STAT3 in mediating the cell growth, differentiation, and survival signals relayed through the IL-6 family of cytokine receptors. Oncogene 2000;19:2548–56.
86. Nonas SA, Finigan JH, Gao L, et al. Functional genomics insights into acute lung injury: role of ventilators and mechanical stress. Proc Am Thorac Soc 2005;2: 188–94.
87. Fishman D, Faulds G, Jeffrey R, et al. The effect of novel polymorphisms in the IL-6 gene on IL-6 transcription and plasma IL-6 levels and an association with systemic onset juvenile chronic arthritis. J Clin Invest 1998;102:1369–76.
88. Marshall RP, Webb S, Hill MR, et al. Genetic polymorphisms associated with susceptibility and outcome in ARDS. Chest 2002;121(Suppl 3):68s–9s.
89. Sutherland AM, Walley KR, Manocha S, et al. The association of interleukin 6 haplotype clades with mortality in critically ill adults. Arch Intern Med 2005; 165:75 82.
90. Kamp R, Sun X. Garcia JGN Making genomics functional: deciphering the genetics of acute lung injury. Proc Am Thorac Soc 2008;5:348–53.
91. Kolliputi N, Waxman AB. IL-6 cytoprotection in hyperoxic acute lung injury occurs via PI3K/Akt-mediated Bax phosphorylation. Am J Physiol Lung Cell Mol Physiol 2009;297:L6–16.
92. Olman MA, White KE, Ware LB, et al. Pulmonary edema fluid from patients with early lung injury stimulates fibroblast proliferation through IL-1β induced IL-6 expression. J Immunol 2004;172:2668–77.
93. Xing Z, Gauldie G, Cox H, et al. IL-6 is an anti-inflammatory cytokine required for controlling local or systemic acute inflammatory responses. J Clin Invest 1998; 101:311–20.
94. Wu C-L, Lin L-Y, Yang J-S, et al. Attenuation of lipopolysaccharide-induced acute lung injury by treatment with IL-10. Respirology 2009;14:511–21.

95. Schottelius AJ, Mayo MW, Sartor RB, et al. IL-10 signaling blocks inhibitor of kappa B kinase activity and nuclear factor kappa B DNA binding. J Biol Chem 1999;274:31868–74.

96. Wang P, Wu P, Siegel MI, et al. IL-10 inhibits nuclear factor kappa B activation in human monocytes. IL-10 and IL-4 suppress cytokine synthesis by different mechanisms. J Biol Chem 1995;270:9558–63.

97. Fan J, Ye RD, Malik AB. Transcriptional mechanisms of acute lung injury. Am J Physiol Lung Cell Mol Physiol 2001;281:1037–50.

98. Galani V, Chondrogiannis G, Kastamoulas M, et al. TNF-alpha, IL-1β, IL-13, and IFNγ effects on the cell death of the A540 lung carcinoma cells. FEBS J 2009; 276(Suppl 1):310.

99. Lentsch AB, Shanley TP, Sarma V, et al. In vivo suppression of NF-kappa B and preservation of I kappa B alpha by interleukin-10 and interleukin-13. J Clin Invest 1997;100:2443–8.

100. Ware LB, Fang X, Matthay MA. Protein C and thrombomodulin in human acute lug injury. Am J Physiol Lung Cell Mol Physiol 2003;285:L514–21.

101. Gunther A, Mosavi P, Heinemann S, et al. Alveolar fibrin formation caused by enhanced procoagulant and depressed fibrinolytic capacities in severe pneumonia. Comparison with the acute respiratory distress syndrome. Am J Respir Crit Care Med 2000;161:454–67.

102. Schultz MJ, Millo J, Levi M, et al. Local activation of coagulation and inhibition of fibrinolysis in the lung during ventilation associated pneumonia. Thorax 2004;59: 130–5.

103. Zarbock A, Singbartl K, Ley K. Complete reversal of acid-induced acute lung injury by blocking of platelet–neutrophil aggregation. J Clin Invest 2006;116: 3211–9.

104. Kiefmann R, Heckel K, Schenkat S, et al. Platelet–endothelial cell interaction in pulmonary microcirculation: the role of PARS. Thromb Haemost 2004;91: 761–70.

105. Belperio JA, Keane MP, Lynch JP, et al. The role of cytokines during the pathogenesis of ventilator-associated and ventilator-induced lung injury. Semin Respir Crit Care Med 2006;27:350–64.

106. Bozza FA, Shah AM, Weyrich AS, et al. Amicus or adversary platelets in lung biology, acute injury, and inflammation. Am J Respir Cell Mol Biol 2009;40:123–34.

107. Baja MS, Tricomi SM. Plasma levels of the three endothelial specific proteins von Willebrand factor, tissue factor pathway inhibitor and thrombomodulin do not predict the development of acute respiratory distress syndrome. Intensive Care Med 1999;25:1259–66.

108. Prabhukaran P, Ware LB, White KE, et al. Elevated levels of plasminogen activator inhibitor-1 in pulmonary oedema fluid are associated with mortality in acute lung injury. Am J Physiol Lung Cell Mol Physiol 2003;285:L20–8.

109. Hofstra JJ, Juffermans NP, Schultz MJ. Pulmonary coagulopathy as a new target in lung injury—a review of available pre-clinical models. Curr Med Chem 2008; 15(6):588–95.

110. Looney MR, Esmon CT, Matthay MA. Role of coagulation pathways and treatment with activated protein C in hyperoxic lung injury. Thorax 2009;64(2): 114–20.

111. Bernard GR, Vincent JL, Laterre PF, et al. Efficacy and safety of recombinant human activated protein C for severe sepsis. N Engl J Med 2001;344:699–709.

112. Liu KD, Levitt J, Zhuo H, et al. Randomized clinical trial of activated protein C for the treatment of acute lung injury. Am J Respir Crit Care Med 2008;78(6):618–23.

113. Wang L, Bastarache JA, Wickersham N, et al. Novel role of the human alveolar epithelium in regulating intra-alveolar coagulation. Am J Respir Cell Mol Biol 2007;36:497–503.

114. Laterre PF, Abraham E, Janes JM, et al. ADDRESS (ADministration of DRotrecogin alfa [activated] in early stage severe Sepsis) long-term follow-up: one-year safety and efficacy evaluation. Crit Care Med 2007;35(6):1457–63.

115. Nadel S, Goldstein B, Williams MD, et al. Drotrecogin alfa (activated) in children with severe sepsis: a multicentre phase III randomised controlled trial. Lancet 2007;369(9564):836–43.

116. Silva E, de Figueiredo LF, Colombari F. PROWESS SHOCK trial: a protocol overview and perspectives. Shock 2010;34(Suppl 1):48–53.

117. The PROWESS SHOCK Steering Committee, Thompson BT, Ranieri VM, et al. Statistical analysis plan of PROWESS SHOCK study. Intensive Care Med 2010;36(11):1972–3.

118. Bachofen M, Weibel ER. Structural alterations of lung parenchyma in the adult respiratory distress syndrome. Clin Chest Med 1982;3:35–56.

119. Moss M, Gillespsie MK, Ackerson L, et al. Endothelial cell activity varies in patients at risk for the adult respiratory distress syndrome. Crit Care Med 1996;24:1782–6.

120. Donnelly SC, Haslett C, Dransfield I, et al. Role of selectins in development of adult respiratory distress syndrome. Lancet 1994;344:215–9.

121. Okalima K, Harada N, Sakurai G, et al. Rapid assay for plasma soluble E-selectin predicts the development of acute respiratory distress syndrome in patients with systemic inflammatory response syndrome. Transl Res 2006;148:295–300.

122. Berthiaume Y, Lesur O, Dagenais A. Treatment of adult respiratory distress syndrome: plea for rescue therapy of the alveolar epithelium. Thorax 1999;54:150–60.

123. Atabai K, Ishigaki M, Geiser T, et al. Keratinocyte growth factor can enhance alveolar epithelial repair by nonmitogenic mechanisms. Am J Physiol Lung Cell Mol Physiol 2002;283:L163–9.

124. Desari TJ, Cardoso WV. Growth factors in lung development and disease: friends or foe? Respir Res 2002;3:2–5.

125. Lindsay C. Novel therapeutic strategies for acute lung injury induced by lung damaging agents: The potential role of growth factors as treatment options. Hum Exp Toxicol 2010. [Epub ahead of print].

126. Verghese GM, McCormick-Shannon K, Mason RJ, et al. Hepatocyte growth factor and keratinocyte growth factor in the pulmonary edema fluid of patients with acute lung injury. Biologic and clinical significance. Am J Respir Crit Care Med 1998;158(2):386–94.

127. Ware LB, Matthay MA. Keratinocyte and hepatocyte growth factors in the lung: roles in lung development, inflammation, and repair. Am J Physiol Lung Cell Mol Physiol 2002;282(5):L924–40.

128. Naldini L, Vigna E, Narismhan R, et al. HGF stimulates the tyrosine kinase activity of the receptor encoded by the proto-oncogene c-MET. Oncogene 1991;6:501–4.

129. Fan S, Ma YX, Wang JA, et al. The cytokine HGF inhibits apoptosis and enhances DNA repair by a common mechanism involving signaling through phosphatidylinositol-3'-kinase. Oncogene 2000;19:2212–23.

130. Thickett DR, Armstrong L, Chrsitie SJ, et al. VEGF may contribute to increased vascular permeability in acute respiratory distress syndrome. Am J Respir Crit Care Med 2001;164:1601–5.

131. Maitre B, Boussat S, Jean D, et al. VEGF synthesis in the acute phase of experimental and clinical lung injury. Eur Respir J 2001;18:100–6.
132. Thickett DR, Armstrong L, Millar AB. A role for VEGF in acute and resolving lung injury. Am J Respir Crit Care Med 2002;166:1332–7.
133. Abadie Y, Bregeon F, Papazian L, et al. Decreased VEGF concentration in lung tissue and vascular injury during ARDS. Eur Respir J 2005;25:139–46.
134. Ware LB, Kaner RJ, Crystal RG, et al. VEGF levels in the alveolar compartment do not distinguish between ARDS and hydrostatic pulmonary oedema. Eur Respir J 2005;26:101–5.
135. van der Heijden M, van Nieuw Amerongen GP, Koolwijk P, et al. Angiopoietin-2 permeability oedema, occurrence and severity of ALI/ARDS in septic and non-septic critically ill patients. Thorax 2008;63:903–9.
136. Ong T, McClintock DE, Kallett RH, et al. Ratio of angiopoietin-2 to angiopoietin-1 as a predictor of mortality in acute lung patients. Crit Care Med 2010;38(9):1845–51.
137. Eklund L, Oslen BR. Tie receptors and their angiopoietin ligands are context-dependent regulators of vascular remodeling. Exp Cell Res 2006;312:630–41.
138. Eisner MD, Parson P, Matthay MA, et al. Plasma surfactant protein levels and clinical outcomes in patients with acute lung injury. Thorax 2003;58:983–8.
139. Calfee CS, Ware LB, Eisner MD, et al. Plasma receptor for advanced glycation end-products and clinical outcomes in acute lung injury. Thorax 2008;63:1083–9.
140. Donahue JE, Flaherty SL, Johanson CE, et al. RAGE, LRP-1, and amyloid-beta protein in Alzheimer's disease. Acta Neuropathol 2006;112:405–15.
141. Ghavami S, Rashedi I, Dattilo BM, et al. S100A8/A9 at low concentration promotes tumor cell growth via RAGE ligation and MAP kinase-dependent pathway. J Leukoc Biol 2008;83:1484–92.
142. Aleshin A, Ananthakrishnan R, Li Q, et al. RAGE modulates myocardial injury consequent to LAD infarction via impact on JNK and STAT signaling in a murine model. Am J Physiol Heart Circ Physiol 2008;294:H1823–32.
143. Ishizaka A, Matsuda T, Albertine KH, et al. Elevation of KL-6, a lung epithelial cell marker in plasma and epithelial lining fluid in acute respiratory distress syndrome. Am J Physiol Lung Cell Mol Physiol 2004;286:L1088–94.
144. Inoue Y, Barker E, Daniloff E, et al. Pulmonary epithelial cell injury and alveolar-capillary permeability in berylliosis. Am J Respir Crit Care Med 1997;156:109–15.
145. McClintock DE, Starcher B, Eisner MD, et al. Higher urine desmosine levels are associated with mortality in patients with acute lung injury. Am J Physiol Lung Cell Mol Physiol 2006;291:L566–71.
146. Nathani N, Perkins GD, Tunnicliffe W, et al. Kerbs von den Lungren 6 antigen is a marker of alveolar inflammation but not of infection in patients with acute respiratory distress syndrome. Crit Care 2008;12:R12–9.
147. Lesur O, Langevin S, Berthiaume Y, et al. Outcome value of Clara cell protein in serum of patients with acute respiratory distress syndrome. Intensive Care Med 2006;32(8):1167–74.
148. Maniatis NA, Kotanidou A, Catravas JD, et al. Endothelial pathomechanisms in acute lung injury. Vascul Pharmacol 2008;49:119–33.
149. Moss M, Ackerson L, Gillespie MK, et al. von Willebrand factor antigen levels are not predictive for the adult respiratory distress syndrome. Am J Respir Crit Care Med 1995;151:15–20.

150. Ware LB, Conner ER, Matthay MA. von Willebrand factor antigen is an independent marker of poor outcome in patients with early acute lung injury. Crit Care Med 2001;29:2325–31.
151. Bowler RP, Duda B, Chan ED, et al. Proteomic analysis of pulmonary edema fluid and plasma in patients with acute lung injury. Am J Physiol Lung Cell Mol Physiol 2004;286(6):L1095–104.
152. Bowler RP, Ellison MC, Reisdorph N. Proteomics in pulmonary medicine. Chest 2006;130(2):567–74.
153. Chang DW, Hayashi S, Gharib SA, et al. Proteomic and computational analysis of bronchoalveolar proteins during the course of the acute respiratory distress syndrome. Am J Respir Crit Care Med 2008;178(7):701–9.

Neutrophil gelatinase–associated lipocalin (NGAL) as a Biomarker for Early Acute Kidney Injury

Douglas Shemin, MD*, Lance D. Dworkin, MD

KEYWORDS

• NGAL • Acute kidney injury • Acute tubular necrosis

For many years, an acute and potentially reversible decline in the glomerular filtration rate (GFR) was termed acute renal failure (ARF); acute renal failure was classically thought to be attributable to prerenal factors (an actual or effective decline in the extracellular volume), postrenal factors owing to urinary obstruction, or intrarenal factors owing to a pathologic process occurring in 1 of the 4 loci in the nephron: the glomerulus, the renal vasculature, the interstitium, and the renal tubules.[1] Although hundreds of causes of ARF have been described, in clinical observational studies, the vast majority of patients with ARF were found to have 1 of 2 etiologies: prerenal failure, and tubular injury owing to ischemic or nephrotoxic factors, or ATN.[2,3]

In the past several years, there have been 2 major changes in the description and definition of ARF. First, the term ARF itself has been discarded in the nephrology literature; the term for an acute and potentially reversible decline in the GFR is now called acute kidney injury (AKI). The term "kidney" more directly describes the location of the pathologic process than "renal," and the term "injury" is more comprehensive than "failure," and includes even small declines in the GFR. This terminology change is based on data that strongly suggest that even tiny increases in the serum creatinine level over baseline values are associated with clinically significant morbid and mortal outcomes, including progression to chronic kidney disease (CKD). In more than 80,000 elderly patients studied after a myocardial infarction, for example, patients whose serum creatinine levels rose by 0.1 mg/dL over the course of a hospitalization had a 14% higher mortality rate and a 45% higher rate of progression to end-stage renal disease (ESRD) than patients whose serum creatinine level did not change.[4]

The authors have nothing to disclose.
Division of Kidney Diseases and Hypertension, Rhode Island Hospital, Alpert Medical School of Brown University, 593 Eddy Street, Providence, RI 02903, USA
* Corresponding author.
E-mail address: Dshemin@lifespan.org

Crit Care Clin 27 (2011) 379–389
doi:10.1016/j.ccc.2010.12.003   criticalcare.theclinics.com

The second change has been in the definition of AKI, which historically had been defined in multiple different studies in multiple different ways. In 2002, a consensus panel devised the RIFLE classification, which divided declines in renal function over at least a 7-day period into 5 categories: Risk, Injury, Failure, Loss, and End Stage.[5] The RIFLE criteria were further modified by another consensus panel, which devised the Acute Kidney Injury Network (AKIN) criteria, published in 2007. This defined AKI as an abrupt (within 48 hours) reduction in kidney function; reduction in kidney function was further defined either as an absolute increase in the serum creatinine by 0.3 mg/dL (25 μm/L), or by 50% of the baseline value, or oliguria, with a urine output less than 0.5 mL/kg/h for at least 6 hours in the setting of appropriate volume expansion. AKI is subdivided into 3 stages, according to severity.[6]

The AKIN criteria, like the RIFLE criteria and the many idiosyncratic criteria for AKI in the past, relies heavily on the serum creatinine level as a biochemical indicator of renal function. The change in the serum creatinine, however, cannot differentiate between changes in renal function owing to volume depletion, hemodynamic changes in renal perfusion, urinary obstruction, or actual renal injury, and there is also good evidence that the change in creatinine may not occur until hours or days after the onset of renal injury.[7] The blood urea nitrogen (BUN) level is even less reliable than the serum creatinine level in diagnosis; it is dependent upon, among other factors, dietary protein intake, hepatic function, and renal tubular avidity for sodium. Urinary sodium, fractional excretion of sodium, and urinary microscopic findings do not reliably predict AKI.[8]

BIOMARKERS IN THE DIAGNOSIS OF AKI

These concerns about diagnostic accuracy in testing for AKI have led to efforts to identify reliable biomarkers for AKI, much as troponin is a biomarker for acute coronary syndrome. The ideal biomarker for AKI is one that can be objectively and reliably measured, is sensitive and specific in diagnosis of AKI, is able to detect AKI at or near the onset of injury, is predictive of severity, and can be used to monitor the effects of treatment.[9] Of all of these characteristics, the most important is early detection; a large number of experimental therapies for AKI seem to be most beneficial when administered very early in the course of injury, before the onset of a rise in the serum creatinine.[7]

Based on studies in experimental models of AKI and in humans, a number of biomarkers have been proposed: cystatin C, soluble tumor necrosis factor (TNF) receptors, N-acetyl-beta-D-glucosaminidase, kidney injury molecule 1, isoform 3 of the sodium-hydrogen exchanger, interleukin (IL)-16, IL-18, matrix metalloproteinase-9, and neutrophil gelatinase–associated lipocalin (NGAL).[9] This review focuses on the biomarker NGAL and its potential utility in the diagnosis, prognosis, and treatment of AKI.

NGAL is a 25-kD protein that was originally described covalently bound to matrix metalloprotein-9 (MMP-9) in animal neutrophils.[10] It has a barrel-shaped structure with a hydrophobic calyx that binds small, lipid, and lipophilic molecules.[11] NGAL is synthesized in renal tubular, intestinal, hepatic, and pulmonary tissue, and synthesis is markedly upregulated in tissue injury. NGAL synthesis is also increased in cancer: NGAL binds to MMP-9, preventing MMP degradation, and the resulting increase MMP-9 in activity promotes cancer progression.[12] Under physiologic conditions, NGAL is expressed in low concentrations in kidney, lung, and gastrointestinal tissue. Circulating NGAL is filtered by the glomerulus, and reabsorbed in the proximal tubule. It is secreted in low concentrations by the thick ascending limb of the renal tubule and the normal urinary level of NGAL is very low (<5 ng/mL).[13] In proximal tubular injury, NGAL synthesis is increased and reabsorption may decrease so that urinary levels increase.[12] In distal tubular injury there is increased distal renal tubular expression and synthesis of NGAL and NGAL secretion increases, increasing urinary levels as well.[14] NGAL is protease resistant[15] and does not seem to be degraded or metabolized after synthesis and secretion into the tubule lumen.

NGAL is synthesized by normal intestinal, hepatic, and pulmonary tissue and can be detected in the plasma; the normal plasma level, in healthy adults, is 50 to 90 ng/mL.[16,17] The kidney is not considered to be a significant source for plasma NGAL. In one experimental study of unilateral renal ischemia, NGAL was not immediately present in the renal vein or the circulation, but was present in the ureter of the ischemic kidney.[14] In AKI, plasma NGAL levels rise, either related to concomitant hepatic, pulmonary, or intestinal tissue injury, coupled with decreased glomerular filtration of NGAL.

NGAL AS A PREDICTOR OF THE DEVELOPMENT OF AKI

Beginning about 10 years ago, experimental studies demonstrated that NGAL gene expression was markedly and immediately upregulated after renal ischemia/reperfusion injury in mice,[18] after ischemia/reperfusion injury and mercuric chloride administration in rats,[19] after cisplatin-induced renal injury in mice,[15] and in cultured human proximal tubular cells subjected to hypoxic injury.[15] In both mouse and rat models of acute kidney injury, NGAL has been shown to be detectable within an hour after onset of injury, which precedes the urinary appearance of beta-2 microglobulin and many other markers of tubular injury.[15]

Clinical studies have confirmed these experimental findings. In 2005, a landmark trial by Mishra and colleagues[13] examined 71 pediatric patients undergoing open-heart surgery and cardiopulmonary bypass. Urinary and plasma samples of NGAL were sequentially measured, and their values were compared with conventional criteria for the diagnosis of AKI, defined as a 50% increase in the serum creatinine level. Twenty percent of the children developed conventional clinical evidence for AKI within 24 to 72 hours after cardiopulmonary bypass. Elevations of both the urine and plasma NGAL level correlated very strongly with the subsequent development of AKI. In those patients in whom 50% increases in serum creatinine eventually developed, urinary NGAL levels significantly rose (to values over 100 times the baseline value) and serum levels significantly rose, to values 10 times the baseline value, both within 2 hours of cardiopulmonary bypass.

In addition to these data, there are now a large number of clinical trials that have examined the predictive value of NGAL in the urine and plasma, in pediatric and in adult populations, as correlated with the subsequent development of clinically evident AKI (usually defined, per the AKIN criteria, as a 50% increase in the serum creatinine level or an arithmetic increase of at least 0.3 mg/dL over a 48-hour period) in patients at risk for AKI. Rather than using a strict cutoff for an abnormal urinary or serum level of NGAL, these studies tend to measure sensitivity and specificity for a wide variety of threshold values with an area under the receiver operating characteristic curve (AUC ROC). An AUC ROC value of 0.90 to 1.00 may indicate excellent, 0.80 to 0.89 good, 0.70 to 0.79 fair, 0.60 to 0.69 poor, and 0.50 to 0.59 no useful performance for discrimination of an outcome being evaluated.[20] The following tables summarize these studies on the predictive value of one NGAL measurement on the subsequent risk for AKI, using the AKIN or RIFLE criteria for AKI. **Tables 1** and **2** list studies examining urinary NGAL levels; **Table 1** in adult populations, and

Table 1
Sensitivity and specificity of elevations in urinary NGAL levels in predicting development of AKI: adult populations

References	Clinical Setting	Number of Patients	Sensitivity	Specificity	AUC ROC (95% CI)
Wagener et al,[21] 2006	Cardiothoracic surgery patients	81	73%	78%	0.80 (0.57–1.03)
Parikh et al,[22] 2006	Kidney transplant recipients	63	90%	83%	0.90 (0.70–0.92)
Koyner et al,[23] 2008	Cardiothoracic surgery	72	49%	79%	0.69 (0.57–0.82)
Xin et al,[24] 2008	Cardiothoracic surgery	33	71%	73%	0.88
Bennett et al,[25] 2008	Cardiothoracic surgery	196	82%	90%	0.93
Portilla et al,[26] 2008	Cardiothoracic surgery	40	100%	100%	1.00
Ling et al,[27] 2008	Cardiac catheterization	40	77%	71%	0.73 (0.54–0.93)
Nickolas et al,[28] 2008	Emergency room patients	635	90%	99%	0.95 (0.88–1.00)
Tuladhar et al,[29] 2009	Cardiothoracic surgery	50	93%	Not reported	0.96 (0.9–1.0)
Siew et al,[30] 2009	Critically ill adults	451	Not reported	Not reported	0.71 (0.63–0.78)
Makris et al,[31] 2009	Multiple trauma	31	91%	95%	0.98 (0.82–0.98)
McIllroy et al,[32] 2010	Cardiothoracic surgery	426	76%	34%	0.61 (0.54–0.68)
Hall et al,[33] 2010	Kidney transplant recipients	91	77%	74%	0.81 (0.70–0.92)
Yang et al,[34] 2010	Hospitalized inpatients	256	88%	81%	0.88
Martensson et al,[35] 2010	Patients with septic shock	65	Not reported	Not reported	0.67

Abbreviations: AKI, acute kidney injury; AUC ROC, area under the receiver operating characteristic curve; CI, confidence interval; NGAL, neutrophil gelatinase–associated lipocalin.

Table 2
Sensitivity and specificity of elevations in urinary NGAL in predicting development of AKI in a 48-hour period: pediatric studies

References	Clinical Setting	Number of Patients	Sensitivity	Specificity	AUC ROC (95% CI)
Mishra et al,[13] 2005	Pediatric cardiopulmonary bypass	71	100%	98%	0.99
Hirsch et al,[36] 2007	Pediatric cardiac catheterization	91	73%	100%	0.92
Zappitelli et al,[37] 2007	Pediatric critical care	150	77%	72%	0.78 (0.62–0.95)

Abbreviations: AKI, acute kidney injury; AUC ROC, area under the receiver operating characteristic curve; CI, confidence interval; NGAL, neutrophil gelatinase–associated lipocalin.

Table 2 in pediatric populations. **Tables 3** and **4** list studies examining serum NGAL levels; **Table 3** in adult populations and **Table 4** in pediatric populations.

Clinical data on the efficacy of urinary or plasma NGAL levels in prediction of AKI were recently summarized in a large meta-analysis.[13] This analysis suggested that in critical care settings, urinary NGAL has a slightly higher predictive value than serum NGAL. Studies in pediatric patients seem to yield higher sensitivities, specificities, and AUC ROC values than studies in adults, and studies in which AKI resulted from a single

Table 3
Sensitivity and specificity of elevations in serum NGAL levels in predicting development of AKI in a 48-hour period: adult studies

References	Clinical Setting	Number of Patients	Sensitivity	Specificity	AUC ROC (95% CI)
Koyner et al,[23] 2008	Cardiothoracic surgery	72	Not reported	Not reported	0.54 (0.40–0.67)
Haase-Fielitz et al,[38] 2009	Cardiothoracic surgery	100	79%	78%	0.80 (0.63–0.96)
Tuladhar et al,[29] 2009	Cardiothoracic surgery	80	80%	67%	0.85 (0.73–0.97)
Malyszko et al,[39] 2009	Diabetics undergoing cardiac catheterization	91	73%	100%	0.91
Constantin et al,[40] 2009	Adult ICU patients	88	82%	97%	0.92 (0.85 – 0.97)
Cruz et al,[16] 2010	Adult ICU patients	301	73%	81%	0.78 (0.65–0.90)
Niemann et al,[41] 2009	Liver transplant recipients	59	68%	80%	0.79
Martensson et al,[35] 2010	Patients with septic shock	65	Not reported	Not reported	0.67
Bagshaw et al,[42] 2010	Critically ill patients	83	Not reported	Not reported	0.71

Abbreviations: AKI, acute kidney injury; AUC ROC, area under the receiver operating characteristic curve; CI, confidence interval; ICU, intensive care unit; NGAL, neutrophil gelatinase–associated lipocalin.

Table 4
Sensitivity and specificity of elevations in serum NGAL levels in predicting development of AKI in a 48-hour period: pediatric studies

References	Clinical Setting	Number of Patients	Sensitivity	Specificity	AUC ROC (95% CI)
Mishra et al,[13] 2005	Pediatric cardiopulmonary bypass	71	70%	94%	0.91
Dent et al,[43] 2007	Pediatric cardiothoracic surgery	120	84%	94%	0.96 (0.94–0.99)
Wheeler et al,[17] 2008	Pediatric critical care	143	86%	39%	0.68 (0.56–0.79)

Abbreviations: AKI, acute kidney injury; AUC ROC, area under the receiver operating characteristic curve; CI, confidence interval; NGAL, neutrophil gelatinase–associated lipocalin.

nephrotoxic injury (for example, hypotension during cardiopulmonary bypass) seem to show a higher predictive effect of urinary or serum NGAL than studies in which patients had multiple and prolonged nephrotoxic injury (for example, in intensive care units [ICUs] in the setting of septic shock).

Urinary or serum NGAL values are most predictive when the diagnosis of AKI is based on more severe declines in the GFR. In one study, if AKI was defined as an increase in the serum creatinine of more than 25% above baseline, the mean AUC ROC value was 0.65; when AKI was defined as an increase in the serum creatinine of more than 50% above baseline, the mean AUC ROC was 0.79.[38] In addition, and very importantly, the predictive value of an NGAL increase is greatest in patients whose kidney function is normal at baseline. In one large prospective trial of patients undergoing cardiac surgery, urinary NGAL did not significantly change in patients with stage III, IV, and V chronic kidney disease (CKD) and a baseline estimated GFR of lower than 60 mL/min, who developed AKI. In contrast, it changed significantly in patients who had a preoperative estimated GFR higher than 90 mL/min and developed AKI.[32] In other series of patients with established CKD or chronic renal allograft dysfunction[44] and in heart transplant recipients,[45] the serum NGAL level inversely correlated with the GFR, confirming a high baseline level of NGAL in individuals with established CKD.

There is some variability among these studies regarding the method used to measure the urinary or serum NGAL level. Most investigators use an enzyme-linked immunosorbent (ELISA) assay; a minority use an immunoblot technique. Individual studies varied in the level of NGAL that was associated with injury. With the ELISA tests, a urinary NGAL level of >150 ng/mL seemed to correlate best with the subsequent development of AKI, with a slightly lower cutoff (>150 ng/mL) for pediatric populations[43]; plasma levels of >100 ng/mL seemed to correlate with subsequent development of AKI.[16]

Finally, and as the above tables indicate, virtually all the studies examining NGAL as a marker for the development of AKI have been performed in critical care settings, particularly after cardiopulmonary bypass, or in the setting of intra-arterial contrast administration. There are a handful of exceptions: one small recently published study showed that urinary NGAL excretion predicted AKI in patients with solid tumors receiving cis platinum[46] and another study showed that urinary NGAL levels predicted AKI in a multicenter cohort of children with diarrhea-associated hemolytic uremic syndrome.[47] There is some evidence that NGAL might play an important role in the diagnosis of delayed graft function following renal transplantation. In a pediatric transplant study, an increase in NGAL expression in renal tissue detected within 1 hour of renal perfusion after implantation was strongly correlated with the subsequent elevation of the serum creatinine after transplantation and the clinical development of delayed graft function.[48] Other studies confirm that urinary[21,32] and plasma[49] elevations in NGAL levels after renal transplantation correlate with the subsequent development of delayed graft function.

NGAL AS A PREDICTOR OF THE SEVERITY OF AKI

Most of the clinical trials summarized previously are inadequately powered to evaluate the predictive value of NGAL levels in determining the risk for requiring renal replacement therapy (RRT) or the risk of mortality associated with AKI; RRT rates and mortality rates are too low in these series. This caveat notwithstanding, it appears that there is a relationship between the magnitude of the elevation in NGAL levels and the severity of AKI. In 3 studies of plasma NGAL measurements, the initial plasma NGAL level directly predicted the severity of AKI, as assessed by the RIFLE and AKIN criteria.[16,38,40] In a study of 301 adults admitted to a single ICU, mean peak plasma NGAL levels were 162 ng/mL in patients who did not develop AKI, and 230 ng/mL, 332 ng/mL, and 804 ng/mL in patients who met the criteria for risk, injury, and failure respectively in the RIFLE classification scheme.[16] A study of 88 ICU patients showed that no patients with a preliminary plasma NGAL level of lower than 155 ng/mL needed RRT for AKI; 15% of patients with a plasma NGAL level higher than 155 ng/mL required RRT.[40] A meta-analysis published in 2009 suggested that early urinary and plasma NGAL levels correlated directly with requirement for RRT in AKI and with in-hospital mortality.[43] **Tables 5** and **6** summarize studies that have examined the relationship between NGAL levels in the plasma and urine, in patients who required RRT for AKI as compared with patients who did not require RRT, and in patients who died with AKI as compared with patients who survived.

Table 5
Mean urinary levels of NGAL and outcomes (RRT and death) in patients with AKI

Study	Clinical Setting	NGAL Measurement	Mean (or Median) NGAL Levels
Bennett et al,[25] 2008	196 patients undergoing cardiothoracic surgery	Urine NGAL 2 hours after cardiopulmonary bypass	RRT data (in ng/mg creatinine) 5081 ± 320 with RRT 1850 ± 197 no RRT (P<.01) Mortality data: not reported
Siew et al,[30] 2009	451 critically ill adults	Urine NGAL within 24 hours of admission to ICU	RRT data (in ng/mg creatinine) 548 (IQR 156–4665) with RRT 61 (IQR 17–232) no RRT (P<.001) Mortality data: 223 (IQR 36–1074) dead 56 (IQR 16–195) alive (P<.001)
Bagshaw et al,[42] 2010	83 adults in intensive care units	Urine NGAL within 12 and 24 hours of admission to ICU	RRT data (in ng/mg creatinine) 423 (247–1088) with RRT 143 (28–283) no RRT (P<.03) Mortality data: 418 (201–1068) dead 106 (30–883) alive (P = .078)

Abbreviations: AKI, acute kidney injury; ICU, intensive care unit; IQR, interquartile range; NGAL, neutrophil gelatinase–associated lipocalin; RRT, renal replacement therapy.

Table 6
Mean plasma levels of NGAL and outcomes (RRT and death) in patients with AKI

Study	Clinical Setting	NGAL Measurement	Mean (or Median) NGAL Levels
Bagshaw et al,[42] 2010	83 adults in intensive care units	Urine NGAL within 24 and 48 hours of admission to ICU	RRT data (in ng/mL) 445 (336–869) with RRT 269 (133–401) no RRT ($P = .051$) Mortality data: 496 (192–750) dead 264 (122–437) alive ($P = .019$)

Abbreviations: AKI, acute kidney injury; ICU, intensive care unit; NGAL, neutrophil gelatinase–associated lipocalin; RRT, renal replacement therapy.

LIMITATIONS OF NGAL

A number of limitations to the value of NGAL as a predictor of AKI and its severity remain. As discussed previously, NGAL levels appear to be most sensitive and specific in predicting AKI in studies of homogeneous patients with single, acute, easily identifiable, and predictable nephrotoxic insults, such as cardiopulmonary bypass or intravenous contrast. NGAL appears to be less sensitive and specific in more heterogeneous cohorts with multifactorial causes for AKI. It is also unclear whether NGAL levels can differentiate potentially reversible causes of AKI such as prerenal azotemia from more severe kidney injury. NGAL levels seem to predict AKI in children with better accuracy than with adults, who make up the vast majority of patients with AKI. Plasma NGAL levels are also higher in patients with underlying CKD,[32] and most of the clinical trials of NGAL discussed earlier excluded patients with CKD from analysis. This exclusion is an important confounding issue, because CKD is a major risk factor for AKI, particularly in the critical care setting. Of note, in a recent prospective study of more than 25,000 patients with AKI, over 30% had underlying CKD.[50]

Baseline plasma NGAL levels are higher in patients with malignancies and systemic bacterial infections and these may be confounding factors. Urinary NGAL levels may also be elevated in the setting of urinary tract infections, and in one study levels were even used to diagnose early urinary tract infections in the absence of AKI.[51] Finally, most studies of NGAL have used research laboratory–based enzyme-linked immunosorbent assays (ELISAs) with variable and potentially lengthy turnaround times. Because NGAL elevations need to be detected early if they are to have any clinical benefit, assays need to provide results rapidly and in a point-of-care setting. Rapid, point-of-care assays for urinary and plasma NGAL are now available[11] but have not been tested in large clinical trials.

SUMMARY

Based on the information to date, although limitations in the accuracy of NGAL in predicting AKI persist, the preponderance of published studies demonstrate that NGAL, when measured in the plasma and in the urine, is a reliable biomarker for the subsequent development of clinically apparent AKI, much as troponin is a biomarker for the development of acute coronary syndrome. Significant increases in NGAL levels above baseline antedate other clinical markers of AKI such as the rise in the serum creatinine level, by 24 to 48 hours. A less extensive data set suggests that the magnitude of the NGAL elevation, in the plasma and urine, correlates with the severity of AKI, with the eventual requirement for RRT, and the risk of mortality.

Studies of NGAL in AKI need to be conducted in larger series involving multiple centers and in settings other than cardiothoracic ICUs. The NGAL assays need to be standardized assays and methods developed to provide results rapidly and at the point of care. Finally, early detection of AKI is only important and clinically relevant if it facilitates interventions that can improve outcomes. If very early detection of AKI, via the measurement of plasma or urinary NGAL, can be followed by effective treatment to abort the development or limit the severity of AKI, and therefore decrease the rate of RRT, length of hospitalization stay, and/or mortality risk, NGAL measurement will become a critically important diagnostic tool in critical care medicine, pediatrics, and surgery. Those trials have yet to be performed.

REFERENCES

1. Nolan CR, Anderson RJ. Hospital acquired acute renal failure. J Am Soc Nephrol 1998;9:710–8.
2. Hou SH, Bushinksy DA, Wish JA, et al. Hospital acquired renal insufficiency: a prospective study. Am J Med 1983;74:243–8.
3. Mehta RL, Pascual MT, Soroko S, et al. Spectrum of acute renal failure in the intensive care unit: the PICARD experience. Kidney Int 2004;66:1613–21.
4. Newsome BB, Warnock DG, McClellan WM, et al. Long term risk of mortality and end stage renal disease among the elderly after small increases in serum creatinine level during hospitalization for acute myocardial infarction. Arch Intern Med 2008;168:609–16.
5. Bellomo R, Ronco C, Kellum JA, et al. Acute Renal Failure: definition, outcome measures, animal models, fluid therapy and informational technology needs. The Second International Consensus Conference of the Acute Dialysis Quality Initiative (ADQI) Group. Crit Care 2004;8:R204–12.
6. Mehta RL, Kellum JA, Shah SV, et al. Acute kidney injury network (AKIN): report on an initiative to improve outcomes in acute kidney injury. Crit Care 2007;11:R31.
7. Schrier RW. Need to intervene in established acute renal failure. J Am Soc Nephrol 2004;15:2756–8.
8. Bagshaw SM, Langenberg C, Bellomo R. Urinary biochemistry and microscopy in septic acute renal failure: a systematic review. Am J Kidney Dis 2006;48:695–705.
9. Zhou H, Hewitt SM, Yuen PS, et al. Acute kidney injury biomarkers: needs, present status, and future promise. Nephrol Self Assess Program 2006;5:63–71.
10. Kjeldsen L, Cowland JB, Borregaard N. Human neutrophil gelatinase-associated lipocalin and homologous proteins in rat and mouse. Biochim Biophys Acta 2000; 1482:272–83.
11. Devarajan P. Review: neutrophil gelatinase-associated lipocalin: a troponin-like marker for human acute kidney injury. Nephrology (Carlton) 2010;15:419–28.
12. Devarajan P. Neutrophil gelatinase-associated lipocalin: new paths for an old shuttle. Cancer Ther 2007;5:463–70.
13. Mishra J, Dent C, Tarabishi R, et al. Neutrophil gelatinase-associated lipocalin (NGAL) as a biomarker for acute renal injury after cardiac surgery. Lancet 2005;365:1231–8.
14. Schmidt-Ott KM, Mori K, Li JY, et al. Dual action of neutrophil gelatinase associated lipocalin. J Am Soc Nephrol 2007;18:407–13.
15. Mishra J, Ma Q, Prada A, et al. Identification of neutrophil gelatinase associated lipocalin as a novel early urinary biomarker for ischemic renal injury. J Am Soc Nephrol 2003;10:2534–43.

16. Cruz DN, de Cal M, Garzotto F, et al. Plasma neutrophil gelatinase-associated lipocalin is an early biomarker for acute kidney injury in an adult ICU population. Intensive Care Med 2010;36:444–51.

17. Wheeler DS, Devarajan P, Ma Q, et al. Serum neutrophil gelatinase associated lipocalin as a marker of acute kidney injury in critically ill children with septic shock. Crit Care Med 2008;36:1297–303.

18. Supavekin S, Zhang W, Kucherlapati R, et al. Differential gene expression following early renal ischemia/reperfusion. Kidney Int 2003;63:1714–24.

19. Yuen PS, Jo SK, Holly MK, et al. Ischemic and nephrotoxic acute renal failure are distinguished by their broad transcriptomic responses. Physiol Genomics 2006; 25:375–86.

20. Haase M, Bellomo R, Devarajan P, et al. Accuracy of neutrophil gelatinase associated lipocalin (NGAL) in diagnosis and prognosis in acute kidney injury: a systematic review and meta analysis. Am J Kidney Dis 2009;54:1012–24.

21. Wagener G, Jan M, Kim M, et al. Association between increases in urinary neutrophil associated lipocalin and acute renal dysfunction after adult cardiac surgery. Anesthesiology 2006;105:485–91.

22. Parikh CR, Jani A, Mishra J, et al. Urine NGAL and IL-18 are predictive biomarkers for delayed graft function following kidney transplantation. Am J Transplant 2006;6:1639–45.

23. Koyner J, Bennett M, Worcester E, et al. Urinary cystatin C as an early biomarker for acute kidney injury following adult cardiothoracic surgery. Kidney Int 2008;74: 1059–69.

24. Xin C, Yulong X, Yu C, et al. Urine neutrophil gelatinase associated lipocalin and interleukin 18 predict acute kidney injury after cardiac surgery. Ren Fail 2008;30: 904–13.

25. Bennett M, Dent CL, Ma Q, et al. Urine NGAL predicts severity of acute kidney injury after cardiac surgery: a prospective study. Clin J Am Soc Nephrol 2008; 3:665–73.

26. Portilla D, Dent C, Sugaya T, et al. Liver fatty acid binding protein as a biomarker for acute kidney injury after cardiac surgery. Kidney Int 2008;73:465–72.

27. Ling W, Zhahoui N, Ben H, et al. Urinary IL-18 and NGAL as early predictive biomarkers in contrast induced nephropathy after coronary angiography. Nephron Clin Pract 2008;108:176–81.

28. Nickolas TL, O'Rourke MJ, Yang J, et al. Sensitivity and specificity of a single emergency department measurement of urinary neutrophil gelatinase associated lipocalin for diagnosing acute kidney injury. Ann Intern Med 2008;148:810–9.

29. Tuladhar SM, Puntmann VO, Soni M, et al. Rapid detection of acute kidney injury by plasma and urinary neutrophil gelatinase associated lipocalin after cardiopulmonary bypass. J Cardiovasc Pharmacol 2009;53:261–6.

30. Siew ED, Wre LB, Gebretsadik T, et al. Urine neutrophil gelatinase associated lipocalin moderately predicts acute kidney injury in critically ill adults. J Am Soc Nephrol 2009;20:1823–32.

31. Makris K, Markou N, Evodia E, et al. Urinary neutrophil gelatinase associated lipocalin (NGAL) as an early marker of acute kidney injury in critically ill multiple trauma patients. Clin Chem Lab Med 2009;47:79–82.

32. McIllroy DR, Wagener G, Lee HT. Neutrophil gelatinase associated lipocalin and acute kidney injury after cardiac surgery: the effect of baseline renal function on diagnostic performance. Clin J Am Soc Nephrol 2010;5:211–9.

33. Hall IE, Yarlagadda SG, Coca SG, et al. IL-18 and urinary NGAL predict dialysis and graft recovery after kidney transplantation. J Am Soc Nephrol 2010;21:189–97.

34. Yang HN, Boo CS, Kim MG, et al. Urine neutrophil gelatinase associated lipocalin: an independent predictor of adverse outcomes in acute kidney injury. Am J Nephrol 2010;6:501–9.
35. Martensson J, Bell M, Oldner A, et al. Neutrophil gelatinase associated lipocalin in adult septic patients with and without kidney injury. Intensive Care Med 2010; 36:1333–40.
36. Hirsch R, Dent C, Pfrim H, et al. NGAL is a early predictive biomarker of contrast-induced nephropathy in children. Pediatr Nephrol 2007;22:2089–95.
37. Zappitelli M, Washburn KM, Arikan AA, et al. Urine NGAL is an early marker of acute renal injury in critically ill children. Crit Care 2007;11:R84.
38. Haase-Fielitz A, Bellomo R, Devarajan P, et al. Novel and conventional serum biomarkers predicting acute kidney injury in adult cardiac surgery—a prospective cohort study. Crit Care Med 2009;37:553–60.
39. Malyszko J, Bachorewska-Gajewska H, Poniatowski B, et al. Urinary and serum biomarkers after cardiac catheterization in diabetic patients with stable angina and without severe chronic kidney disease. Ren Fail 2009;31:910–9.
40. Constantin JM, Futier E, Perbet S, et al. Plasma neutrophil gelatinase associated lipocalin is an early marker of acute kidney injury in adult critically ill patients: a prospective study. J Crit Care 2009;25(176):1–6.
41. Niemann CU, Walla A, Waldman J, et al. Acute kidney injury during liver transplantation as determined by neutrophil gelatinase associated lipocalin. Liver Transpl 2009;15:1852–60.
42. Bagshaw SM, Bennett M, Haase M, et al. Plasma and urine neutrophil gelatinase associated lipocalin in septic versus non-septic acute kidney injury in critical illness. Intensive Care Med 2010;36:452–61.
43. Dent CL, Ma Q, Dastrala S, et al. Plasma NGAL predicts acute kidney injury, morbidity and mortality after pediatric cardiac surgery: a prospective uncontrolled cohort study. Crit Care 2007;11:R127.
44. Malyszko J, Malyszko JS, Baochorewska-Gajewska H, et al. Neutrophil gelatinase associated lipocalin is a new and sensitive marker of kidney function in chronic kidney disease patients and renal allograft recipients. Transplant Proc 2009;41:158–61.
45. Przbylowski P, Malyszko M, Malyszko JS. Serum neutrophil gelatinase associated lipocalin correlates with kidney function in heart allograft recipients. Transplant Proc 2010;42:1797–802.
46. Gaspari F, Cravedi P, Mandala M, et al. Predicting cisplatin-induced acute kidney injury by urinary neutrophil gelatinase associated lipocalin excretion: a pilot prospective case control study. Nephron Clin Pract 2010;115:154–60.
47. Trachtman H, Christen E, Canaan A, et al. Urinary neutrophil gelatinase associated lipocalin in D+ HUS: a novel marker of renal injury. Pediatr Nephrol 2006; 21:989–94.
48. Mishra J, Ma Q, Kelly C, et al. Kidney NGAL is a novel early marker of acute injury following transplantation. Pediatr Nephrol 2006;21:856–63.
49. Kusaka M, Kuroyanagi Y, Mori T, et al. Serum neutrophil gelatinase associated lipocalin as a predictor of organ recovery after kidney transplantation from donors after cardiac death. Cell Transplant 2008;17:129–34.
50. Uchino S, Kellum JA, Bellomo R, et al. Acute renal failure in critically ill patients: a multinational multicenter study. JAMA 2005;294:813–8.
51. Yilmaz A, Sevketoglu E, Gedikbasi A, et al. Early prediction of urinary tract infection with urinary neutrophil gelatinase associated lipocalin. Pediatr Nephrol 2009; 60:2772–81.

Multimarker Panels in Sepsis

Brian Casserly, MD[a],*, Richard Read, MD[b], Mitchell M. Levy, MD[b]

KEYWORDS
• Multimarker panels • Sepsis • Biomarkers • Statistics
• Systemic inflammatory response syndrome

A biomarker has been defined as "a characteristic that is objectively measured and evaluated as an indicator of normal biologic processes, pathogenic processes, or pharmacologic responses to therapeutic intervention."[1] Often, the term biomarker is commonly restricted to a quantifiable parameter that is measured from a biologic sample such as blood or urine. However, a biomarker can describe any measurable biologic parameter that provides insight into biologic processes in health or disease.[2] Biomarkers derive their value from their ability to differentiate between 2 or more biologic states. This ability to discriminate separates biomarkers from simple measurements.[3] The theoretic advantage of combining several biomarkers into a single classification rule is that it should help to improve their classification accuracy and, therefore, their clinical usefulness. The search for multimarker panels that fulfill this criterion will continue in complex diseases, such as sepsis, where it seems unlikely that any single marker will allow for precise disease specification.[4]

The critical care literature is replete with studies using multiple biomarkers.[5–7] However, when several markers are measured, they are often considered separately, irrespective of the additional information contained in their joint interpretation. This does not constitute a multimarker panel.[8] This distinction is important, because these studies typically describe a list of different biomarkers with potential diagnostic or prognostic values that are used as individual predictors of disease or clinical outcome. Another common confusion is the term multiplex assay, which is a type of laboratory procedure that simultaneously measures multiple analytes (dozens or more) in a single assay. It is distinguished from procedures that measure 1 or a few analytes at a time.[9] In contrast, a multimarker panel involves each biomarker representing the inputs to a multivariable, computational prediction or classification model. Multimarker panels can be further subdivided into homogeneous and heterogeneous panels, depending on the diversity of their source data.[10] An example of a homogeneous panel would be if the source data was exclusively gene expression

[a] Division of Pulmonary and Critical Care Medicine, The Memorial Hospital of Rhode Island, 111 Brewster Street, Pawtucket, RI 02048, USA
[b] Rhode Island Hospital, Alpert Medical School of Brown University, Providence, RI, USA
* Corresponding author.
E-mail address: brian_casserly@brown.edu

Crit Care Clin 27 (2011) 391–405
doi:10.1016/j.ccc.2010.12.011   criticalcare.theclinics.com
0749-0704/11/$ – see front matter © 2011 Elsevier Inc. All rights reserved.

microarray analysis, whereas heterogeneous source data might include a clinical variable (eg, lung injury score) with microarray analysis.

The recent advances in high-throughput technology in genomics (gene expression arrays and single nucleotide polymorphisms) and proteomics (protein expression using mass spectrometry or antibody arrays) will result in the simultaneous identification of a vast array of potential new biomarkers.[11] This development will allow biomedical researchers to combine multiple biomarkers for disease classifications (detection, diagnosis, and prognosis). However, there are also challenges. The increasing number of available potential biomarker candidates will greatly increase the number of ways of combining multiple biomarkers.[12,13] Future challenges will not be the discovery of new markers. More than 100 distinct molecules have been proposed as useful biologic markers of sepsis.[14] The real challenge will be the optimal selection and validation of a subgroup of clinically useful markers from the large pool of potential candidates.[15] Searching for the optimal combination of biomarkers will significantly increase the complexity of the statistical modeling and increase the computational demands.[16]

The effective use of multimarker panels in routine clinical practice will depend on the ability of future studies to adequately distill the information regarding the complex assessment of multimarker panels into readily digestible information for practicing clinicians. This increased complexity is only useful if it informs clinical decision making. Clinicians need to understand, and not be overwhelmed by, the increasing complexity.

The process of converting multiple reliable predictors into a practical clinical test is particularly daunting. As a consequence, multimarker panels in sepsis are presently underdeveloped. Furthermore, the appropriate methodologies for the clinical and statistical evaluation of multimarker panels have not yet been systematically defined.[17] Molecules are often described as biomarkers before they have gone through the crucial validation steps.[18] This review provides some insights into the assessment of multimarker panels and some context to the increasingly important role that statistical rigor will play in the development of multimarker panels.[19,20]

THE SYNDROME OF SEPSIS: A DIFFICULT PHENOTYPE

The complexity and redundancy of the host immune response makes it unlikely that a single biomarker can adequately describe and stratify the sepsis syndrome.[21] Ideally, multimarker panels will add to diagnostic accuracy and risk assessment in sepsis.

Sepsis is the innate host response to infection.[22] However, various definitions and terminologies are often used interchangeably, leading to problems of accurate assessment of the identification, incidence, and prognosis in sepsis.[23] New understanding of inflammatory mediators and pathways, immunity, and genetic variability in sepsis suggests that the current definitions of systemic inflammatory response syndrome (SIRS), sepsis, serious sepsis, and septic shock are oversimplified.[24] These definitions rely on the presence of a nonspecific physiologic host response to infection rather than a discrete pathologic process.[25] Therefore, there is no objective pathologic gold standard that can be used to confirm the presence or absence of sepsis.

An example of this conundrum is the use of bacterial cultures as the current gold standard for the detection of infection. Blood cultures have low rates of positive results in septic patients, especially in patients treated with antibiotics.[26,27] Detection of ubiquitous, highly conserved sequences within the 16S rRNA of bacteria using universal primers and clone libraries has shown that the number of microbes identified by blood culture represents only a small fraction of those present.[28,29] Furthermore, the detection of a low abundance of anaerobic organisms is difficult.[30] This is further compounded by many organisms that are commensals in healthy individuals undergoing a pathogenic shift resulting in the ability to cause disease in the immunocompromised. These changes in bacterial properties are not adequately described by culture-dependent techniques.[31] Despite these limitations, there is a growing body of literature suggesting that procalcition (PCT) is a specific marker for severe bacterial infection using blood cultures as the gold standard and, in the appropriate clinical context, may distinguish patients who have sepsis from patients who have SIRS.[32–38] The improvement in techniques based on polymerase chain reaction (PCR) have resulted in the ability to detect very low levels of bacterial DNA,[39,40] which achieves a significant increase in sensitivity and contributes to earlier detection of bacteria. To validate the ability of PCT to discriminate bacterial infection will require more than blood cultures as the gold standard. Ironically, if PCR technology is validated, the use of a biomarker to detect bacterial infection will likely have limited clinical usefulness.

Therefore, the rate-limiting step for biomarker development and validation still remains our limited ability to define the clinical phenotypes of sepsis; the so-called phenome. Currently, we lack the capacity to accurately separate distinct populations of patients in sepsis with specific disease characteristics. As our ability to discriminate the various patient subsets in sepsis improves so will our ability to accurately validate biomarkers and, paradoxically, it will simultaneously reduce the need for biomarkers.

COMBINING BIOMARKERS: TRIAL DESIGN CONSIDERATIONS

The principles of clinical validation are well established in, for example, randomized controlled trials.[41] The consumers of clinical trial reports have been educated to be skeptical of exhaustive searches for statistical significance. They are wary of subset analysis and trials with multiple endpoints, knowing that the chance of an erroneous conclusion increases with any departure from a single primary endpoint.[42] However, studies using newer technologies and high-throughput approaches like gene expression analysis are often less structured with no written protocol, no eligibility criteria, and no a priori hypothesis.[43] There is substantial confusion about what it means to validate biomarkers.[44] Furthermore, the assessment of models using multiple input variables raises unique issues. For example, the possibility of assay inconsistencies is amplified. Any biases encountered at this point of the study will be hardwired into the data and cannot be removed by statistical analysis. Therefore, any classifier derived from multiple variables has a higher chance of including such a wired-in bias and, as a consequence, has a higher chance of failing in a subsequent validation study.[18]

Ultimately, the assessment of multimarker panels should rely on the same principles as evaluating any observational trial.[45] The key question is always whether the study is valid. The control group should reflect true diagnostic uncertainty. Comparing healthy volunteers with patients in septic shock will increase the likelihood of artificial case/control differences, which is known as spectrum bias.[46] Other sources of potential bias include specimen samples being used as controls that were historically collected. Therefore, the controls were unlikely to be drawn from the same population from which the cases were selected. Other relevant questions that need to be asked include- do the sample of patients, controls, or other comparison groups truly represent the patient population of interest? Is the prevalence of disease in the samples used to build a model similar to the prevalence of disease in the target patient population? Were the patients equal at baseline? It is often overlooked that proteins are known to vary widely in different individuals because of variables such as age, gender, medications, and the presence of various diseases. Verification bias results when the accuracy of a test is evaluated among only those with known disease status (excluding the unknown or indeterminate).[47] Were the samples handled the same way? Details of the storage methods might reveal differences in the way specimens were collected or handled. Were there any differences in the timing of the blood draws, and were all assays measured in all patients recruited to the study? If not, this suggests that the samples were collected as convenient samples rather than through a randomized protocol. These factors represent major sources of false-positive biomarker predictions.[48]

Other barriers to reproducibility, including technical variation, can be addressed through replication, ensuring data reliability and accuracy. Measurement error may result if a true reference standard is absent or an imperfect standard is used for comparison.[49] Biologic variation reflects the variability in the population of interest, and the appropriate statistical analysis needs to be used to take the biologic variance into account. As with all case-control studies, they require independent replication and eventual confirmation in large prospective cohort studies.

COMBINING BIOMARKERS: STATISTICAL CONSIDERATIONS

There are some commonly used statistical approaches to validate multimarker panels. Rather than recapitulating the principles outlined in earlier reviews (see the article by Gerlach and colleagues elsewhere in this issue for further exploration of this topic). This article will emphasize the statistical approaches that are especially pertinent to multimarker panels. There is a sound basis to the strategy for combining multiple biomarkers.[50] If each tested biomarker behaves independently as a predictor of disease, then testing many biomarkers simultaneously provides the opportunity to improve both sensitivity and specificity.[49] The key questions are what is the value added to the existing data by the addition of a new marker?[2] Does this new information justify the increase in complexity? The competing forces within a multimarker panel (namely maximizing total information and minimizing complexity) need to be carefully balanced.

The first statistical pitfall that needs to be considered is that the ability to identify predictive patterns is increased with the number of measurements that are made. These predictive patterns may be unique to the data set from which they were derived and not survive external validation (ie, overfitting the data). This problem can be avoided by using the appropriate statistical methods for multiple variables and verifying any discoveries on independent validation sets.[51] Therefore, findings from studies with multiple variables in their multimarker panel, derived from small sample sizes, should be treated as exploratory and in need of external validation.[52]

Sample size requirements for validating a new biomarker are demanding. The sample size requirements that allow identification of a benefit beyond existing markers are even more demanding. As a general principle, models tend to perform better in their derivation data sets than they do in independent validation.[53] Therefore, a careful assessment is required to ensure that a panel truly performs better than its constituent individual biomarkers, hence avoiding false hopes.[54] The appropriate experimental and statistical design and the demonstration of external validation are the most important factors for ensuring that these concerns are addressed appropriately.[55] In assessing clinical studies using multimarker panels, a key observation is whether the patients in the study were used to create the prediction model or validate the prediction model. Many of the published clinical studies, thus far, have created prediction models with no accompanying internal validation (using a test data set that played no role in model development) or external validation (using data from a completely different study).

COMBINING BIOMARKERS: MODEL BUILDING

The data analysis starts by building a discrimination model that separates the groups as well as possible, by identifying which combinations of variables in the groups are most distinct. Often there is little a priori knowledge about which biomarkers to include in the model.[56] The temptation is to simply select the variables that survive univariate analysis or, alternatively, to use an automated procedure such as stepwise regression. This method often leads to the model capturing patterns that are idiosyncratic features of that particular data set.[57] However, the subsequent use of all possible variables can suppress or reduce the performance of the prediction algorithm. Selection of discriminatory features is critical to the accuracy prediction.[58] To create classification rules, there has to be some preliminary selection of the variables based on the performance of each variable separately.[59] It is important to know what methods were used to construct the model performing the classification task because, in the development of a prediction model, the most important question still concerns the ability of the model to predict results using independent samples.[57] Complex algorithms may create complicated boundaries from the training sample that can not be generalized to other data sets (ie, overfitting the data).[60] Ideally, one should use the smallest number of classification rules for consideration in the training sample.[61] This needs to be reconciled with the many methods that can be applied to define biomarker panels.

Some classifications can be generated by simple "and/or" rules, but more complicated rules are generally applied. The threshold methods have the advantage of simple boundaries that reduce the risk of overfitting the training data.[62] They are easy to interpret and well suited to biomarker panel data, in which class boundaries of a single marker can often be represented as single cutoff points. Decision trees are similar to threshold-based methods, but they can create more complex boundaries. A boosting algorithm iteratively combines multiple predictors. In each iteration it downweights the observations that are correctly classified by the existing classifier, and upweights the observations that are not. Therefore, the focus shifts to the previously misclassified observations and to improving their classification. A new predictor is added to the current classifier depending on its ability to improve the existing classification.[19]

In its simplest form, logistic regression uses a linear boundary to classify variables. It uses a mathematical formulation that yields a globally optimal solution. Logistic regression and linear and nonlinear discriminate analyses identify the linear combinations of markers that yield the highest sensitivity and specificity.[13] These models derive a score, in contrast with decision trees, Bayesian decision making, and neural networks, which devise a specific decision rule.[12] The recent proliferation of statistical studies addressing the problem of combining correlated diagnostic tests to maximize discriminatory power highlights the lack of consensus about what is the best and most appropriate test to use.[63]

However, the key to assessing the usefulness of these algorithms is that, once the panel is defined, its performance must be evaluated and validated. A common statistical practice is to internally validate the data by splitting them into training and test samples.[64] The training set is used to build the model and the test sample is used to validate it. Therefore, internal validation has the advantage of not requiring collection of data beyond the original study.[57] For internal validation to be valid, the testing data should only be used during validation procedures and should play no role in model development.

If not enough subjects are available to split the data, randomization techniques, such as permutation tests, cross validation, and bootstrapping can help assess the validity of the classifier model.[65] When using a data set with small number of samples but a large number of variables, it may be possible to find two arbitrary groups that can be well separated. However, in that case, the good discrimination in the classifier model may be a coincidence and may not be significant.

The ultimate validation is to reproduce the experiment on a different data set not derived from the original investigation (ie, external validation). As with internal validation, external validation can only be performed once, and only to validate. It is not legitimate to subsequently reevaluate the model using this external data set. External validation represents the gold standard but is vanishingly rare in the clinical literature because of funding and timing constraints.[66] The creation of biomarker subtrials within randomized controlled trials is a possible solution that could be considered. However, subtrials have to be carefully constructed with due statistical consideration given to analyzing multiple primary outcomes.[67]

COMBINING BIOMARKERS: INTERPRETING RESULTS

Regarding the assessment of the results of a multimarker panel, no single test can characterize the overall performance and usefulness.[68] The interpretation of diverse performance quality measures is recommended.[69] These, in turn, should be context specific (eg, the area under the curve [AUC] would not be the most suitable choice when risk assessment is the main focus). Also, in determining the usefulness of new biomarkers, it is important to adjust the risk for established markers (covariant or possible confounders) to decide whether the new marker adds additional diagnostic discrimination.[70] The way these established markers are treated is also significant. For example, if a biomarker was only tested in an elderly population, then the effect of age on the outcome of that population would be reduced, which may give the false impression that the new biomarker gives additional prognostic information beyond what is contained in the patient's age. However, it may not be possible to generalize this biomarker to patient populations of all ages. It is also important to draw a distinction between validating patient populations and patient-level predictions. Individual predictions are more difficult and variable, but ultimately define the usefulness of the multimarker panel.

There are 2 principal types of errors in disease classification: identifying disease where it is not present (a false positive) and failing to identify disease when it is present (false negative). Therefore, to be able fully characterize performance, measures of performance should contain 2 components related to the 2 types of classification errors. Odds ratios are only a single measure of association and, as such, cannot meaningfully describe the ability of a marker to classify patients.[71] In the ideal test, the probabilities of both types of errors, a false positive and a false negative, are small. At any particular data point, this can be estimated using the likelihood ratio. Likelihood ratios are particularly useful in multimarker panels because they can be used in series (eg, posttest probability from the first marker becomes the pretest probability for the second marker).

Receiver operator characteristic (ROC) curves can be useful in determining the discriminatory capacity of a biomarker, identifying optimal cutoff points for decision making, and evaluating the trade-off between sensitivity and specificity.[72] Each point on the ROC curve represents a likelihood ratio. The AUC may be presented with 95% confidence intervals to indicate whether the curve crosses or approaches the nonsignificant 0.5 value at any point.[47]

MULTIMARKER PANELS IN SEPSIS: CLINICAL EXAMPLES

There is a limited number of studies using multimarker panels in the sepsis literature. A couple of examples are described here to illustrate how multimarker panels are developing. Kofoed and colleagues[73] compared the ability of 4 composite biomarkers including a 3-marker panel (soluble urokinase-type plasminogen activator receptor [V-suPAR], soluble triggering receptor expressed on myeloid cells-1[sTREM-1], and macrophage inhibiting factor [MIF]), V-suPAR and age, sTREM and age, and the 3-marker panel and age to predict 30-day and 180-day mortality in patients presenting with community acquired infection with 2 criteria of SIRS. The 3-marker panel plus age outperformed the 3 other composites with an area under the ROC curve of 0.93 for predicting 30-day mortality and an area under the ROC curve of 0.87 for predicting 180-day mortality.

The strength of this study was the ability of the 3-marker panel and age to predict an objective endpoint, namely mortality, in the patients who would not necessarily be regarded as high risk (ie, patients with SIRS). Duplicate measures of the soluble receptors and cytokines were performed and within-assay coefficients of variation (CV), as well between-assay CVs, were reported and within acceptable ranges. However, only 19 of the total 151 patients died within 180 days; the small numbers limit the ability of the study to make definitive conclusions. Also, not all blood samples were collected within 24 hours, making reproducibility more difficult. Furthermore, the use of patients with SIRS ensured a wide patient spectrum in that it did not include patients who required direct admission to the intensive care unit (ICU).

The same group previously performed some pioneering experiments developing and validating a multiplex add-on assay for sepsis biomarkers.[74] This technology allows multiplexing of analytes in solution with flow cytometry. Using color coded microspheres, this technology has the ability to produce 100 distinctly colored bead sets that can be conjugated with a different capture antibody. Using this technology, they compared a 6-marker panel including V-suPAR, sTREM-1, MIF, C-reactive protein (CRP), PCT, and neutrophil count with a 3-marker panel including neutrophil count, CRP, and PCT, and with each component of the 6-marker panel individually.[75] The primary endpoint of the study was to assess which marker could identify most accurately the patients with SIRS who developed bacterial infection. The 6-marker panel outperformed the 3-marker panel and each of its individual components, with an AUC of 0.88. The study suggests some interesting points. Of the 96 patients classified as having bacterial infection, 32 patients were culture negative and classified solely by expert opinion, which highlights the difficulty validating the use of biomarkers to predict the presence of bacterial infection.

Selberg and colleagues[76] compared the combination of PCT and activated complement 3 (C3a) in a sepsis score with the performance of PCT, interleukin (IL)-6, C3a, elastase, and CRP individually in discriminating between patients with SIRS and patients with sepsis. The sepsis score outperformed the individual biomarkers with an area under the ROC curve of 0.93. The sepsis score was derived using a complicated logistic regression equation that identified 28.6 as the optimal cutoff between patients with SIRS and with sepsis. However, the usefulness of this cutoff was not validated prospectively and was not able to discriminate well in patients who had scores between 27.22 and 29.99. Given that this score was generated in a cohort of 33 patients, the likelihood of it surviving external validation is reduced.

Harbath and colleagues[35] found that the addition of PCT to a clinical predictive model improved its ability to distinguish between SIRS and sepsis syndrome (confirmed sepsis severe sepsis and septic shock). However, the clinical model only contained temperature, heart rate, blood pressure, and white blood cell count and, as expected, had limited discriminatory value in differentiating patients with sepsis syndrome from patients with SIRS (AUC 0.77). The poor performance of the clinical model alone may have amplified the effect of adding PCT. However, the combination did achieve an impressive AUC of 0.94. Conversely, PCT in this study was inferior to IL-6 in predicting sepsis-related mortality, which is a more objective clinical outcome and illustrates the limitations of using AUC for risk classification.

A study by Punyadeera and colleagues[77] showed that combined measurement of matrix metalloproteinases (MMP-3), IL-10, IL-1α, IP-10, sIL-2R, sFas, soluble tumor necrosis receptor 1(sTNF-R1), sRAGE, granulocyte myeloid colony stimulating factor (GM-CSF), IL-1β, and eotaxin allows for a good separation of patients with SIRS or sepsis who survived from those who died (mortality prediction with a sensitivity of 79% and specificity of 86%). This study gives an insight into future studies. In the plasma samples that were obtained, 28 biomolecules were analyzed using the Luminex system (USA): 10 cytokines (TNF-α, IL-1β, eotaxin, IL-13, MIP-1α, IL-10, IL-1α, IP-10, GM-CSF and IFN-γ), 8 matrix metalloproteinases (MMP-1, -2, -3, -7, -8, -9, -10, and -13), and 10 soluble factors (GP130, IL-2R, ICAM, E-selectin, Fas, TNF-R1, TNF-R2, RAGE, VCAM, and MIF). This study is noteworthy for several reasons. There was a small number of patients in the study. In total, 118 samples were collected from the 16 patients mentioned earlier. Six of these patients died and 10 survived. Although this ratio of patients to sample number is unusual, thus far, in clinical studies using multimarker panels, these types of ratios are commonly seen in studies of gene expression analysis. As a consequence, they are likely to become more common in the future and, therefore, statistical analysis will have to be adjusted accordingly. In this study, a support vector machine was trained on some observations and tested on others. They applied a leave-one-out scheme to internally validate the classifier that they had constructed. They also used the Bonferroni correction for multiple testing. The determination of whether a patient was SIRS versus sepsis was made on a daily basis, which is particularly important because SIRS can persist in patients after infection has cleared. Therefore, even an unbiased expert opinion, that only classifies patients into one of these groups based on their hospital stay as a whole, cannot account for this possible misclassification bias. Also, blood samples were drawn daily, allowing for assessment of biomarker velocity (ie, an assessment of the perfomance of the biomarker over a period of time, rather than just once).

Lukaszeki and colleagues recruited on admission 92 patients in ICUs who had undergone procedures that increased the risk of developing sepsis. Blood samples were taken daily until either a clinical diagnosis of sepsis was made or until the patient was discharged from the ICU. The levels of expression of IL-1, IL-6, IL-8, and IL-10, tumor necrosis factor-α, FasL, and CCL2 mRNA were measured by real-time reverse transcriptase PCR. Neural networks using cytokine and chemokine data were able to correctly predict patient outcomes in an average of 83.09% of cases between 4 and 1 days before clinical diagnosis with high sensitivity and selectivity (91.43% and 80.20%, respectively). The neural network had an improved predictive accuracy of 94.55% when data from 22 healthy volunteers were analyzed in conjunction with the ICU patient data. However, comparing healthy volunteers with patients in septic shock will increase the likelihood of artificial case/control differences creating a spectrum bias. This pilot study may represent an example of the type of statistical approaches that will be used in the future to develop predictive models.

Dhainault and colleagues[78] created a composite coagulopathy score based on a retrospective analysis of the PROWESS trial. The composite coagulopathy score in combination with the APACHE II score outperformed the APACHE II score alone in predicting patients who would develop multiple organ failure (AUC 0.61 APACHE II alone vs AUC 0.65 APACHE II and composite coagulopathy score in combination) and patients who would die in 28 days (AUC 0.69 APACHE II alone vs AUC 0.74 APACHE II and composite coagulopathy score in combination). The composite coagulopathy score included 4 parameters: antithrombin measurement at baseline, decrease in antithrombin measurement in time, the lack of a decrease in prothrombin time measurement in time, and a lack of decrease in D-dimer measurement in time. Logistic regression was used to select the optimal cutoffs for the ability of these measurements to predict mortality. This study suggests a temporal relationship between coagulopathy and the development of organ failure but, as acknowledged by the investigators, this hypothesis needs to be confirmed in future studies. The coagulopathy score requires further validation.

In what is probably the largest study using multimarker panels in the critical care literature, Shapiro and colleagues[79] showed that a biomarker panel of neutrophil gelatinase-associated lipocalin, protein C, and IL-1 receptor antagonist could be used to develop a sepsis score. The AUC for the sepsis score 0.80 for severe sepsis, 0.77 for septic shock and 0.79 for death. This was a multicenter study with a total of 971 patients with suspected infection or SIRS enrolled from the emergency department. The sepsis score was devised from 9 potential biomarkers with the 3 biomarkers used in the score being selected from/by/because their performance in a multivariate logistic regression model. Models with more than 3 biomarkers were shown not to improve accuracy as determined by AUC. The model underwent cross validation and overfitting was estimated to be less than 1% of the ROC curve. Furthermore, these investigators built new multivariate models using demographic, clinical, and laboratory information to adjust for important covariates and potential confounders. The sepsis score remained significant. As discussed by the investigators, the sepsis score will require validation on an independent data set, ideally in a prospective clinical trial. However, the study does provide a template on which future studies using multimarker panels can be based. The large number of patients, the multicenter design, and the rigorous statistical interrogation suggest that the investigators have uncovered a multimarker panel that could survive the test of time.

MULTIMARKER PANELS: FUTURE APPROACHES

The identification and testing of new candidate markers has been dominated by targeted approaches in which candidates derived from biologic knowledge are evaluated for their correlations with biologic conditions. This approach has yielded many useful biomarkers. However, the power of high-throughput methodology will make this stepwise approach increasingly impractical because of the large number of new markers to be evaluated.[80] Many people believe that these new unbiased search strategies, unencumbered by the constraints of current biologic knowledge, are better suited to the development of novel biomarkers.[81,82] Using the hypothesis-driven approach has resulted in the selection of biomarkers from well-studied functional pathways. As a consequence, multimarker models tend to include correlated biomarkers, which may in turn reduce the classification ability of such models. The ability to use markers that reflect distinct biologic processes to provide incremental clinical information will be increasingly difficult. Therefore, the use of unbiased proteomic techniques will increasingly yield potential markers with poorly described, or even unknown, biologic functions.[83,84]

The solution may be take a systems-orientated view.[85] In complex disease, it is necessary to assess the overall network and its changed dynamics rather than individual pathways. Because the network contains extensive cross talk between pathways, as well as important feedback loops, it is crucial to represent it in the form of a computational model that allows a global analysis.[86] A systems-orientated view maintains that the properties of complex systems consist of many components that interact with each other in nonlinear, nonadditive ways and cannot be understood by focusing exclusively on the components.[87] Instead of pathways in which signaling is linear and definable, the reality is a large, interconnected network of proteins that regulate the host response to infection. Alterations in this network occur in unpredictable ways. Using a combination of DNA microarray data and protein-protein interaction information, prognostic forecasting will include the use of subnetworks of the protein-protein interaction network as predictors, rather than collections of individual genes.[88] Incorporation of modern postgenomic bioinformatics and functional genomics can determine associations between disease for phenotype and gene/protein expression.[89] The Inflammation and Host Response to Injury Large Scale Collaborative Research Program has already taken advantage of this approach by developing a structured network knowledge-base analysis of genome-wide transcriptional responses in human subjects receiving bacterial endotoxin.[90] This was achieved by assessing changes in blood leukocyte gene expression patterns and thereby providing insight into their regulation in response to an inflammatory stimulus.

The systems biology approach can utilize the advances in computational biology by using artificial neural networks to analyze large data sets and complex changes in multiple pathways simultaneously.[91] Practical biomarker panels can be constructed from biomarkers that are as independent as possible and reflective of the overall phenotype.[92] This development will require an understanding of new mathematical models capable of combining linearities and nonlinearities. Neural networks can be trained to recognize the relevant patterns in data (linear and nonlinear), whereas older statistical models requires prior knowledge of the relationships between the factors being investigated.[93]

SUMMARY

The most fundamental barrier to the creation of clinically useful multimarker panels and sepsis is the limited understanding of the biology of sepsis. The complex nature of biomarker development means that no individual has sufficient breadth of knowledge to be expert in the many domains involved in their creation, assessment, and validation. Accurate and robust biomarkers should not be rejected because the underlying biology is not understood. The performance of the model is paramount, and although transparency is a virtue, simplicity cannot be sacrificed for complexity at the expense of clinical usefulness. The acceptance of multimarker panels has been hindered by the lack of data sharing (for technical or strategic reasons). This problem can only be overcome by improved collaboration and communication between clinicians, basic researchers, and biostatisticians, and this will be required to achieve real progress in multimarker panels.

REFERENCES

1. Biomarkers Definitions Working Group. Biomarkers and surrogate endpoints: preferred definitions and conceptual framework. Clin Pharmacol Ther 2001;69:89.
2. Allen LA. Use of multiple biomarkers in heart failure. Curr Cardiol Rep 2010; 12:230.

3. LaBaer J. So, you want to look for biomarkers (introduction to the special biomarkers issue). J Proteome Res 2005;4:1053.
4. Marshall JC, Reinhart K. Biomarkers of sepsis. Crit Care Med 2009;37:2290.
5. Bozza FA, Salluh JI, Japiassu AM, et al. Cytokine profiles as markers of disease severity in sepsis: a multiplex analysis. Crit Care 2007;11:R49.
6. Hartemink KJ, Groeneveld AB, de Groot MC, et al. Alpha-atrial natriuretic peptide, cyclic guanosine monophosphate, and endothelin in plasma as markers of myocardial depression in human septic shock. Crit Care Med 2001;29:80.
7. Parikh CR, Devarajan P. New biomarkers of acute kidney injury. Crit Care Med 2008;36:S159.
8. Robin X, Turck N, Hainard A, et al. Bioinformatics for protein biomarker panel classification: what is needed to bring biomarker panels into in vitro diagnostics? Expert Rev Proteomics 2009;6:675.
9. Khan SS, Smith MS, Reda D, et al. Multiplex bead array assays for detection of soluble cytokines: comparisons of sensitivity and quantitative values among kits from multiple manufacturers. Cytometry B Clin Cytom 2004;61:35.
10. Azuaje F, Devaux Y, Wagner D. Computational biology for cardiovascular biomarker discovery. Brief Bioinform 2009;10:367.
11. Schiess R, Wollscheid B, Aebersold R. Targeted proteomic strategy for clinical biomarker discovery. Mol Oncol 2009;3:33.
12. McIntosh MW, Pepe MS. Combining several screening tests: optimality of the risk score. Biometrics 2002;58:657.
13. Pepe MS, Thompson ML. Combining diagnostic test results to increase accuracy. Biostatistics 2000;1:123.
14. Marshall JC. Sepsis: rethinking the approach to clinical research. J Leukoc Biol 2008;83:471.
15. Allen LA, Felker GM. Multi-marker strategies in heart failure: clinical and statistical approaches. Heart Fail Rev 2010;15:343.
16. Wishart DS. Computational approaches to metabolomics. Methods Mol Biol 2010;593:283.
17. Chau CH, Rixe O, McLeod H, et al. Validation of analytic methods for biomarkers used in drug development. Clin Cancer Res 2008;14:5967.
18. Ransohoff DF. Bias as a threat to the validity of cancer molecular-marker research. Nat Rev Cancer 2005;5:142.
19. Feng Z, Prentice R, Srivastava S. Research issues and strategies for genomic and proteomic biomarker discovery and validation: a statistical perspective. Pharmacogenomics 2004;5:709.
20. Feng Z, Yasui Y. Statistical considerations in combining biomarkers for disease classification. Dis Markers 2004;20:45.
21. Carrigan SD, Scott G, Tabrizian M. Toward resolving the challenges of sepsis diagnosis. Clin Chem 2004;50:1301.
22. Russell JA. Management of sepsis. N Engl J Med 2006;355:1699.
23. Catenacci MH, King K. Severe sepsis and septic shock: improving outcomes in the emergency department. Emerg Med Clin North Am 2008;26:603.
24. Bone RC, Balk RA, Cerra FB, et al. Definitions for sepsis and organ failure and guidelines for the use of innovative therapies in sepsis. The ACCP/SCCM Consensus Conference Committee. American College of Chest Physicians/ Society of Critical Care Medicine. Chest 1992;101:1644.
25. Marshall JC, Vincent JL, Fink MP, et al. Measures, markers, and mediators: toward a staging system for clinical sepsis. A report of the Fifth Toronto Sepsis

Roundtable. Toronto, Ontario, Canada, October 25–26, 2000. Crit Care Med 2003;31:1560.

26. Brun-Buisson C, Doyon F, Carlet J. Bacteremia and severe sepsis in adults: a multicenter prospective survey in ICUs and wards of 24 hospitals. French Bacteremia-Sepsis Study Group. Am J Respir Crit Care Med 1996;154:617.

27. Brun-Buisson C, Doyon F, Carlet J, et al. Incidence, risk factors, and outcome of severe sepsis and septic shock in adults. A multicenter prospective study in intensive care units. French ICU Group for Severe Sepsis. JAMA 1995;274: 968.

28. Suau A, Bonnet R, Sutren M, et al. Direct analysis of genes encoding 16S rRNA from complex communities reveals many novel molecular species within the human gut. Appl Environ Microbiol 1999;65:4799.

29. Weng L, Rubin EM, Bristow J. Application of sequence-based methods in human microbial ecology. Genome Res 2006;16:316.

30. Kollef MH, Sherman G, Ward S, et al. Inadequate antimicrobial treatment of infections: a risk factor for hospital mortality among critically ill patients. Chest 1999; 115:462.

31. Claus RA, Otto GP, Deigner HP, et al. Approaching clinical reality: markers for monitoring systemic inflammation and sepsis. Curr Mol Med 2010;10:227.

32. Assicot M, Gendrel D, Carsin H, et al. High serum procalcitonin concentrations in patients with sepsis and infection. Lancet 1993;341:515.

33. Castelli GP, Pognani C, Meisner M, et al. Procalcitonin and C-reactive protein during systemic inflammatory response syndrome, sepsis and organ dysfunction. Crit Care 2004;8:R234.

34. Dahaba AA, Hagara B, Fall A, et al. Procalcitonin for early prediction of survival outcome in postoperative critically ill patients with severe sepsis. Br J Anaesth 2006;97:503.

35. Harbarth S, Holeckova K, Froidevaux C, et al. Diagnostic value of procalcitonin, interleukin-6, and interleukin-8 in critically ill patients admitted with suspected sepsis. Am J Respir Crit Care Med 2001;164:396.

36. Jensen JU, Heslet L, Jensen TH, et al. Procalcitonin increase in early identification of critically ill patients at high risk of mortality. Crit Care Med 2006;34: 2596.

37. Muller B, Becker KL, Schachinger H, et al. Calcitonin precursors are reliable markers of sepsis in a medical intensive care unit. Crit Care Med 2000;28:977.

38. Nobre V, Harbarth S, Graf JD, et al. Use of procalcitonin to shorten antibiotic treatment duration in septic patients: a randomized trial. Am J Respir Crit Care Med 2008;177:498.

39. Lehmann LE, Hunfeld KP, Emrich T, et al. A multiplex real-time PCR assay for rapid detection and differentiation of 25 bacterial and fungal pathogens from whole blood samples. Med Microbiol Immunol 2008;197:313.

40. Mussap M, Molinari MP, Senno E, et al. New diagnostic tools for neonatal sepsis: the role of a real-time polymerase chain reaction for the early detection and identification of bacterial and fungal species in blood samples. J Chemother 2007;19(Suppl 2):31.

41. Leon AC. Implications of clinical trial design on sample size requirements. Schizophr Bull 2008;34:664.

42. Simon R. Patient subsets and variation in therapeutic efficacy. Br J Clin Pharmacol 1982;14:473.

43. Ransohoff DF. Rules of evidence for cancer molecular-marker discovery and validation. Nat Rev Cancer 2004;4:309.

44. Ghosh D, Poisson LM. "Omics" data and levels of evidence for biomarker discovery. Genomics 2009;93:13.
45. Mehta T, Tanik M, Allison DB. Towards sound epistemological foundations of statistical methods for high-dimensional biology. Nat Genet 2004;36:943.
46. Lijmer JG, Mol BW, Heisterkamp S, et al. Empirical evidence of design-related bias in studies of diagnostic tests. JAMA 1999;282:1061.
47. Soreide K. Receiver-operating characteristic curve analysis in diagnostic, prognostic and predictive biomarker research. J Clin Pathol 2009;62:1.
48. Simon R. Lost in translation: problems and pitfalls in translating laboratory observations to clinical utility. Eur J Cancer 2008;44:2707.
49. Vitzthum F, Behrens F, Anderson NL, et al. Proteomics: from basic research to diagnostic application. A review of requirements & needs. J Proteome Res 2005;4:1086.
50. Williams FM. Biomarkers: in combination they may do better. Arthritis Res Ther 2009;11:130.
51. Pepe MS, Etzioni R, Feng Z, et al. Phases of biomarker development for early detection of cancer. J Natl Cancer Inst 2001;93:1054.
52. Lassere MN. The Biomarker-Surrogacy Evaluation Schema: a review of the biomarker-surrogate literature and a proposal for a criterion-based, quantitative, multidimensional hierarchical levels of evidence schema for evaluating the status of biomarkers as surrogate endpoints. Stat Methods Med Res 2008;17:303.
53. Ambroise C, McLachlan GJ. Selection bias in gene extraction on the basis of microarray gene-expression data. Proc Natl Acad Sci U S A 2002;99:6562.
54. Molenberghs G, Burzykowski T, Alonso A, et al. A perspective on surrogate endpoints in controlled clinical trials. Stat Methods Med Res 2004;13:177.
55. Pepe MS, Feng Z, Janes H, et al. Pivotal evaluation of the accuracy of a biomarker used for classification or prediction: standards for study design. J Natl Cancer Inst 2008;100:1432.
56. Smit S, van Breemen MJ, Hoefsloot HC, et al. Assessing the statistical validity of proteomics based biomarkers. Anal Chim Acta 2007;592:210.
57. Taylor JM, Ankerst DP, Andridge RR. Validation of biomarker-based risk prediction models. Clin Cancer Res 2008;14:5977.
58. Zervakis M, Blazadonakis ME, Tsiliki G, et al. Outcome prediction based on microarray analysis: a critical perspective on methods. BMC Bioinformatics 2009;10:53.
59. Boulesteix AL, Strobl C. Optimal classifier selection and negative bias in error rate estimation: an empirical study on high-dimensional prediction. BMC Med Res Methodol 2009;9:85.
60. Wiemer JC, Prokudin A. Bioinformatics in proteomics: application, terminology, and pitfalls. Pathol Res Pract 2004;200:173.
61. Shariat SF, Lotan Y, Vickers A, et al. Statistical consideration for clinical biomarker research in bladder cancer. Urol Oncol 2010;28:389.
62. Subtil F, Rabilloud MA. Bayesian method to estimate the optimal threshold of a longitudinal biomarker. Biom J 2010;52:333.
63. Scotch M, Duggal M, Brandt C, et al. Use of statistical analysis in the biomedical informatics literature. J Am Med Inform Assoc 2010;17:3.
64. Omenn GS. Strategies for plasma proteomic profiling of cancers. Proteomics 2006;6:5662.
65. Smit S, Hoefsloot HC, Smilde AK. Statistical data processing in clinical proteomics. J Chromatogr B Analyt Technol Biomed Life Sci 2008;866:77.
66. Eldridge S, Ashby D, Bennett C, et al. Internal and external validity of cluster randomised trials: systematic review of recent trials. BMJ 2008;336:876.

67. James Hung HM, Wang SJ. Challenges to multiple testing in clinical trials. Biom J 2010;52:747–56.
68. Cook NR. Use and misuse of the receiver operating characteristic curve in risk prediction. Circulation 2007;115:928.
69. Sylvester RJ. Combining a molecular profile with a clinical and pathological profile: biostatistical considerations. Scand J Urol Nephrol Suppl 2008;218:185.
70. Levinson SS. Weak associations between prognostic biomarkers and disease in preliminary studies illustrates the breach between statistical significance and diagnostic discrimination. Clin Chim Acta 2010;411:467.
71. Baker SG. The central role of receiver operating characteristic (ROC) curves in evaluating tests for the early detection of cancer. J Natl Cancer Inst 2003;95:511.
72. Thompson ML, Zucchini W. On the statistical analysis of ROC curves. Stat Med 1989;8:1277.
73. Kofoed K, Eugen-Olsen J, Petersen J, et al. Predicting mortality in patients with systemic inflammatory response syndrome: an evaluation of two prognostic models, two soluble receptors, and a macrophage migration inhibitory factor. Eur J Clin Microbiol Infect Dis 2008;27:375.
74. Kofoed K, Schneider UV, Scheel T, et al. Development and validation of a multiplex add-on assay for sepsis biomarkers using xMAP technology. Clin Chem 2006;52:1284.
75. Kofoed K, Andersen O, Kronborg G, et al. Use of plasma C-reactive protein, procalcitonin, neutrophils, macrophage migration inhibitory factor, soluble urokinase-type plasminogen activator receptor, and soluble triggering receptor expressed on myeloid cells-1 in combination to diagnose infections: a prospective study. Crit Care 2007;11:R38.
76. Selberg O, Hecker H, Martin M, et al. Discrimination of sepsis and systemic inflammatory response syndrome by determination of circulating plasma concentrations of procalcitonin, protein complement 3a, and interleukin-6. Crit Care Med 2000;28:2793.
77. Punyadeera C, Schneider EM, Schaffer D, et al. A biomarker panel to discriminate between systemic inflammatory response syndrome and sepsis and sepsis severity. J Emerg Trauma Shock 2010;3:26.
78. Dhainault JF, Shorr AF, Macias WL, et al. Dynamic evolution of coagulopathy in the first day of severe sepsis: relationship with mortality and organ failure. Crit Care Med 2005;33:341.
79. Shapiro NI, Trzeciak S, Hollander JE, et al. A prospective, multicenter derivation of a biomarker panel to assess risk of organ dysfunction, shock, and death in emergency department patients with suspected sepsis. Crit Care Med 2009;37:96.
80. Ginsburg GS, Seo D, Frazier C. Microarrays coming of age in cardiovascular medicine: standards, predictions, and biology. J Am Coll Cardiol 2006;48:1618.
81. Gillette MA, Mani DR, Carr SA. Place of pattern in proteomic biomarker discovery. J Proteome Res 2005;4:1143.
82. Zhang Z, Chan DW. Cancer proteomics: in pursuit of "true" biomarker discovery. Cancer Epidemiol Biomarkers Prev 2005;14:2283.
83. Gerszten RE, Accurso F, Bernard GR, et al. Challenges in translating plasma proteomics from bench to bedside: update from the NHLBI Clinical Proteomics Programs. Am J Physiol Lung Cell Mol Physiol 2008;295:L16.
84. Wang P, Whiteaker JR, Paulovich AG. The evolving role of mass spectrometry in cancer biomarker discovery. Cancer Biol Ther 2009;8:1083.
85. Foteinou PT, Calvano SE, Lowry SF, et al. Translational potential of systems-based models of inflammation. Clin Transl Sci 2009;2:85.

86. Laubenbacher R, Hower V, Jarrah A, et al. A systems biology view of cancer. Biochim Biophys Acta 2009;1796:129.
87. Hurst RE. Does the biomarker search paradigm need re-booting? BMC Urol 2009;9:1.
88. Kohl P, Crampin EJ, Quinn TA, et al. Systems biology: an approach. Clin Pharmacol Ther 2010;88:25.
89. Volonte C, D'Ambrosi N, Amadio S. Protein cooperation: from neurons to networks. Prog Neurobiol 2008;86:61.
90. Calvano SE, Xiao W, Richards DR, et al. A network-based analysis of systemic inflammation in humans. Nature 2005;437:1032.
91. Friend SH. The need for precompetitive integrative bionetwork disease model building. Clin Pharmacol Ther 2010;87:536.
92. Azuaje F, Devaux Y, Wagner DR. Coordinated modular functionality and prognostic potential of a heart failure biomarker-driven interaction network. BMC Syst Biol 2010;4:60.
93. Fogel GB. Computational intelligence approaches for pattern discovery in biological systems. Brief Bioinform 2008;9:307.

Biomarkers: The Future

Steven P. LaRosa, MD[a,b,*], Steven M. Opal, MD[a,c]

KEYWORDS

- Sepsis • Biomarkers • Theragnostics • Genomics
- Gene expression • Proteomics

The current care of critically ill patients is often based on categorizing patients into groups based on clinical syndromes. Patients are described and treated as having a systemic inflammatory response syndrome (SIRS) caused by surgery, trauma, or burns or by an infection known as sepsis. This approach tends to result in similar treatment strategies in all patients within a category even though patients are often misclassified. This approach does not take into account the individual genetic uniqueness, changes that occur during critical illness, or interplay of multiple biologic pathways over time.

The immediate future use of biomarkers in the care of critically ill patients will involve those that can be used to tailor treatment. Assays that help select and guide therapeutic decisions are known as theragnostics. This article reviews the future of biomarkers as theragnostics. Specific biomarkers that suggest a particular pathophysiologic perturbation or indicate a depletion of a protective protein are discussed. The ability to detect individual single nucleotide polymorphisms (SNPs) and haplotypes to gauge an individual's risk for severe illness and potential response to a given therapy are highlighted. The potential value of gene expression in helping to differentiate populations of critically ill patients and to guide therapy over time is addressed. Functional and expressional proteomics could lead to the identification of new biomarkers as well as organ-specific therapies.

ENDOTOXIN ACTIVITY ASSAY

Endotoxin, an outer membrane component of gram-negative bacteria, is a well-described mediator of severe sepsis. Endotoxin given in small doses to healthy human

Financial Disclosures: Drs Opal and LaRosa receive investigator grants from Eisai Medical Research (maker of Eritoran) as members of the Ocean State Clinical Coordinating Center.
[a] Warren Alpert School of Medicine, Brown University, 171 Meeting Street, Providence, RI 02912, USA
[b] Division of Infectious Diseases, Rhode Island Hospital, POB Suite #330, 593 Eddy Street, Providence, RI 02903, USA
[c] Division of Infectious Diseases, Memorial Hospital, 111 Brewster Street, Pawtucket, RI 02860, USA
* Corresponding author. Division of Infectious Diseases, Rhode Island Hospital, POB Suite #330, 593 Eddy Street, Providence, RI 02903.
E-mail address: slarosa@lifespan.org

volunteers can generate the clinical, inflammatory, and coagulopathic features of sepsis.[1] Endotoxemia has been described in sepsis caused by all pathogen classes probably as a result of endogenous release from the liver and spleen because of splanchnic hypoperfusion.[2] Until recently, endotoxin levels were measured using a limulus amebocyte lysate assay. This assay is time consuming, and false-negative test results can occur because of plasma protein inhibition,[3] whereas false-positive reactions can occur because of fungal elements.[4] A new rapid endotoxin assay (endotoxin activity assay [EAA]) is approved by the Food and Drug Administration for assessing the risk of developing severe sepsis in patients in the intensive care unit (ICU). This assay must be performed within 3 hours of blood collection and takes about 1 hour to perform. This chemiluminescent assay compares the respiratory burst by endotoxin in the test sample to the maximum burst when the sample is spiked with excess lipopolysaccharide (LPS). Endotoxin activity of 0.4 is approximately equivalent to 25 to 50 pg/mL. In one study, elevated endotoxin levels were found in 58% of patients admitted to a mixed surgical-medical ICU, irrespective of the reason for admission, and in 85% of the patients with severe sepsis.[5] A recent study performed by Klein[6] found a mortality of 14% in patients with septic shock with an EAA level less than 0.4, a mortality of 17% in patients with EAA levels 0.4 to 0.6, and a mortality of 27% in those with EAA levels greater than 0.6.

The EAA's real-time capability and ability to stratify risk of sepsis and mortality make it amenable to use in clinical trials. Numerous failed clinical trials have been performed with antiendotoxin strategies. These trials involved experimental agents that were either not potent or were used before the approval of the EAA assay. Two promising therapeutic antiendotoxin strategies are currently in human testing. Eritoran is a molecule that competes with endotoxin for the MD2–toll-like receptor (TLR) 4 complex and blocks the inflammatory response.[7] A phase 2 clinical trial showed a trend toward benefit in patients with severe sepsis, with a high predicted risk of mortality in eritoran-treated severe patients. The molecule is currently in a phase 3 registration trial.[8] Toraymyxin is a filter with polymyxin bound and immobilized to polystyrene fibers that has been shown to bind endotoxin. A patient's blood is hemoperfused over the filter during a 2-hour session on 2 consecutive days. A meta-analysis of the clinical trials to date suggested benefit with this treatment,[9] and a phase 3 trial is about to begin in the United States using EAA level as one of the inclusion criteria. It is possible that the EAA device could help guide therapy with both these therapies in the future.

ANGIOPOIETIN-1 AND ANGIOPOIETIN-2

A common clinical feature in human sepsis is the development of capillary leak resulting in hypotension and the noncardiogenic pulmonary edema of acute lung injury. This capillary leak is a manifestation of a disrupted endothelial barrier.[10] Angiopoietin-1 and angiopoietin-2 are proteins critical to the state of the endothelium. Angiopoietin-1 is a ligand for the tyrosine kinase receptor with immunoglobulin and epidermal growth factor domains (Tie2) and stabilizes the endothelium, inhibiting vascular leakage and inflammatory gene expression, and prevents recruitment and transmigration of leukocytes.[11] Angiopoietin-2 competes with angiopoietin-1 for the Tie 2 receptor, which results in destabilization of the endothelium, increased capillary permeability, endothelial apoptosis, and increased expression of adhesion molecules.[12,13] Numerous studies have now demonstrated increased angiopoietin-2 levels in the setting of sepsis. Angiopoietin-2 levels have positively correlated well with organ dysfunction scores, lactate levels, and Acute Physiology and Chronic Health Evaluation II scores and inversely correlated with impaired oxygenation as measured by the partial pressure of oxygen to fraction of inspired oxygen ratio.[14,15] Angiopoietin-2 levels less than 11 ng/mL have been associated with a good prognosis in critically ill subjects.[14,15]

Angiopoietin-2 in animal and in vitro models has been demonstrated to be a mediator of endothelial injury and not just a biomarker. Serum from septic patients or angiopoietin-2 applied to a human cell monolayer caused endothelial destruction and increased permeability. Mice injected with angiopoietin-2 developed increased pulmonary vascular congestion as well as increased intestinal and liver weight compared with control animals.[16] The potential then exists for identifying individuals with excessively high levels of angiopoietin-2 and targeting the Tie2 receptor. Angiopoietin-1 administration in a murine endotoxin model was found to be protective.[17] Activated protein C, a molecule currently clinically available for the treatment of sepsis, was recently found in an in vitro model to increase the expression of angiopoietin-1 and the Tie 2 receptor while inhibiting angiopoietin-2.[18]

GELSOLIN

Gelsolin is a cytoplasmic and secreted plasma protein that is involved as an actin scavenger. Actin released during tissue injury is noted to be toxic to pulmonary endothelial cells and the microvaculature.[19] Gelsolin severs and caps actin filaments. Gelsolin is also noted to bind to inflammatory mediators, including endotoxin, platelet-activating factor, and lysophosphatidic acid. Normal plasma gelsolin levels are between 150 and 300 mg/L, and severe depletion has been noted in many clinical conditions, including sepsis, trauma, major surgery, burns, extensive surgery, liver failure, and myocardial infarction.[20] In a critically ill surgical population composed of trauma and burn patients, gelsolin levels remained low compared with control patients for 5 days, and at a cutoff level of 61 mg/L, an area under the receiver operating curve (ROC) of 0.905 for predicting survivorship was observed in these patients.[21] In medical patients with sepsis, actin could be detected in 81% of patients, and at a plasma gelsolin level of 113.6 mg/L, there was an area under the ROC of 0.86 for determining survivorship.[22]

Animal models of sepsis have raised the possibility of gelsolin as a theragnostic. Lee and colleagues[23] examined the effects of LPS challenge and cecal ligation and perforation on actin and plasma gelsolin levels as well as the effects of exogenously given plasma gelsolin in mice. Endotoxin infusion caused plasma gelsolin levels to decrease to a median of 80 µg/mL or to 50% of that in healthy controls, whereas the cecal ligation and puncture (CLP) model decreased levels to 41 µg/ml or to 25% of that in healthy controls. In mice administered with gelsolin exogenously to maintain levels greater than 200 µg/mL, the survivorship was 88% in the LPS model and 30% in the CLP model compared with 0% in the placebo treated animals in both models. Gelsolin seemed to lead to an increase in the solubilization of actin in these animal models and decreased the release of proinflammatory cytokine in the LPS but not the CLP model.

Many important hurdles remain in developing gelsolin as a theragnostic. The optimal assay would have to be determined and would need to be reasonably easy to perform. Studies performed using an enzyme-linked immunosorbent assay have demonstrated lower gelsolin levels than those using an actin nucleation assay. The optimal gelsolin cutoff as an inclusion criteria for a therapeutic study would need to be determined, as would the optimal target concentration.

INTER-ALPHA INHIBITOR PROTEINS

Inter-alpha inhibitor proteins (IαIps) are human plasma serine protease inhibitors that consist of a complex of a light chain (known as bikunin) covalently bound to 1 or 2 heavy chains.[24] Iαlps are secreted by the liver into the plasma and are found at relatively high concentrations of 600 to 1200 mg/L.[25] Lim and colleagues[25] demonstrated that nonsurviving patients with severe sepsis had significantly lower levels of Iαlp than survivors (498 ± 196 mg/L vs 687 ± 300, P = .0103). Individuals with Iαlp levels less than 600 mg/L had a mortality of more than 50%. Iαlp levels inversely correlated with disease severity measurements and correlated with consumption of coagulation factors. In a second study by Opal and colleagues,[26] levels of Iαlp were lower on average at 290 ± 15 μg/mL in patients with severe sepsis compared with 614 ± 197 μg/ml in healthy volunteers. When followed-up for 5 days of illness, nonsurvivors were unlikely to recover plasma levels more than 300 μg/mL, and even levels in survivors remained less than those found in normal healthy controls.

The in vitro and in vivo actions of Iαlp suggest that the molecule could serve as a theragnostic. Iαlp is known to inhibit the proteolytic enzymes, complement component C5a, cathepsin, human leukocyte elastase, and granzyme K.[27] Bikunin is also capable of decreasing LPS-mediated cytokine release.[28] In addition, Iαlp in association with TSG-6 bind to hyaluronan and protect the extracellular matrix.[29] Iαlps have been protective in several animal models of sepsis when given up to 20 hours after the infectious challenge.[25,30,31] The challenge in developing Iαlp as a theragnostic will, as in the case of gelsolin, be in developing a standardized feasible assay and determining the cutoff value to target in patients.

MONOCYTIC HLA-DR EXPRESSION

Numerous clinical conditions, including sepsis, trauma, burns, and pancreatitis, are categorized by an initial hyperinflammatory state followed by a compensatory antiinflammatory state known as immunoparalysis.[32] The expression of HLA-DR on monocytes has been found to be a marker of the capacity of monocytes to generate proinflammatory cytokines in response to a stimulus such as that by LPS. Prolonged periods with decreased mHLA-DR (monocytic HLA-DR) expression have been associated with a poor outcome in sepsis.[33] An early clinical trial with gamma interferon demonstrated an ability to reverse monocyte nonresponsiveness.[34] Large multicenter trials to study the effects of reversing immunoparalysis were hampered by the lack of a standardized assay of monocyte HLA-DR expression. The type of flow cytometer as well as its settings and the specimen handling were found to dramatically affect the results.

The development of a standardized assay for mHLA-DR expression has facilitated its development as a potential theragnostic. The Becton Dickinson QuantiBRITE assay (Becton Dickinson, NJ, USA), which uses an anti–HLA DR antibody conjugated 1:1 with phycoerythrin, allows the measurement of antibodies bound per cell (AB/cell) that is not affected by the flow cytometer or settings.[35] Pilot studies have suggested that 16,844 AB/cell (13,255–20,890) are typical of healthy volunteers.[36] A study in patients who had undergone cardiopulmonary bypass demonstrated that less than 5000 AB/cell predicted patients who were likely to develop postoperative infections.[37] In a study by Lukaszewicz and colleagues[36] using this assay on day 7, mean mHLA-DR expression was not different in those with infection versus those without infection, but the slope of HLA-DR expression recovery was flatter in the infected patients. In a pilot study, placebo-controlled trial of 38 patients with sepsis and mHLA-DR expression less than 8000 AB/cell for 2 days, granulocyte-macrophage colony-stimulating factor (GM-CSF)-administered subjects compared with placebo-treated subjects had statistically significant increases in mHLA-DR expression and proinflammatory cytokine production and trends toward improvement in the ICU and hospital stay as well as duration of mechanical ventilation.[38]

Larger trials of GM-CSF and gamma interferon should be performed using the standardized assay with examination of different cutoff values for mHLA-DR response in terms of the development of secondary infection. Several novel immunomodulators that regulate the interactions between monocyte/macrophage cells and dendritic cells with CD4+ and CD8+ T lymphocytes and regulatory T cells are in preclinical and clinical development at present.[39] A rapid and reliable assay for the assessment of the functional immune status of individual patients and the mHLA-DR assay would be invaluable in the clinical development of targeted immunoadjuvants for the treatment of sepsis-induced immunosuppression.

GENOME-BASED BIOMARKERS FOR SEPSIS

The ultimate goal of personalized medicine is to use evidence-based medical decision making and the systems biology approach to guide informed clinical decisions most likely to benefit, and least likely to harm, individual patients based on their unique characteristics. Central to this approach is the availability of genome-wide information about potential genetic risks, vulnerabilities, and responsiveness.[40] At least one of the long-term goals of so-called P4 medicine (personalized, preventive, participatory, and predictive) is fast becoming reality with the advent of novel high-throughput DNA sequencing methods.[41–43] It may be possible to perform genome-wide sequencing of individuals for a reasonable cost ($1000/genome) in the foreseeable future.[44] This possibility would revolutionize medicine, providing clinicians with rapid access to information about genetic risk likelihood ratios, predicted genetic-environmental interactions, vaccine responsiveness, and pharmacogenomic information for guiding drug dosage and drug-drug interactions and possible drug toxicities.[44,45]

Thus far, the genomic age has had only a modest effect in clinical medicine, primarily in the fields of oncology, rare genetic diseases, and pharmacogenomics. The clinical utility of genome-based information in the care of critically ill patients with sepsis has largely been absent because sepsis is complex, rapidly evolving, incompletely understood, and heavily driven by predisposing elements and environmental factors (site of injury, infectious source, type of pathogen, immunosuppressive medications). The seminal work of Sorensen and colleagues[46] over 20 years ago indicates that deaths from infectious diseases have a strong heritable basis. Detection of the specific genetic substrate that accounts for susceptibility to infection and to disease severity has been complicated by pathogen-specific events, competing and compensatory pathways, gender and age-dependent associations, and small sample size studies with poor reproducibility between studies.[47,48]

Despite these limitations, progress has been made in the detection and gene loci and nonsynonymous coding SNPs (SNPs that mediate amino acid changes in translated gene products). A detailed understanding of the mouse genome and the comparative genetics of the mammalian host immune system has been greatly facilitated by rapid genome sequencing methods.[49,50] An enlarging catalog of SNPs within the human genome is already available,[51,52] and linkage maps with haplotype maps with genes in linkage disequilibrium affecting immune response genes, coagulation factor genes, and regulatory elements are being developed.[53] Genomic information relating to genes that affect drug metabolism (ie, cytochrome p450 isoenzymes), excretion, and toxicity has proven to be particularly valuable and is increasingly available for clinical use.[54]

Genomic information specifically related to sepsis pathophysiology is expected to rapidly expand in the near future as ongoing clinical studies with large consortia with established biobanks from septic patients. Data mining and interrogation of the DNA sequences for large numbers of septic patients should yield a large number of novel genes that alter the outcome in sepsis.

As computational methods in modeling inflammatory pathways and interacting links between signaling networks of immune response genes become more sophisticated, the value of genomics as a biomarker for sepsis risk, response predictions, and therapeutic options will become more apparent. Carrying the entire genome sequence and linkage map on a portable disk or a smart phone to the hospital when care is required is not that far off in the future. The promise of systems biology to improve individual patient care is likely to become a reality within the next decade.[48,55] A current survey of selected candidate SNPs in gene loci that might influence the outcome in sepsis is given in **Table 1**.[40,56–59]

GENE EXPRESSION ASSAYS AS BIOMARKERS FOR SEPSIS

Considerable effort has been expended in an attempt to understand the complexity of the host response to sepsis at the level of transcription of messenger RNA (mRNA) and exploit this information for the early recognition of sepsis.[60,61] Analysis of transcription profiles of upregulated and downregulated genes can now be accomplished with relative ease using microarrays commonly referred to as gene chips. These arrays are designed to capture signature oligonucleotides from specific mRNA transcripts by complementation from synthetic oligonucleotides aligned in silico on a microarray plate.[60,62] These microarrays simultaneously identify and quantify specific transcripts that are upregulated or downregulated after a specific stimulus. Essentially, changes in the entire transcriptome (universe of all mRNA species transcribed from the human genome) are compared at baseline and after the onset of sepsis. Alternatively, changes in the transcript profiles can be analyzed during periods of systemic inflammation (noninfectious SIRS, trauma, major surgery, or burns) by comparing patients who develop severe sepsis with those who do not develop systemic infection and severe sepsis/septic shock.[63] It is now possible to isolate RNA from peripheral blood leukocytes, hybridize the RNA, analyze the RNA on microarray chips, quantify the RNA changes, and then align these changes into a signal pathway analysis within a few hours. The data are usually displayed in a figure with color code, with red representing upregulation of mRNA levels, black representing no change, and green representing downregulation of mRNA at a specific gene locus.[61]

Initial enthusiasm for transcriptome analysis for the diagnosis of severe sepsis and septic shock has been dampened somewhat by several complications, including (1) interindividual variation in the host response genes, (2) lack of ability to distinguish the nature of the pathogen based on the transcription profile from the infected host, (3) marked variations in the transcriptome over time in the same individual over the course of systemic inflammation and sepsis, (4) differential gene expression from one target organ to another, (5) high frequency of false discovery rates with changes in RNA expression, (6) complexity of redundant circuitry of inflammatory and antiinflammatory networks, and (7) frequent dyssynergy between cytokine ligands and cognate receptor expression. Despite all these complexities and challenges, transcriptome analysis has begun to yield discernable patterns within specific sets of genes. These emerging discoveries of interacting transcription pathways of sets of immune response genes in sepsis and septic shock may yet prove to have diagnostic utility as a biomarker in sepsis.

Genes that regulate the innate and adaptive immune responses are heavily affected during systemic inflammation and sepsis. The alterations in gene transcript frequency

Table 1		
Selected gene association studies with susceptibility to infection and sepsis		
Gene Product	**SNP/Amino Acid Changes**	**Clinical Findings**
TLR4	Asp299Gly in peptide sequence	Possible increased susceptibility to gram-negative bacteria and aspergillosis, lower risk of legionellosis
TLR2	SNPs in TLR2 gene coding regions	Associated with increased risk of infection from gram-positive bacteria
CD14	C-159T promoterpolymorphism	TT homozygotes at position −159 reported to have increased levels of soluble CD14 and increased risk of septic mortality
MBL	SNPs in exon 1 of MBL gene	Associated with low MBL levels and increased risk of severe infection
IL-6	−174 G/Cpolymorphism	Conflicting reports that this promoter polymorphism alters IL-6 levels and increases incidence of sepsis
TNF-α	G-A polymorphism at position −308	Polymorphism in promoter region of TNF-α gene associated with increased risk of sepsis in some studies
Protein C	−1654C/T or −1641G/A	Polymorphisms in this noncoding region associated with increased risk of death from sepsis
PAI-1	SNP in promoter region	Increased production of PAI-1 leads to reduced fibrinolysis and poor outcome in meningococcal sepsis
Mal[57]	Polymorphism in coding region S180L	Serine/leucine heterozygotes at position 180 are protected from pneumococcal disease and sepsis
C-reactive protein	Haplotype 1, 184C, 2, 911C	May be protective from nasal carriage and infection by *Staphylococcus aureus*
IRAK 4[58]	Loss-of-function exon mutations	Predisposition to severe pneumococcal and staphylococcal infection in childhood
CISH[59]	SNP in the promoter region −292	Alterations in cytokine synthesis and IL-2 levels, increasing susceptibility to bacteremic infection

Abbreviations: Asp, aspartic acid; C/T, cytosine/thymine; CISH, cytokine-inducible SRC homology domain protein; Gly, glycine; G/A, guanine/adenine; IRAK, interleukin 1 receptor–associated kinase; Mal, myeloid differentiation factor adaptor like; MBL, mannose-binding lectin; PAI-1, plasminogen activator inhibitor 1; TNF-α, tumor necrosis factor α.

Data from Sutherland AM, Walley R. Bench-to-bedside review: association of genetic variation with sepsis. Crit Care 2009;13:210; and van der Poll T, Opal SM. Pathogenesis, treatment, and prevention of pneumococcal pneumonia. Lancet 2009;374:1543–56.

that affect cytokine synthesis, cytokine receptor expression, T-cell differentiation, protein synthesis regulation, and regulators of apoptosis are readily observed in severely septic patients.[61] Genes involved in the proinflammatory response are often significantly reduced over time in sepsis, whereas genes that regulate apoptosis are often highly expressed in severe sepsis. These transcriptional profiles lend further support for evidence of widespread sepsis-induced immune suppression after an initial septic insult.[39]

Johnson and colleagues[63] have analyzed differential gene expression in severely ill patients after major trauma and used transcriptome analysis to distinguish sterile inflammation from sepsis in this patient population. SIRS criteria are almost uniformly present in patients with severe trauma, without any evidence of infection. Distinguishing trauma-induced SIRS from infection-related SIRS after major trauma is critically important from a clinical and therapeutic perspective. Sepsis indicates the need for appropriate antimicrobial therapy and often surgical intervention for drainage of abscesses or excision of infected tissue. This distinction is not readily apparent at the bedside in many severely traumatized patients. The investigators performed a daily assessment of gene transcript profiles of their severely ill patients in a shock/trauma unit and then correlated changes in transcript profiles with early predictors for systemic infection and severe sepsis. The investigators found up to 459 specific genes that were either upregulated (86%) or downregulated (14%) within 2 days of the onset of severe sepsis. They developed a gene array system that could potentially identify individuals who have noninfectious SIRS from those with systemic infection and sepsis. If this type of analysis can be confirmed in other centers and with other types of transcriptome analysis, this technique could provide a much-needed novel biomarker for distinguishing sterile inflammation from sepsis.[63]

This group subsequently reported a specific analysis of TLR gene expression that varied from sterile inflammation in patients who subsequently developed a diagnosis of sepsis within the next 24 hours.[64] The MD2-TLR4 (the primary LPS receptor), TLR1 (signaling partner with TLR2 for several gram-positive bacterial mediators), and TLR 5 (the bacterial flagellin receptor) genes are upregulated along with several intracellular signaling pathways related to TLR signal transduction. Moreover, TLR8 (recognition receptor for single-stranded RNA) was also upregulated during the early phases of severe sepsis. It is anticipated that further analysis of the changes in the transcriptome during the evolution of sepsis provides new insights into patterns of signal activation and deactivation within inflammatory networks during sepsis. This information could potentially be exploited to direct early interventions to block the progression to severe sepsis.

PROTEOMICS AS A BIOMARKER TOOL IN SEVERE SEPSIS

Proteomics is the global assessment of the nature of synthesized proteins and their relative abundance in biologic fluids in health and disease.[65] The advantage of studying the proteome in severe sepsis is that secreted proteins are the primary circulating signaling system that translates genetic signals into direct changes in enzymatic activity and signal transduction throughout the host tissues in sepsis. It is fully anticipated that advances in systems biology and technical aspects of proteome analysis will provide a new level of understanding of sepsis within the next few decades.[66–68]

Several technical challenges exist in plasma protein analysis that have impeded rapid progress in this emerging field of systems biology. Protein sequences are not as readily identified as are changes in sequences in nucleic acids. Watson-Crick complementary base pairing has proven to be exceedingly valuable in the rapid sequencing of the primary structure of nucleic acids. Similar mechanisms are not available to analyze individual amino acids along a peptide sequence, making protein analysis more difficult and more challenging. Peptide sequencers are available but are more time consuming and expensive than nucleic acid sequence analysis. Proteins also undergo extensive posttranslational modifications, and these modifications can markedly alter the tertiary structure and activity of specific proteins. In addition, the range of protein concentrations and size of protein sequences vary drastically in the human plasma. The protein concentrations may vary by up to 12 orders of magnitude between one rare peptide and common proteins, such as albumin, making for a major analytic challenge when studying plasma proteomics. Direct cell-to-cell interactions and nonprotein-based signaling, such as lipid mediators and neuroendocrine signaling, in severe sepsis are not readily detectable using proteomic methods.[65]

Proteomics methods applied to the diagnosis of sepsis are expressional proteomics and functional proteomics. Expressional proteomics deal with those proteins that are expressed within accessible biologic fluids, such as plasma, urine, or amniotic fluid. Functional proteomics is an analysis of proteins that undergo specific changes after a given stimulus, such as severe sepsis or other forms of systemic inflammation. The identification of proteins is generally based on their physical and chemical characteristics and molecular mass using mass spectrometry. Two systems are primarily used at present: matrix-assisted laser desorption/ionization time-of-flight mass spectrometry (MALDI-TOF MS) or surface-enhanced laser desorption/ionization coupled to time-of-flight mass spectrometry (SELDI-TOF MS). MALDI-TOF MS is usually combined with 2-dimensional gel electrophoresis, which is readily available but time consuming and is not able to pick up small peptides (<10 kDa) or very large proteins (>200 kDa). SELDI-TOF MS is an automated system with a high throughput process, but the system is limited to only those proteins recognized by the chip and reproducibility and reliability remain to be firmly established.[65]

Other methods that could be useful in the future include microarray technology by which proteins are identified by an array of monoclonal antibodies with subsequent detection by surface plasmon spectrometry. This system might prove very useful in the near future, but it is currently limited by the number of known monoclonal antibodies with high-affinity binding to specific proteins. As this technology improves, the reliability and accessibility of proteomics will increase and could become a clinical tool for biomarker detection for sepsis.

At present, early experience with proteomics and systems biology in sepsis have already revealed several interesting findings.[66,68–70] Usage of a variety of analytic techniques and numerous changes in plasma protein profiles have been observed in sepsis both in experimental models and in specific patient populations. Experimental animal models have shown marked changes in mitochondrial protein activity, heat shock proteins, antioxidants, lipid metabolism enzyme, and energy conservation in intracellular chaperone proteins.[71] Actin and myosin-binding protein found in the plasma may have pathophysiologic consequences.[19] Organ-specific measures of cellular injury, such as proteins that are unique to the kidney, can also be detected using proteomic techniques.

Plasma proteins that are upregulated or downregulated in sepsis include many cytokines and signaling molecules that have already been described in sepsis along with a large group of other proteins of unknown function that are significantly altered in sepsis. The roles of these other proteins need to be further characterized and provide new insights into novel markers and mediators in the pathophysiology of sepsis.[70,71]

Tissue-specific proteomic analysis such as amniotic fluid analysis to predict the onset of neonatal sepsis,[72] bronchoalveolar lavage fluid analysis for the diagnosis of acute lung injury, and acute respiratory distress syndrome and urinary protein analysis have all shown promise as rapid diagnostic techniques and biomarkers for the detection of infection and systemic inflammation from these tissues.[65]

Two other areas of particular interest in sepsis are the proteomics of endothelial cells, a central player in the pathogenesis of septic shock,[10] and the proteome of platelets.[73] Platelets are anucleated cells that have a documented role in the pathophysiology of septic shock and have proven to be excellent predictors of adverse outcome in sepsis.[74] Analysis of the proteins found in platelets could be readily accessible and highly informative proteome to investigate in severe sepsis.

ACKNOWLEDGMENTS

The authors would like to thank Nicole Lundstrom for assistance with article preparation and formatting.

REFERENCES

1. Santos AA, Wilmore DW. The systematic inflammatory response: perspective of human endotoxemia. Shock 1996;6:S50–6.
2. Opal SM, Scannon PJ, Vincent JL, et al. Relationship between plasma levels of lipopolysaccharide (LPS) and LPS-binding protein in patients with severe sepsis and septic shock. J Infect Dis 1999;180:1584–9.
3. Cohen J. The detection and interpretation of endotoxemia. Intensive Care Med 2000;26:S51–6.
4. Bates DW, Parsommet J, Ketchum PA, et al. Limulus amebocyte lysate assay for detection of endotoxin in patients with sepsis syndrome. Clin Infect Dis 1998;27: 582–91.
5. Marshall JC, Walker PM, Foster DM, et al. Measurement of endotoxin activity in critically ill patients using whole blood neutrophil dependent chemiluminescence. Crit Care 2002;6:342–8.
6. Klein D. Clinical assessment does not predict endotoxemia in septic shock [abstract 469]. In: Programs and abstracts of the Society of Critical Care Medicine. Miami (FL), January 9–13, 2010.
7. Lynn M, Rossignol DP, Wheeler JL, et al. Blocking of responses to endotoxin by E5564 in healthy volunteers with experimental endotoxemia. J Infect Dis 2003; 187:631–9.
8. Tidswell M, Tillis W, LaRosa SP, et al. Phase 2 trial of eritoran tetrasodium (E5564), a toll-like receptor 4 antagonist, in patients with severe sepsis. Crit Care Med 2010;38:72–83.
9. Cruz DN, Perazella MA, Bellomo R, et al. Effectiveness of polymyxin B-immobilized fiber column in sepsis: a systematic review. Crit Care 2007;11:R47.
10. Aird WC. The role of the endothelium in severe sepsis and multiple organ dysfunction. Blood 2003;101:3765–77.
11. Gamble JR, Drew J, Trezise L, et al. Angiopoietin-1 is an antipermeability and anti-inflammatory agent in vitro and targets cell junctions. Circ Res 2000;87: 603–7.
12. Scharpfenecker M, Fiedler U, Reiss Y, et al. The Tie-2 ligand angiopoietin-2 destabilizes quiescent endothelium through an internal autocrine loop mechanism. J Cell Sci 2004;118:771–80.

13. Fiedler U, Reiss Y, Scharpfenecker M, et al. Angiopoietin-2 sensitizes endothelial cells to TNF-alpha and has a crucial role in the induction of inflammation. Nat Med 2006;12:235–9.
14. Siner JM, Bhandari V, Engle KM. Elevated serum angiopoietin 2 levels are associated with increased mortality in sepsis. Shock 2009;31:348–53.
15. Kumpers P, Lukasz A, David S, et al. Excess circulating angiopoietin-2 is a strong predictor of mortality in critically ill medical patients. Crit Care 2008;12:R147.
16. Parikh SM, Mammoto T, Schultz A, et al. Excess circulating angiopoietin-2 may contribute to pulmonary vascular leak in sepsis in humans. PLoS Med 2006;3:e46.
17. Witzenbichler B, Westermann D, Knueppel S, et al. Protective role of angiopoietin-1 in endotoxic shock. Circulation 2005;111:97–105.
18. Minhas N, Xue M, Fukudome K, et al. Activated protein C utilizes the angiopoietin/Tie2 axis to promote endothelial barrier function. FASEB J 2010;24:873–81.
19. Haddad JG, Harper KD, Guoth M, et al. Angiopathic consequences of saturating the plasma scavenger system for actin. Proc Natl Acad Sci U S A 1990;87: 1381–5.
20. Bucki R, Levental I, Kulakowska A, et al. Plasma gelsolin: function, prognostic value, and potential therapeutic use. Curr Protein Pept Sci 2008;9:541–51.
21. Lee PS, Drager LR, Stossel TP, et al. Relationship of plasma gelsolin levels to outcomes in critically ill surgical patients. Ann Surg 2006;243:399–403.
22. Lee PS, Patel SR, Christiani DC, et al. Plasma gelsolin depletion and circulating actin in sepsis—a pilot study. PLoS One 2008;3:e3712.
23. Lee PS, Waxman AB, Cotich KL. Plasma gelsolin is a marker and therapeutic agent in animal sepsis. Crit Care Med 2007;35:849–52.
24. Salier J, Rouet P, Raguenez G, et al. The inter-alpha-inhibitor family: from structure to regulation. Biochem J 1996;315:1–9.
25. Lim YP, Bendelja K, Opal SM, et al. Correlation between mortality and the levels of inter-alpha inhibitors in the plasma of patients with severe sepsis. J Infect Dis 2003;188:919–26.
26. Opal SM, Lim YP, Siryaporn E, et al. Longitudinal studies of inter-alpha inhibitor proteins in severely septic patients: a potential clinical marker and mediator of severe sepsis. Crit Care Med 2007;35:387–92.
27. Fries E, Blum A. Bikunin-not just a plasma proteinase inhibitor. Int J Biochem Cell Biol 2000;32:125–37.
28. Wakahara K, Kobayashi H, Yagyu T, et al. Bikunin suppresses lipopolysaccharide-induced lethality through down-regulation of tumor necrosis factor-α and interleukin-1β in macrophages. J Infect Dis 2005;191:930–8.
29. Fries E, Kaczmarczyk A. Inter-α-inhibitor, hyaluronan and inflammation. Acta Biochim Pol 2003;50:735–42.
30. Yang S, Lim YP, Zhou M, et al. Administration of human inter-a-inhibitors maintains homodynamic stability and improves survival during sepsis. Crit Care Med 2002; 30:617–22.
31. Wu R, Cui X, Lim YP, et al. Delayed administration of human inter-α inhibitor proteins reduces mortality in sepsis. Crit Care Med 2004;32:1747–52.
32. Volk HD, Reinke P, Docke WD. Clinical aspects: from systemic inflammation to immunoparalysis. Chem Immunol 2000;74:162–77.
33. Volk HD, Reinke P, Krausch D, et al. Monocyte deactivation-rationale for a new therapeutic strategy in sepsis. Intensive Care Med 1996;22:S474–81.
34. Kox WJ, Bone RC, Krausch D, et al. Interferon gamma-1b in the treatment of compensatory anti-inflammatory response syndrome. Arch Intern Med 1997; 157:389–93.

35. Docke WD, Hoflich C, Davis KA. Monitoring temporary immunodepression by flow cytometric measurement of monocytic HLA-DR expression: a multicenter standardized study. Clin Chem 2005;51:2341–7.

36. Lukaszewicz AC, Grienay M, Resche-Rigon M, et al. Monocytic HLA-DR expression in intensive care patients: interest for prognosis and secondary infection prediction. Crit Care Med 2009;37:2746–52.

37. Strohmeyer JC, Blume C, Meisel C. Standardized immune monitoring for the prediction of infections after cardiopulmonary bypass surgery in risk patients. Cytometry B Clin Cytom 2003;53:54–62.

38. Meisel C, Schefold JC, Pschowski R, et al. Granulocyte-microphage colony-stimulating factor to reverse sepsis-associated immunosuppression. Am J Respir Crit Care Med 2009;180:640–8.

39. Hotchkiss RS, Opal SM. Immunotherapy for sepsis: a new approach against an ancient foe. N Engl J Med 2010;363(1):87–9.

40. Sutherland AM, Walley R. Bench-to-bedside review: association of genetic variation with sepsis. Crit Care 2009;13:210.

41. Ashley EA, Butte AJ, Wheeler MT, et al. Clinical assessment incorporating a personal genome. Lancet 2010;375:1525–35.

42. Choi M, Scholl UI, Ji W, et al. Genetic diagnosis by whole exome capture and massively parallel DNA sequencing. Proc Natl Acad Sci U S A 2009;106: 19096–101.

43. Pushkarev D, Neff NF, Quake SR. Single-molecule sequencing of an individual human genome. Nat Biotechnol 2009;27:847–52.

44. Samani NJ, Tomaszewski M, Schunkert H. The personal genome—the future of personalized medicine. Lancet 2010;375:1497–8.

45. Ormond KE, Wheeler MT, Hudgins L, et al. Challenges in the clinical application of whole-genome sequencing. Lancet 2010;375:1749–51.

46. Sorensen TI, Nielson GG, Andersen PK, et al. Genetic and environmental influences on premature death in adult adoptees. N Engl J Med 1988;318:727–32.

47. Burgner D, Levin M. Genetic susceptibility to infectious diseases. Pediatr Infect Dis J 2003;22:1–6.

48. Varmus H. Ten years on-the human genome and medicine. N Engl J Med 2010; 362(21):2028–9.

49. Akey JM, Eberle MA, Rieder MJ, et al. Population history and natural selection shape patterns of genetic variation in 132 genes. PLoS Biol 2004;2:e286.

50. Luyendyk JP, Schabbauer GA, Tencati M, et al. Genetic analysis of the role of the P13K-Akt pathway in lipopolysaccharide-induced cytokine and tissue factor gene expression in monocytes/macrophages. J Immunol 2008;180:4218–26.

51. Stenson PD, Mort M, Ball EV, et al. The human gene mutation database: 2008 update. Genome Med 2009;1:13.

52. Jegga AG, Gowrisankar S, Chen J, et al. PolyDoms: a whole genome database for the identification of non-synonymous coding SNPs with the potential to impact disease. Nucleic Acids Res 2007;35:D700–6.

53. The International HapMap Consortium. A haplotype map of the human genome. Nature 2005;437:1299–320.

54. Klein TE, Chang JT, Cho MK, et al. Integrating genotype and phenotype information: an overview of the PharmGKB project. PharmaGKB project. Pharmacogenetics Research Network and Knowledge Base. Pharmacogenomics J 2001;1: 167–70.

55. Feero WG, Guttmacher AE, Collins FS. Genomic medicine—an updated primer. N Engl J Med 2010;362:2001–11.

56. van der Poll T, Opal SM. Pathogenesis, treatment, and prevention of pneumococcal pneumonia. Lancet 2009;374:1543–56.
57. Khor CC, Chapman SJ, Vannberg FO, et al. A Mal functional variant is associated with protection against invasive pneumococcal disease, bacteremia, malaria and tuberculosis. Nat Genet 2007;39:523–8.
58. Ku CL, Bernuth H, Picard C, et al. Selective predisposition to bacterial infections in IRAK-4-deficient children: IRAK-4-dependent TLRs are otherwise redundant in protective immunity. J Exp Med 2007;204:2407–22.
59. Khor CC, Phil D, Vannberg FO, et al. CISH and susceptibility to infectious diseases. N Engl J Med 2010;362:2092–101.
60. Cobb JP, Stormo GD, Morrissey JJ, et al. Sepsis gene expression profiling: murine splenic compared with hepatic responses determined by using complementary DNA microarrays. Crit Care Med 2002;30(12):2711–21.
61. Tang BM, McLean AS, Dawes IW, et al. Gene-expression profiling of peripheral blood mononuclear cells in sepsis. Crit Care Med 2009;37(3):882–8.
62. Calvano SE, Xiao W, Richards DR, et al. A network-based analysis of systemic inflammation in humans. Nature 2005;437:1032–7.
63. Johnson SB, Lissauer ME, Bochicchio GV, et al. Gene expression profiles differentiate between sterile SIRS and early sepsis. Ann Surg 2007;245(4):611–21.
64. Lissauer ME, Johnson SB, Bochicchio GV, et al. Differential expression of toll-like receptor genes: sepsis compared with sterile inflammation 1 day before sepsis diagnosis. Shock 2009;31(3):238–44.
65. Karvunidis T, Mares J, Thongboonkerd V, et al. Recent progress of proteomics in critical illness. Shock 2009;31:545–52.
66. Nguyen A, Yaffe MB. Proteomics and systems biology approaches to signal transduction in sepsis. Crit Care Med 2003;31(Suppl 1):S1–6.
67. Sigdel TK, Sarwal MM. The proteogenomic path toward biomarker discovery. Pediatr Transplant 2008;12:737–47.
68. Hodgetts A, Levin M, Kroll JS, et al. Biomarker discovery in infectious diseases using SELD1. Future Microbiol 2007;2:35–49.
69. Paugam-Burtz C, Albuquerque M, Baron G, et al. Plasma proteome to look for diagnostic biomarkers of early bacterial sepsis after liver transplantation: a preliminary study. Anesthesiology 2010;112:926–35.
70. Service RF. Proteomics. Will biomarkers take off at last? Science 2008;321:1760.
71. Kalenka A, Feldmann RE Jr, Otero K, et al. Changes in the serum proteome of patients with sepsis and septic shock. Anesth Analg 2006;103:1522–6.
72. Buhimschi CS, Bhandari V, Hamar BD, et al. Proteomic profiling of the amniotic fluid to detect inflammation, infection and neonatal sepsis. PLoS Med 2007; 4(1):e18.
73. Macquire PB, Fitzgerald DJ. Platelet proteomics. J Thromb Haemost 2003;1: 1593–601.
74. Levi M, Opal SM. Coagulation abnormalities in critically ill patients. Crit Care 2006;10:222–8.

Index

Note: Page numbers of article titles are in **boldface** type.

A

Acute kidney injury (AKI)
    described, 379–380
    diagnosis of, biomarkers in, 380–381
    early, NGAL as biomarker in, **379–389**. See also *Neutrophil gelatinase–associated lipocalin (NGAL), as biomarker in early AKI.*
Acute lung injury (ALI)
    biomarkers in, **355–377**
        Ang-2/Ang-1, 361, 367
        cytokines, 356–365
        growth factors, 361, 366–367
        HGF, 361, 366
        ideal properties of, 356
        IL-1ß, 357
        IL-4, 360, 364
        IL-6, 359, 362
        IL-8, 359, 362–364
        IL-10, 359–360
        IL-13, 360, 364
        IL-18, 359
        in coagulation, 358–360, 365–366
        in fibrinolysis, 358–360, 365–366
        KGF, 361, 366
        of alveolar epithelial/endothelial injury, 361, 367–368
        PAI-1, 360, 365
        protein C, 360
        RAGE, 361, 367
        sIL-6R, 359
        sTNFr-1 and 2, 358, 363
        surfactant D, 361, 367
        TGF-ß, 360, 364
        thrombomodulin, 361
        TNF-α, 357, 358, 362–363
        VEGF, 361, 366–367
        VWF, 361, 368
    described, 355–356
    inflammatory responses in, 356–365
Acute renal failure (ARF). See *Acute kidney injury (AKI).*
    described, 379
Adrenomedullin, 333
AKI. See *Acute kidney injury (AKI).*

Crit Care Clin 27 (2011) 421–428
doi:10.1016/S0749-0704(11)00011-X
0749-0704/11/$ – see front matter © 2011 Elsevier Inc. All rights reserved.

criticalcare.theclinics.com

Moving?

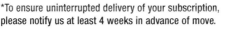

Make sure your subscription moves with you!

To notify us of your new address, find your **Clinics Account Number** (located on your mailing label above your name), and contact customer service at:

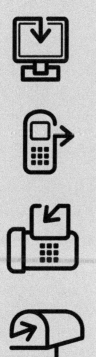

Email: journalscustomerservice-usa@elsevier.com

800-654-2452 (subscribers in the U.S. & Canada)
314-447-8871 (subscribers outside of the U.S. & Canada)

Fax number: 314-447-8029

Elsevier Health Sciences Division
Subscription Customer Service
3251 Riverport Lane
Maryland Heights, MO 63043

*To ensure uninterrupted delivery of your subscription, please notify us at least 4 weeks in advance of move.

Printed and bound by CPI Group (UK) Ltd, Croydon, CR0 4YY

21/10/2024

01776965-0003